# BEHAVIOR PATHOLOGY OF CHILDHOOD AND ADOLESCENCE

# BEHAVIOR PATHOLOGY OF CHILDHOOD AND ADOLESCENCE

EDITED BY

# SIDNEY L. COPEL

**BASIC BOOKS, INC.**

*Publishers*  NEW YORK

Library of Congress Catalog Card Number: 72–89276
SBN: 465–00624–8
Manufactured in the United States of America
73  74  75  76  77    10  9  8  7  6  5  4  3  2  1

For My Wife Joan and My Children Val and Kenny

# The Authors

JULES C. ABRAMS, Ph.D., is Director of the Institute for Learning, Professor of Psychiatry, Head of the Section of Psychology, Hahnemann Medical College and Hospital, Philadelphia. He is also Lecturer in Educational Psychology, Temple University, Philadelphia and Director of the Parkway Day School, Philadelphia, Pennsylvania.

HERMAN S. BELMONT, M.D., is Professor and Director, Division of Child Psychiatry, Hahnemann Medical College and Hospital, Philadelphia, Pennsylvania. He is also on the Faculty of the Institute of the Philadelphia Association for Psychoanalysis.

GERALD R. CLARK, M.D., is President, Elwyn Institute, Elwyn, Pennsylvania. He is also Professor of Psychiatry and Pediatrics, University of Pennsylvania, Philadelphia; and Senior Physician, Children's Hospital, Philadelphia.

SIDNEY L. COPEL, Ed.D., is Chief Psychologist at the Youth Psychotherapy Center, The Bryn Mawr Hospital, Bryn Mawr, Pennsylvania. He is also a Consulting Psychologist for the Chester Public Schools, Chester, Pennsylvania.

A. SCOTT DOWLING, M.D., is Chief Psychiatrist, Bellefaire Residential Treatment Center for Children, Cleveland, Ohio; Clinical Assistant Professor of Child Psychiatry and Clinical Assistant Professor of Psychiatry in Pediatrics at Case Western Reserve University School of Medicine, Cleveland. He is also on the Faculty of the Cleveland Psychoanalytic Institute.

THOMAS J. EDWARDS, Ph.D., is Professor of Education in the Faculty of Educational Studies and is Director of the Learning Center, State University of New York at Buffalo.

GEORGE W. GENS, Ph.D., is Director of the Speech and Hearing Clinic and Professor of Special Education, Newark State College, Union, New Jersey.

JOHN R. KLEISER, Ph.D., is Director of Clinical Services, The Woods Schools and Treatment Center, Langhorne, Pennsylvania.

HAROLD KOLANSKY, M.D., is Associate Professor of Psychiatry, University of Pennsylvania School of Medicine. He is also President, Regional Council of Child Psychiatry (Pennsylvania, Southern New Jersey, and Delaware); and Chairman, Child Analysis Curriculum Committee, Institute of the Philadelphia Association for Psychoanalysis.

REGINALD S. LOURIE, M.D., is Director, Department of Psychiatry, Children's Hospital of the District of Columbia; Medical Director, Hillcrest Children's Center, Washington, D.C. He is also Professor of Child Health and Development at George Washington University School of Medicine, and President, Joint Commission for Mental Health of Children.

RALPH A. LUCE, M.D., is Medical Director of the Concord Mental Health Center, Concord, New Hampshire; Consultant Psychiatrist, New Hampshire Hospital, Concord, New Hampshire. He is also Consultant Psychiatrist, Franklin Regional Hospital, Franklin, New Hampshire.

ROBERT C. PRALL, M.D., is Director, Children's Unit, Eastern Pennsylvania Psychiatric Institute, Philadelphia; and is Clinical Professor of Child Psychiatry, The Medical College of Pennsylvania in Philadelphia. He is also Supervisor of Child Analysis and is on the Faculty of the Philadelphia Psychoanalytic Institute and the Faculty-by-Invitation of the Pittsburgh Psychoanalytic Institute.

JONAS ROBITSCHER, J.D., M.D., is Henry R. Luce Professor of Law and the Behavioral Sciences, Emory University, Atlanta, Georgia.

MARVIN ROSEN, Ph.D., is Director of Psychology, Elwyn Institute, Elwyn, Pennsylvania. He is also an Instructor at the Pennsylvania State Uni- Continuing Education Department.

PHILIP E. ROSENBERG, Ph.D., is Professor of Audiology, Temple University Hospital Health Sciences Center, Philadelphia, Pennsylvania.

STANLEY H. SHAPIRO, M.D., is Professor of Child Psychiatry, Hahnemann Medical College and Hospital, Philadelphia, Pennsylvania. He is also Supervising Child Analyst and is on the Faculty of the Philadelphia Association for Psychoanalysis.

WILLIAM STENNIS, M.D., is a Psychiatric Consultant for the School System of Bucks County, Pennsylvania and for the Los Alamos School System, Los Alamos, New Mexico.

SIDNEY L. WERKMAN, M.D., is Associate Professor of Psychiatry, University of Colorado School of Medicine, Denver, Colorado.

JEAN H. YACOUBIAN, M.D., is on the Faculty of the Washington Psychoanalytic Institute and is Associate Clinical Professor, Department of Psychiatry, at George Washington University, Washington, D.C.

# *Preface*

This book had its origins in a project that was started some five years ago. At that time it was felt that it would be useful to bring out a current "state-of-the-art" summary in the field of childhood psychopathology. The focus of professional attention was then, and still is, directed toward social phenomena and group processes to a point where the needs and understanding of the individual patient are being largely ignored.

All sciences seem to have their fads and the behavioral sciences are particularly vulnerable in this respect. The present interest in disordered social conditions and all of the undesirable consequences that follow from them has given rise to mechanistic therapeutic approaches in which external manipulation of the individual and his surroundings is emphasized. The dilemma posed by our social problems has led to a search for quick and easy solutions which could be applied en masse to just about every kind of difficulty related to human adjustment. A mechanistic approach has its origins in the nature of the American character and in our country's history of having solved massive objective problems through technology.

The theoretical point of view in this book is psychoanalytic. Psychoanalysis offers no panaceas for our social ills. It does, however, furnish us with a body of comprehensive theory and a framework within which human behavior can be understood. It leads us to consider inner psychological experience as paramount and to regard the main determinants of human behavior as unconscious processes. It does not neglect environmental forces, but sees these as selectively interweaving with our constitutional givens to mold psychosexual development and character formation. These processes can often be most advantageously observed during the early years and this is another reason why child therapy is so important.

A psychoanalytic approach to mental health must, of necessity, be a conservative one. It regards the workings of the human mind as highly involved and makes no attempt to oversimplify what is a complicated psychological process. To do so would be to distort reality. Psychoanalysis does help to set our task in perspective. It does give us a method for understanding the psychological make-up of the individual. As this knowledge becomes more broadened, it may hopefully lead to the development of truly intelligent social and educational planning.

None of this should be taken to mean that mechanistic therapies have no place. They certainly can make a valuable contribution in selected areas of habilitation. In this volume, the use of behavioral techniques for training the retarded child is one example of this.

The preparation of a work of this kind involves the combined effort of many people, all of whom could not possibly be enumerated here. I would like to make my main acknowledgment to the various authors—all of whom gave generously of their time and energy to get this work through to completion. Finally, I would like to thank my secretary, Mrs. Margaret Clark, who transformed our rough notes into an expertly typed manuscript.

SIDNEY L. COPEL

*Bryn Mawr, Pennsylvania*
1973

# Contents

# BEHAVIOR
# PATHOLOGY OF
# CHILDHOOD
# AND
# ADOLESCENCE

# 1

# An Overview of Child Psychiatry

HAROLD KOLANSKY, M.D.

## Introduction

Formal training in child psychiatry in the United States began in the 1930s. Knowledge of children was limited at that time, and medicine sought help from the behavioral disciplines of psychology and social work. After that, organizations, including the American Orthopsychiatric Association, the Commonwealth Fund, and the American Association of Psychiatric Clinics for Children, gradually established training standards. The early child psychiatry clinics were community agencies in which there was enormous pressure to help many children. The physician in such a clinic often began his training with the major disadvantage of studying psychopathology before he had a firm grasp of normal development. As Dr. William Stennis and I have stated, "For many years, medicine, in general, and psychiatry, in particular, failed to recognize child psychiatry as a separate specialty with its own training and certification requirements" (11). Only as recently as 1959 was a Committee on Certification in Child Psychiatry of the American Board of Psychiatry and Neurology established. This brought a major impetus toward upgrading training standards. To understand current trends, it is important to retrace the child psychiatrist's historical background.

## History

The eighteenth century was characterized by a humanistic movement, but there had been little study of children prior to the nineteenth century when educators focused their attention on children. At that time Pestalozzi and Rousseau stressed the development of children's abilities and opposed rigid training. They encouraged native powers of observation and the sense of perception, while laying the basis for modern elementary education. Following that, Froebel founded the first kindergarten. Again there was a resurgence of stress on education.

In the nineteenth century, there developed an era of interest in child foster homes and in orphanages, and with this came an increasing emphasis on the education of the child. During this century, Darwin and James Sully (a psychologist) made very important observations on children. Men-

Reprinted with permission of the *Journal of the Albert Einstein Medical Center.*

tal illnesses in children were described for the first time by Paul Moreau and by Manheimer.

Next came the study of mentally defective children and the contributions of psychologists studying them. In fact, these contributions were perhaps more important than the contribution from the educators. Itard, a leading Parisian psychologist, started to train the so-called "wild boy from Aveyron." It was in this educational process that we see the beginning efforts to work directly, and in this instance individually, with a mentally retarded child. Seguin, his pupil, gave private instructions to the retarded and then came to the United States to start schools for the feeble-minded. By 1904, Binet, in France, began testing children, and Terman adopted this method for the United States by 1916. In 1917, of course, a tremendous impetus was given to testing by the large-scale testing of draftees for the war.

The problem of the dependent child also made a contribution to our field. Under slavery, children were the property of their owners. With increased economic progress, dependent children left the estates but became burdens to society, and, therefore, alms houses were created for them. In England, dependent children were at first indentured. By the mid-nineteenth century, foster homes were established in New York for immigrant children. In 1909, Theodore Roosevelt—in a White House conference on the care of dependent children—brought much of the country's attention to this problem. Also, at the same time the psychologist G. Stanley Hall studied delinquents, and medical scientific child psychiatry had its origin, especially with the work of William Healey in Chicago.

It is surprising to realize that little effort was made to differentiate children from adults in any area; for instance, through the centuries, in art and history children were largely portrayed as miniature adults, very often in adult costumes.

In 1891, Hall introduced the pedagogical seminar and the first journal of child psychology, which contributed much to our knowledge of adolescence. A pupil of his, Goddard, established the Vineland Training School in New Jersey.

Freud's work, introduced in this country by Hall, was a monumental contribution to the understanding of children. Freud and Adolph Meyer went far beyond the then prevalent Kraeplinian views on description alone. Children were still not being seen to any extent by psychiatrists, but retrospective studies were being done which emphasized child development. Klaparade, Watson, and Piaget (who is still active) also observed and wrote about children at the turn of the century.

One might say, as Kanner (9) has, that the twentieth century has been characterized by the study of the individual child, even though in some parts of the country there is a disturbing trend today away from the intensive study of the individual child. At times there is a tendency to treat children in groups before understanding the individual dynamics. The advent of community psychiatry, with its many potential advantages, can simultaneously take us away from the study of the individual child unless each child psychiatrist takes special care to keep the individual child in very definite focus in all community psychiatry centers.

During the early part of the twentieth century the child guidance movement began; juvenile courts were established in Illinois and in Colorado. William Healey made a survey for the Juvenile Court of Cook County, Chicago, in 1908, of existing mental facilities for children. He found that only Witmer's Clinic at the University of Pennsylvania in Philadelphia (which had been established in 1896 for the study and care of mentally defective children) and the Vineland Training School under Goddard were in existence. These were the only two facilities at this very recent point in our history, and both were in the Philadelphia area. Thus the child guidance movement was started as a new form of social service with a team, and although at first the child psychiatrist was primarily responsible, his role gradually became subsumed by the team in many clinics. There has been a gradual change in recent years, and with the establishment of certification in child psychiatry in 1959, further impetus was given for the child psychiatrist to be in charge of the diagnosis and the treatment of children in child psychiatry settings. This allowed for a continuation of very able and necessary assistance from the psychologist, social worker, and educator, but with less emphasis in some centers on the team as such.

Going back to origins again, the Boston group with William James, G. Stanley Hall, Adolph Meyer, and Goddard gave the first impetus to these child guidance clinics. There was a union of psychologists and psychiatrists at that time, and the Juvenile Psychopathic Institute in Chicago was established in 1909 under Healey. It still exists, though now as an important research institution with the name of the Illinois Institute for Juvenile Research. Juvenile offenders were studied there at first, and later Healey went to Boston and founded the famous Judge Baker Foundation in 1917. Child psychiatry in that period began to have an influence on sociology, social work, education, law, anthropology, psychology, and general psychiatry. By 1911, Yale had established its famed Child Development Center under Gesell, and the mental health movement in America followed.

Regarding treatment for children, the child guidance team and the approach to the child through the team gained their main impetus again in Philadelphia under the leadership of Dr. Frederic Allen who utilized the Commonwealth Fund to establish a Demonstration Clinic (now the Child Guidance Clinic of Philadelphia) in 1925. At that time he had with him the psychologist Dr. Phyllis Blanchard, who was a very important contributor with Dr. Allen to the literature in child psychiatry. Dr. Blanchard later trained as an analyst and became one of the country's few lay analysts to enjoy national esteem. She contributed much to the child analytic literature. She worked at the Philadelphia Child Guidance Clinic with

Dr. Allen until recently, and while there also helped to train many of us in child analysis.

Anna Freud and the Vienna group began working prior to 1926, and thus the technique of child analysis began to be spelled out in 1926. It was in this same period (1925) that August Aichhorn wrote *Wayward Youth,* describing his important work and contributions on delinquency. Melanie Klein also focused her attention on children at that time.

The transformation of the child guidance clinic from the original status of simply diagnosing and making court disposals of delinquent children into treatment centers for the individual child received very important impetus in the 1930s with the influx of European analysts escaping from the Nazi persecution. The 1930s also saw children's units in psychiatric hospitals, total treatment programs, close collaboration between pediatricians and child psychiatrists, and a laboratory of child research in Bethesda, Maryland. By 1952, an Academy of Child Psychiatry was founded, which set standards in addition to those originally set by the American Orthopsychiatric Association and the American Association of Psychiatric Clinics for Children.

Perhaps the period 1930 to 1940 is most important because of the tremendous influence and impact of analysis and child analysis from Freud, Anna Freud, Berta Bornstein, Gerald Pearson, and many others. In that period the shaping of individual treatment programs, especially for neurotic children, began to be very much in evidence. Of course, Freud's influence is well known (5, 6, 7) in relation to our knowledge of the unconscious, of dreams, and the theory of infantile sexuality. Additionally, of course, his contributions to understanding repression and the analysis of phobias in children deserve special emphasis for child psychiatrists. Among the countless contributions he made, which are still studied and used to shape much of what we do in the individual treatment of neurotic children, are his "Three Essays on the Theory of Sexuality," his many papers on infantile neurosis, and his 1909 paper on the analysis of Hans (5). Melanie Klein and Anna Freud also began to spell out play treatment, but each with very different emphasis. Today, little of Melanie Klein's work is taken with much seriousness, but it was Anna Freud who contributed the basis of child analysis.

Between 1950 and 1960 organizations for training and for standards were established. The National Institute of Mental Health residency programs began, and all of us are the beneficiaries of these.

Psychosomatic medicine and more contributions on the relationship of pediatrics and child psychiatry began to be in evidence, and in the era 1960 to 1965 there was a proliferation of accredited training centers that now number approximately one hundred. It is interesting to note that much of what went on in the earliest period in child psychiatry (and which was, to some extent, lost sight of) has gained considerably new force. For instance, child psychiatry's long neglected entrance into the field of mentally retarded children, child psychiatry's newer interest in the organic deficits of children, and child psychiatry's consideration of the so-called "soft" or subtle neurological signs in children provide partial explanation for such entities as the ego disturbances. This has been an era in which psychoanalysis and child analysis, in concert with our knowledge of neurology, have worked together to form unified pictures of what the child psychiatrist must know, diagnose, and direct or treat in the problems of children. Anna Freud, during this period, produced, in 1965, her book on normality and psychopathology, which is a major addition to a long series of her contributions that have enriched us all. Today, the child psychiatrist expects to be a beginning medical expert on children and their problems by the end of his training.

## Functions of the Child Psychiatrist

Beyond this historical survey, we delve into the functions of the modern child psychiatrist. They are varied. They include, of course, the diagnosis of the individual child and his problems and the planning of therapeutic programs for that child and frequently for the family as well. We even speak today of an individualized psychiatric and educational prescription which the child psychiatrist directs be written for each child he sees in diagnosis. In addition, the child psychiatrist today may avail himself of psychoanalytic training and preparation toward becoming a child psychoanalyst, added to experience in child psychiatry. He now has extremely important relationships to educators who have new respect for the child psychiatrist able to go into their setting, talk their language, and help them plan preventive educational and treatment programs for the children. He has, of course, an important relationship to psychology, to social work, to pediatrics, and to research. He gives consultation in various kinds of agencies. He is involved in training, in administration of so many of the training programs, and in other settings.

## Some Newer Aspects of Training

Among the more recent trends in child psychiatry is the full acceptance that the child psychiatrist does not leave his medical background as he enters the field of child psychiatry. Therefore, in an increasing number of centers, the "team" concept is no longer held in reverence. This does not mean that the social worker and the psychologist do not make major contributions, but rather that the emphasis is on the child psychiatrist's not forgetting that he is, first and foremost, a physician, and that it is his responsibility as a physician to take charge of all things concerning children with psychiatric problems.

Although observation of normal children now plays a distinctly important part in training, this has not always been the case. In the Philadelphia area, which we feel is one of the most progressive in the field today, child observations date back only a few years in training programs. Today we are introducing child observations even to medical students, but only ten years ago the psychiatric resident had very little chance to get any kind of child observational experience.

## Some Comments on Child Observations

Why do we start with child observations? There are many reasons. To know pathology, one must have a firm foundation in normal development. Gerald Pearson (13) emphasized the fact that many developmental problems may look pathological but are not pathological when viewed from the standpoint of normal development. Many pathological conditions are expressions of fixations, so we must see these fixations in the normal child. Regressions are normal to development, and one must be aware of these at various ages and under various conditions. For instance, libidinal and ego regressions are seen in the first phase of latency and in the early phases of adolescence as normally occurring phenomena. Oral disturbances at the onset of school are seen by all pediatricians and certainly in child psychiatry as well. These are regressive phenomena, normal to the child beginning school—the syndrome of abdominal distress, nausea, vomiting, not wanting to go to school at the time of having to leave mother, entering the formal setting of school, and experiencing the regressive tendency back to the oral phase as a consequence of the struggle over leaving mother and yet desiring to be independent.

To see normal children at the outset of training adds conviction to the theory of normal child development. Unlike adult psychiatry, many pathological conditions are related to age alone. For instance, if we do not know normal development, we do not know how to diagnose infantile autism. The severity of a compulsive neurosis in a three-year-old can only be recognized by having seen many three-year-olds and their beginning reaction-formations against anality. The normality of stuttering in the two-year-old can't be understood (except in the literature) unless we see many children of two and know that this is a minor problem that is not in itself pathological in the two-year-old. It is transient and related to the bowel training itself. We cannot understand ego disturbances in adolescence unless we see the "craziness" of adolescence in normal settings. Preventive psychiatry rests on a knowledge of norms. One cannot act as a nursery school adviser without knowledge of norms, gained through observation. One cannot advise parents on feeding and training if one does not see normal children. Again, the expansion of knowledge of the different types of ego disturbances is important because of the countless variations of normal development. We must know, therefore, the ego functions at different ages in children.

As an example, I saw a child at the age of three who was not speaking, who was not involved with peers, who was not in control of his impulses at all, and who made no distinction between reality and unreality. In brief, this child was one who, in addition to all I mention, showed marked perseveration in all of his activities, and I diagnosed him as having infantile autism as described originally by Kanner (8). I planned a therapeutic program for this child including placement in a very special school and direct work with the parents, but not with the child, except for seeing this child at periodic intervals to be certain that we were making progress in all the areas we were working with through educators and through the parents. About the age of five, at a time when this child already had speech but was still using reversals of pronouns, I saw him for one of these periodic checks. I gave him a gift of a small airplane, a red airplane. At this point, the boy began dancing up and down with glee and shouting aloud, "Oh, Jack, say how glad you are! Isn't it wonderful! Look what Dr. Kolansky gave you! Isn't it grand! Isn't it perfect! Say how happy you are, Jack!"

This brief example, in a very disturbed youngster, points to something that we ordinarily take for granted in child development, namely, the introjection of what the mother says, what the mother does, the help the mother gives to the child that goes unnoticed in the normal child's productions. However, by making simultaneous observations of the normal child and of the ego disturbed child, we frequently find silent areas in the normal child that are illuminated by this kind of observational experience with the disturbed child. What was Jack doing? He was showing us that he had progressed to a phase that might have been passed through silently in the normal child at the age of two or two and a half, to a phase at this point where he was verbalizing this struggling, beginning incorporation of what his mother felt and said to him at times of his own pleasure. It was quite obvious that he was very pleased and delighted but still it was not himself speaking. The differentiation of self and nonself was still not wholly possible for this child, and this gives us much illumination on what must occur in normal child development (10).

A similar example: A boy of nine with a very severe ego disturbance was seen in treatment, and one could determine in any therapeutic hour with this child (at any particular moment) who in the child's environment was influencing his thoughts at that particular time; he would scatter himself literally to the winds with expressions that I knew had come directly from the father with the father's voice inflections and mannerisms, or the mother's words, or the teacher's glances, or my way of combing my hair and speaking and dressing. In any one hour one could see all these bits and fragments put together into a disparate mosaic. In the normal child, by comparison, certainly all these factors, these objects in the environment, similarly influence the child, but they influence the child in a much less obvious way. So there is a reciprocal relationship between the observations of normal and of very disturbed children.

The technique of treatment rests, by and large, on knowledge of the norms. If we do not know the norms, we cannot make a diagnosis and we cannot plan a therapeutic program, whether it be individual psychotherapy, drug treatment, educational advances for the child, or so-called family treatment. Whatever the treatment, it cannot be planned without knowing the norms and making the individual diagnosis. Doing psychotherapy or psychoanalysis with neurotic children must be different from the treatment process in adults because of the continuing developmental process in children. For instance, when we see the latency child, we know that he struggles to put away all his impulses, to keep them from consciousness and not to be involved in sexual fantasies that will cause him to masturbate and then to have severe anxiety. We know by observing many latency age children that the latency age child cannot be expected to free associate, because for him free association would be a disaster and a catastrophe that would unnerve him and would throw him back into a kind of snake pit of impulses over which he does not yet have sufficient ego or superego to control except by blotting them out of mind. By observation we can know, in fact, that it isn't until puberty that the child begins to be able to have enough introspective ability, to take a little bit of distance from himself, to really effectively approach giving even the simplest free associations.

As a consequence, Anna Freud's words (1, 2, 3, 4) on not using free association but instead using the child's play, using the child's drawings, using the child's facial expressions, using the differences in verbal expressions from one point in an hour to another, all become highly meaningful for us in the treatment of the individual neurotic child. Certainly by observing children we gain a conviction about the infantile neurosis, about the strength of the sexual and aggressive impulses, and we see (if we have the observational experience) parental interactions between each of the parents or both parents and the child and the part they play in shaping the vicissitudes of some aspects of the child's development and of his pathology.

## Norms of Development Which May Look Pathologic

Pearson's paper on normal development that may look pathological clearly delineates aspects of normality which may be mistakenly diagnosed, if we are not aware of such phenomena (13). In watching the physical maturation of the child from infancy through the preschool years, one is struck by the number of physical findings which are pathologic in older children but which, for particular early age levels, are normal. For example, in relation to the newborn's eyes, fixation is, at first, characteristically monocular, with the other eye wandering at random or being at rest. Binocular conversions are not dominant until the second month when the pupilary reflex is, at first, sluggish for a few days. These things must be known. Otherwise, false neurological conditions in the newborn may be diagnosed. We speak about the normality of the startle reflex, the Moro reflex, the tonic neck reflex, and so on. Other such physical findings include flexed sleeping posture with flexing of the extremities and tense muscles in the infant; still later, one sees the child learning to walk with a forward propulsive gait and with frequent falling. None of these findings is pathologic.

Similarly, there are a number of emotional or psychological findings which, at particular ages, are normal for all children, while at advanced ages these would be indicators of psychopathology, such as generalized anxiety in the infant. In the normal newborn, one observes two primary states of reaction with oscillation between them: the sleep or quiescent state and the active, crying, anxious state (2). When the infant's physical needs (food and oxygen) are fulfilled, he sleeps for long periods of time. When there is internal stimulation due to hunger or the need to be picked up or when painful external stimuli bombard the infant, the quiescent state is interrupted by the state of generalized restless anxiety. External stimuli include such things as a pin prick, excessive warmth or coldness, careless maternal handling, and so on. Internal disease or skin disease will similarly result in this anxious state. The anxious state is characterized by crying, restlessness, and tense extremities difficult for the examiner to move. As internal food or emotional needs are fulfilled by feeding, sucking, rocking, holding, warmth, and patting, and as external painful stimuli are eliminated, the newborn returns to the sleep state. Gradually, the waking state becomes more prolonged, if the mother has responded to the anxious state by prompt care of the infant. If one sees only these two oscillating states with little other response in the infant older than six weeks, one should attempt to investigate the nature of the mother's feelings toward the baby and what interferences there may be. This tense state oscillating with the tranquil state is normal during the first six or eight weeks of the child's life and more moderately for many months, but after the first six or eight weeks, there must be additional aspects of the infant's responses.

To give some additional examples of these states which may look pathological but which are not, there is generally no smile or cooing during the first three, four, or five weeks of life, and we do not view this with alarm in the newborn. This is a normal state. If there is no smiling or cooing at two months, at three, at four months, then we must view this phenomenon with alarm. We must even begin to think of infantile autism and certain other serious conditions of early childhood.

Later in the first year of life, there is a normally occurring fear of strangers. Between eight and twelve months, trips to the doctor's office and strangers in the home lead to considerable anxiety. The baby may cry loudly, turn his head away, and cling to his mother. This lasts for several months or maybe even a year at times, and this follows the child's beginning awareness that his mother is a separate and valued person and with this realization comes the dread that she can leave him. The stranger (we think) who comes and goes perhaps arouses this fear since if the stranger does it, perhaps the mother may do it (not come back) as well. During this period, exposure to strangers should perhaps be somewhat limited until the child feels more secure with this separation of himself from his mother, but here again is a state of normal development which may look pathologic if we are not aware of its occurrence.

Sleep disturbance is another such phenomenon. At eighteen months, there is very rapid ego development. The child is interested in what he can do, feel, and perceive. He is proud of his increasingly complex physical accomplishments, dislikes going to bed, and thereafter to sleep, because of the interruptions in these pleasurable ego maturational activities. Moreover, at this time, he is often taxed by toilet training, and he is in conflict between his desire to remain untrained and the parents' desire for him to be trained. He realizes that as he falls asleep, his conscious control over soiling becomes lessened, so he attempts to remain awake and so not soil and therefore be able to continue to please his mother. As he becomes more certain of his abilities within several months, this problem disappears. This is certainly no occasion for sedation by the pediatrician. Parents should make up their minds to endure several months of broken sleep during this somewhat trying period, but again this represents a normal phenomenon.

There is a sleep disturbance, again quite normal, between the ages of five and a half and seven, wherein the resistance about going to bed has to do with the violent intrapsychic struggle of solving the Oedipus complex and stopping masturbation. The child, at this time, is crystallizing the beginnings of a superego which will aid in helping him repress his passionate, but ambivalent, sexual love for the parent of the opposite sex and the equally passionate love, hate, and fear of the parent of the same sex. To keep these fantasies out of mind, he attempts to refrain from thumb sucking and masturbating, which lead to further fantasies. While alone and falling asleep, his ego is in a state of not as much control as it was previously, and as a consequence, there is more danger that he will masturbate, and he must be on guard that much more. Therefore, he keeps himself awake with frequent calls for water, frequent trips to the parents' room, frequent walks around the house. This is a normal phenomenon once more, which the child must struggle through with support and understanding from the parents.

Negativism is another such phenomenon reflective of the state of the ego during the bowel training period at about eighteen months of age. The child refuses to do what he's told and often does the opposite, not out of hatred, but to assure himself that he is capable of doing for himself and so need not fear his mother's desertion. This is also related to the eighteen-month sleep disturbances already mentioned. He attempts continued new masteries and should be helped to develop new skills such as climbing stairs, placing pots into other pots, and so on. The child should not be reprimanded for the negativism though he may need an assist at times to help him control his impulses.

A word about anger, rage, and jealousy. These reactions, as Pearson (13) has indicated, are seen under special circumstances. If they are prolonged, one should attempt to determine causes. Often they are of short duration. For example, the birth of a sibling will lead to these reactions in a normal child and these episodes will vary in duration. Generally, the parent can ease, but not entirely eliminate, these reactions. Departure of the mother of the young child will lead to angry, impulsive outbursts.

Naughtiness, defiance, and other signs of rebellion, plus peevishness, irritability, whining, and nagging are generally aspects of childhood anxiety and of regression. The behavior reaches a peak between ages three and six. These reactions seem to predominate because of conflicts related to intense oedipal feelings in the child; with the solution of these feelings, the child generally becomes much more practical and reasonable. Associated with this phase, of course, is masturbation, which may be open or secret. Many parents attempt to punish the child for this behavior. He should not be punished nor should he be encouraged to masturbate. If this is an open activity in front of others, one can tell the child that this is not a public activity.

Phobias and nightmares also occur between ages three and six. This is, of course, the phallic-oedipal phase. Most children show phobias at this time. What distinguishes this phobia from the phobia of a neurotic child? Nothing; they are the same, but they are in miniature, they are transient, they are related to rather specific objects, they do not occur daily, but their dynamics have the same regularly occurring themes. The phobias represent first attempts at projecting feelings onto an external object. For example, a boy may feel quite angered toward his father in this phase, but must live with his father. The boy may then fear his father's anger in return. Unconsciously, he turns the reaction around and says in effect, "I don't hate my father. I'm good. My father hates me. What does he have against me? Why is he so mad at me?" He has projected his anger, but this doesn't help him very much. The economy of the mind doesn't set well with this theme because his father still comes home in the evening and now, though he may be comfortable with his hatred toward his father (which he has temporarily dismissed), he is not comfortable with the father's hatred toward him, which is a projection of his own. He still lives in fear each time the father comes home, and economically the mind cannot exist with such profound anxiety on a continuing basis. So what must he do? He must now go through another unconscious intrapsychic process, namely, a displacement onto a phobic object, the choice of which is always determined by his previous life.

The mind is in a much better position with this childhood phobia. Now it has gone through the phase of "I don't hate my father, and he doesn't hate me, but now I only have to fear that dog that's going to bite or hurt or destroy me, and if only I could avoid it or the gorilla on television, then I am safe, and I don't have to be very anxious." If the phobias are not of a bizarre type, are occasional and limited in extent, and are not encroaching on other areas of growth and development, the child can simply be reassured. He should not be taken into bed with the parents nor should they lie down with him in his own bed (which obviously would only increase the conflict, as so often happens in the children we see, because they are stimulated sexually, while trying so hard to avoid masturbation). He should be told that he knows the gorilla stays in the zoo, and although he may feel a little afraid, he will soon be asleep. If the reaction is a severe *pavor nocturnus,* screaming as if in pain with eyes open and not knowing where he is, walking into walls, episodes lasting fifteen to twenty minutes and recurring frequently, then the child is suffering from something more than the usual innocuous phobias and this must be investigated further.

## Method of Normal Child Observations

How do we go about normal observations? We must have frames of reference in mind and we must have some degree of structured knowledge. At the Albert Einstein Medical Center, our framework is psychoanalysis. We are not training people to be psychoanalysts in this residency program, but our framework of understanding normal development and the problems of children is psychoanalytic. Simultaneously, we must use free floating attention in looking at children. We pay attention to the child's physical appearance, his face, his gait, his hand movements, his eyes, and the way he interacts with his peers, the way he plays alone, what he does autoerotically, what he does with the teacher, and what evidence of our theoretical framework we see through play and verbalizations. In brief, we are paying free floating attention while simultaneously having knowledge of normal child development (neurological and psychoanalytic). Therefore, we look at stages of maturation, ego development, libidinal development, state of aggression, interaction with peers, and environment.

We know how frequently obsessional disorders appear during the latency phase of development, partly as a consequence of the parental tendency to enforce the intellectual development and to ignore the child's struggle to keep his oedipal impulses repressed. These impulses are never far removed from consciousness, and this is sufficiently evident if one hears the stories of the latency child in a school setting. Representative of these stories is the following in a third grade class: "Five girls were in a school yard, and one fell. Her mouth fell on a snake's head or tail. The girl didn't have a mouth then. She died. She became a ghost in heaven after the snake bit off her head. The ghost said, 'Mommy, Mommy, I can't see.'" Another story: "The girl had a pet dog, and one day the dog saw her patting a bear. The dog got very angry and bit the bear. One bear ate him up and then began to pat the girl. They got married and lived happily ever after." We must also keep in mind in our observations, especially in some summer day camps, that some adults are sadistic, and they restrict children rather than help them. This then becomes part of what we observe as well: that is, seeing the influence of the adult on the child. The adult may restrict the child's motor, speech, and peer activities, and at least temporary pathological consequences may follow. Under these circumstances, the child is forced back to primary process thinking which undoes repression and increases apprehension.

At one summer day camp, a group of six- and seven-year-old boys was observed at archery. Unfortunately, the instructor was a teenager who understood neither archery nor how to handle children and was himself sadistic and uncomfortable. The children did not know the skills needed in archery. The instructor, with many children waiting on a bench, restricted their motor activity and discussion until their turn with the bow came up. Soon the children lost interest in what was happening. Finally, when it was their turn at the bow, they violated all rules of safety. The counselor then began to nudge with an arrow point to get the child up to take his turn. His comments increased their apprehension while restricting their needed activities: "Be careful with the tips. They're dangerous and can kill you." Anxiety and restlessness increased in the group. Finally, unable to handle their anxiety and restricted in speech and motor activity, the boys began holding and kissing each other. The counselor did not object to this as long as they remained silent and seated. Eventually the group turned on him clutching, pawing, touching, leaning, and irritating him all the more. It was obvious that the boys, who could not release their energies in direct talk and physical activities and in whom heterosexual fantasies of an incestuous type were also restricted due to their age and repressive forces, finally found relief of tension through homosexual activities (10).

## Diagnosis

At the Albert Einstein Medical Center, no diagnosis is made without first doing a searching history of the chief complaint, the present illness, the developmental history, and the family history, followed by interviews with the child, and (where indicated) psychological testing. Here, as in most clinics, the evaluation starts with the telephone screening. Then we see the parents, usually both parents together, followed by the mother alone for several visits, to gather history, followed by one to three interviews with the child. In selected instances, such as learning disturbances, suspected ego disturbance, and questionable borderline conditions, we add psychological testing to aid diagnosis. If our initial impression is of an ego disturbance, we also do a preliminary neurological examination of the child and follow it with a neurological assessment by one of our neurologists. We may also have an electroencephalogram. Our treatment evolves from the nature of the diagnosis.

Some of us feel that the old child guidance approach, in which the child is seen by a trainee and the parent is seen by a social worker, has many disadvantages. In training, it deprives the residents of an opportunity to personally observe and learn about family interaction and to properly develop skills in history taking. We also believe that the traditional approach (the team) did not make proper use of the allied mental health disciplines. Social workers have many skills to offer in working with some parents whose children do not need to be seen directly in a therapeutic way. Thus, in the large number of children needing special educational and family support due to ego deficits, the social worker can frequently act as an effective bridge between child psychiatrist and parent or school, once a diagnosis is established and a therapeutic plan constructed. The psychologist also has major skills to offer beyond his ability to test children. Thus he can be used as a key professional in disturbances in learning processes when these are evident. Using the psychologist selectively for testing and in some therapeutic programs also frees some of his time for much needed research and teaching.

At Einstein Medical Center, we make much less use of the social worker than do most clinics, not because we do not value her work, but because we feel that the resident must be solidly grounded in all aspects of examination and care of the child and of his parents. We are convinced also that a true understanding of a unit of society, such as the community or family, is somewhat inadequate without a thorough knowledge of individual personality development. It is important to stress in these formative years of training especially that the study of the individual child, his development (including the neurological substrata), his intrapsychic conflicts, the results of his problems on the family, and the interaction between the child and the family will offer the resident the rich background necessary to properly treat the child. We note with concern a tendency in some parts of the country to dilute such an approach to the study of the individual child and that, as a consequence, recommendations for treatment often lack specificity. At times in certain centers, a diagnosis is not even established before embarking on courses of treatment. Under the aegis of providing broader community service, there is the danger that the individual child and his problems can be lost. We are convinced that the community is best served through this individual study of children and that, in actuality, recommendations can be carried out on a large scale in individual ways with children.

## Nosology

We have been dissatisfied for a long time with current nosology in child psychiatry and feel it is time to do some updating. As a consequence, Dr. William Stennis and I have developed the following diagnostic schema (11). We classify children in five groups: (a) those with normal development, including the group of children with conditions that may look pathological but which are not; (b) the psychoneuroses and character neuroses;

(c) disturbances in the ego; (d) the prelatency developmental arrests; and (e) overlapping conditions.

In classifying psychoneuroses, we include the acute and chronic states of anxiety, anxiety hysteria, phobias, conversion reactions, regressive and fixed types of obsessional disorders, and also the character neurosis.

When we speak of disturbances in the ego, we refer to disorders which interfere significantly with one or more of the major functions of the ego. Here we are speaking of disturbances in the control of motility, the testing of reality, object relationships, thinking, use of memory, synthetic function, and various other of the major ego functions. Thus the ego disturbances, as described by Anna Marie Weil (14), and all forms of psychosis would be included in our group of ego disturbances. We include Mahler's symbiotic psychosis (12) and Kanner's autistic psychosis (8). Also, since the major psychopathology in severe organic syndromes involving the central nervous system is basically due to disturbances in various ego functions, such as the control of motility, we include the major organic syndromes in this same category. In addition, we include the mentally retarded, since they invariably have defects in the testing of reality, intellectual function, object relations, and control of motility. In grouping these various entities as ego disturbances, we are able to look more intently for specific malfunctions in the ego of each child in this category, and further can search for organic pathology, including the subtle neurological signs.

In the fourth category (prelatency developmental arrests) we classify those disorders which are due to lack of forward movement in the ego or in drives rather than due to internal psychic conflict, as in the neuroses. These differ from the specific ego disorders, often due to organicity. These prelatency disorders include the child who is continuously enuretic or encopretic and also the child who is only interested in immediate gratification of needs and who has extremely low frustration tolerance. Among the characteristic factors in the diagnosis of the prelatency disorder is the high level of narcissistic excitation, the continuous preoccupation with pleasure principle functioning, the seeming lack of conflict, the inordinate degree of awareness of reality but ignoring of reality (if it suits the pleasure principle of the moment). There are, of course, countless adults who also fit into the same category of prelatency fixation. Obviously, many of the college age youngsters and others who are on marijuana and many other drugs would fit into this category.

Regarding our fifth group, there are a number of conditions which others classify separately but which lend themselves to classification under one of the four categories previously mentioned when we examine their development and their major dynamics. Thus delinquency may be due, in one instance, to an organic mental syndrome and would properly be an ego disturbance, or in other instances the delinquency is engaged in primarily out of a sense of guilt. These individuals try to appease their superego by doing things of minor degree that get them into some difficulty, and by so doing may continue to avoid punishment for what they really feel guilty about. In other delinquents who follow the leader into acts that are dangerous and antisocial we are dealing with mentally retarded who fit into the category of ego disturbance. There are still other delinquents who seem to do delinquent acts because they are fixated at early stages of development and fit our category of prelatency developmental arrests.

Similarly, a depression may be due to an ego disturbance or may instead, at times, be primarily due to neurotic conflict. Psychosomatic disorders can also be primarily related to one another of these various categories. Similarly, in looking at learning disturbances and diagnosing them individually, we may classify a child who doesn't learn on the basis of retardation and again he is an ego disturbed child, or we may classify him as a neurotic child who has very specific conflicts about learning certain subjects because of their relation to unconscious conflict; still others may not learn (and these are a very large group in our society today) because they are prelatency fixations who are pleasure-bound and who cannot take the delay in gratification necessary for the learning process.

So, by this classification, we make an effort to include the conditions we see in child psychiatry in a way that is manageable. By thinking of these five large categories in assessing the chief complaint and the history of the present illness, one can begin to classify disorders in major groups and can arrive at a more definitive, descriptive, dynamic, and developmental diagnosis by the end of the study.

We look at diagnosis in three frameworks: the descriptive, the dynamic, and the developmental, and we need to be satisfied on all three diagnostic levels in order to understand what we are dealing with and what our therapeutic plan should be. Dynamically, we consider the child's major fears as fear of the loss of the love object, fear of the loss of the object's love, fear of castration, and fear of the superego. Each child fits descriptively and dynamically into one main category. We also consider the child's symptomatology in relation to developmental age and to factors in the history and clinical interviews which indicate fixation or regression in developmental age.

## Treatment

What is the usefulness of this classification? How does it help us in treatment? We feel that it aids and simplifies our treatment plan considerably. Let's look at some aspects of this for a moment. In a neurotic child, there is intrapsychic conflict, and the main method of treatment is an individual dynamic psychotherapy or psychoanalysis.

For the rest (the largest number in our clinic), we generally do not use psychotherapy, but use other methods which we feel are more effective with the ego disturbed child and the prelatency developmental arrests. Thus, with children who have very severe impairment of specific ego functions as in psychosis, organic syndromes, and mental retardation, our residents develop skills as consultants to the social worker, the psychologist, the teacher, the school counselor, and the tutor, and slowly learn to construct an individual prescription for the specialized education, support, and training of these children and their very specific ego defects. In the prelatency developmental arrests, our work is not primarily with the individual child, but with his parents in helping them to unfreeze their own blocks in allowing development to proceed in a sequential way. This is what is meant by careful attention to diagnosis of the individual child, so that we can, without intense involvement in large group therapy projects, family therapy, etc., still treat large numbers of children and work with them on a continuing basis.

Thus our resident in training sees several hundred children in diagnosis in the two years of residency program at the Albert Einstein Medical Center. Out of this group the resident constructs a therapeutic prescription for each of the children. The resident also treats a group of six or seven children who are psychoneurotic with intensive (two or three times weekly) psychotherapy, under supervision, while most of the other children who are not neurotic are treated through other programs. So in a period of two years the resident here or in any other center may then participate in a therapeutic program for several hundred children.

I will illustrate the therapeutic prescription by borrowing from the Bucks County (Pennsylvania) School System's new project on the "Intensification of Learning." Bucks County was one of six centers in the school systems of the United States to be chosen by the federal government for such new projects. Our Section of Child Psychiatry at the Albert Einstein Medical Center is supplying psychiatric, neurological, and psychological consultants to the project, and participated in the planning and detailing of the project prior to its submission to the federal government. This is an experimental project in which all twenty-five children in one first grade class in the Doyle School (Doylestown, Pennsylvania) were studied intensively, child psychiatrically, neurologically, psychologically, and educationally. Out of our combined studies and with constant communication between educators and child psychiatrists and psychologists, we helped the teachers to develop a program whereby they could keep all twenty-five children in one class. For each of these children, a prescription was developed under the general supervision of Dr. William Stennis. As a result of such fine-tooth screening, we found many different kinds of moderate psychiatric, neurologic, educational, speech, or hearing difficulties. Twenty-five percent of these children showed mild neurological impairment. The object of this study is to supply each child with maximal educational advantage by knowing his specific needs and by supplying these through his own teacher.

With the child who has heart disease, the best therapeutic approach is to know quite definitively how much organic pathology there is in the heart and to get a statement from the cardiologist as to how much physical and school work this child can do, and then work the child to his maximum capacity in order to preserve his psychological soundness. Our premise is similar. If we know all the details about each child, we can help him educationally to realize his maximum potential. This is in line with our feeling that a major role for the child psychiatrist is within the public school system, aiding in the development of children's educational potentials and the prevention of some forms of disorders.

With this as background, I will summarize some aspects of the Bucks County work as a model of the treatment prescription. All the specialists wrote up lengthy descriptions which are currently being computerized for more general application. Assets and deficits are stressed. For instance, a listing of each child's talents, areas of preferred behavior (social, intellectual, or sensory), is made. Thus "spelling" or "math" or "popular with peers" or "reading" is included. Then the child's major interests, as gleaned through contacts with the child and through the histories that we obtained from the parents and the psychological testing, are listed.

Thus, for ——: reading and puzzles, math and medicine

——: art

——: arts and crafts, racing cars, medicine and farming

——: art and math.

Immediately, we may begin to gain a sense of what to emphasize in making education palatable for these children. A child may have listed "need for speech treatment." Moreover, specific language activities that would enhance the education of each child were listed. Role playing, puppets, and dramatization are used for specific children. Reading strength and weakness groups are listed, and here again, weakness in word recognition, phonetic application, and reading comprehension is indicated. Left-right confusion is listed, to aid the teacher in planning special work for these children. Weakness in the realm of memory skills and development of those skills is indicated by special procedures for specific children. Weakness in ability to analyze and synthesize, weakness in the understanding of time sequence, children who need small group approaches, children who need structured approaches (and what kind of structure) are all indicated. Weakness in fine motor skills is included with tasks to be used to develop skill. This is what we mean by a combination of a child psychiatric and educational prescription for the individual child. It is obvious that there needs to be a high degree of cooperation among the specialists in this setting.

# 2

## Disturbances in Development and Childhood Neurosis

STANLEY H. SHAPIRO, M.D.

*Introduction*

HISTORICAL BACKGROUND

Dynamic understanding of the psychopathology of childhood was first approached by Sigmund Freud during his attempt to unravel the mystery of neuroses in his adult patients.

Through reconstruction of the childhood period in the course of analysis of adult neurotics, Freud uncovered the existence of a sexual life in childhood, and further learned that conflicts and disturbances in that early sexual life lay at the root of every neurosis.

Psychoanalytic investigation established the existence of the *infantile neurosis* as the precondition for outbreaks of neurotic disorder at later ages. The nucleus of this disorder was found to be the young child's triadic relationship with his parents. Termed the "Oedipus complex," it comprised the difficulties involved in the child's attempt to resolve the conflict of his ambivalent, erotic, and aggressive feelings toward his mother and father.

The first effort to approach a neurotic disturbance in childhood analytically was recorded by Freud as the case of Little Hans (11), which remains the classic account of an infantile phobia to this day. But at the very beginning period of psychoanalysis Freud was concerned mainly with substantiating the childhood origin of neurosis in adults. The emphasis was on tracing the development of the patient's illness from one period to the other, and stress was placed, therefore, on the similarities between the adult disturbance and its infantile precursor.

When it came to studying the actual pathological disturbances as seen in childhood, it was first thought that these would comprise manifestations of the infantile neurosis that was being reconstructed in the analysis of adult neurotics. But such was not the case. It was discovered that the range of pathology far exceeded that which could be attributed to neurotic conflicts alone. In a recent discussion of this problem, Anna Freud commented that in addition to the psychoses,

. . . there are the (nonorganic) disturbances of vital body needs; i.e. eating-sleeping disorders of the infant; the (nonorganic) excessive delays in acquiring vital capacities, such as control of motility, speech, cleanliness, learning; the primary disturbances of narcissism and of object relations; the states caused by uncontrolled and self-destructive tendencies, or by uncontrolled derivatives of sex and aggression; the retarded and infantile personality. Some of these children never reach the phallic-oedipal phase, which is the true starting point for the infantile neurosis (8).

### PSYCHOANALYTIC DEVELOPMENTAL PSYCHOLOGY

It was obvious that a new approach was needed for an understanding of pathological disturbances in the childhood period itself, one more broadly based than the concept of infantile neurosis as originally conceived. Progress in this direction was forthcoming in the newly emerging field of child psychoanalysis pioneered by Anna Freud. Through the development of the technique of child analysis and by application of analytic concepts in direct observation of children, it became possible to take a closer look at the process of personality formation. Sigmund Freud's basic ideas have been confirmed and extended. Studies of normal development have provided important guidelines in understanding pathological variations. In the critical problem of assessment of pathology, the child's developmental status has moved to the center of the stage.

In 1945 Anna Freud (9), discussing indications for treatment, laid stress on the fact that intervention was to be decided neither on symptomatology nor suffering nor any of the other criteria in use with adults. Rather, the decision for treatment should rest on the assessment as to whether the child's development could proceed or whether there was significant interference present. Dynamic child psychiatry in recent years has, therefore, been moving in the direction of a psychoanalytic developmental psychology. Consequently, a nosology of childhood disorders taking into account the factor of the developmental process is emerging. Thus anxieties, symptoms, and behavior patterns can be understood in the context of the child's total development to that time. In this way the total range, in terms of type and severity, of clinical material in childhood can be made the object of study from an integrated point of view which combines the tools of analysis and understanding of development of the child's personality from infancy onward.

Many of the disturbances frequently seen in children are phase-appropriate manifestations of the inevitable disharmonies in the rate of development of various psychic structures and the sequential unfolding of inborn behavior patterns and drive interests which comprise maturation. In addition to these developmental crises, there is the added disequilibria, similarly inevitable, between the needs of the child and even the most sensitive parental care. It has been pointed out (24) that were such ideal mothering possible and the child not experience any tension at all, it is doubtful that psychological development would take place. It can thus be said that anxiety and defenses against anxiety in the form of symptoms and behavior changes are an inevitable and integral aspect of any child's development. Not all these anxieties and behavior difficulties need be ascribed to neurotic conflicts, as was previously thought. Efforts are currently being made to provide a conceptual framework to facilitate differentiating various types of interference with the developmental process and the resultant pathological as well as normal vicissitudes of which neurosis would be only one eventuality.

In his monograph on infantile neurosis, Nagera (17) suggested four categories of disturbance for the childhood period: developmental interferences, developmental conflicts, neurotic conflicts, and infantile neurosis.

*Developmental interferences.* These comprise the external interferences experienced by the child. They are particularly crucial for development in the first year of life, representing pressures on the child with which he cannot cope because the demands are inappropriate or excessive. Some of these interferences occur in the form of deprivations—failure of the environment to provide adequately for the child's needs.

*Developmental conflicts.* When the demands imposed by the environment are appropriate or when difficulties arise because the child has reached some new developmental level, these difficulties and anxieties are termed developmental conflicts; e.g., as boys move from the anal to the phallic phase, the intense cathexis of the genitals gives rise to the castration anxiety, i.e. fears of damage should they yield to the temptation to touch themselves. Such anxiety reflects a developmental conflict since it is a concomitant of normal psychosexual maturation.

*Neurotic conflicts.* This term is reserved for difficulties arising out of opposition between the drives and internalized prohibitions from the superego or its precursors. Neurotic conflicts may start as phase-appropriate or developmental conflicts, such as the struggle over bowel training with oscillations between the desire to please the mother and the wish to soil. Such conflicts become neurotic when they persist beyond the appropriate time into the next phase of development. One can speak of neurotic conflicts during the pre-oedipal period, but not of an infantile neurosis.

*Infantile neurosis.* This is the most critical of all the developmental conflicts. It represents the regularly observed difficulties in the child as he passes through the phallic-oedipal period of development. In this sense it is part of the human condition. With successful resolution of the Oedipus complex and the onset of latency, the previously anxiety-ridden, irritable, unhappy child suddenly appears quite at peace with himself. Where the conflicts of the Oedipus complex are not adequately resolved and they persist into latency organized within the personality as a pathologic unit, an infantile neurosis can be said to exist.

The term infantile neurosis has undergone considerable change from its original meaning derived from the context of adult analysis. It is still used today to refer to the childhood nuclear conflicts—the genetic components of an adult neurosis. But it became apparent that not all adult neurotics had a history of manifest neurosis. In their analyses, what had to be reconstructed was the crucial phallic-oedipal period of their development. Freud wrote in 1940, "it seems that neuroses are acquired in early childhood (up to the age of 6) even though their symptoms may not make their appearance till much later. A childhood neurosis may become manifest for a short time or even may be overlooked. In every case, the later neurotic illness links up with the prelude in childhood" (12). This second meaning of infantile neurosis is actually, therefore, a synonym for the phallic-oedipal phase of development. The more specific usage referred to above as a fourth category of disturbance makes reference to an actual pathological entity in childhood itself—manifest and requiring treatment.

Referring to the importance of the infantile neurosis in both the normal and pathological sense, Nagera (17a) states,

[it] is, in my view, an attempt to organize all the previous and perhaps manifold neurotic conflicts and developmental shortcomings, with all the conflicts typical of the phallic-oedipal phase, into a single organization, into a single unit of the highest economic significance. This compromise formation is possible at this point because of the relatively high degree reached in several areas, particularly in that of ego's integrative and synthetic functions. For these reasons the "phallic-oedipal" phase is in fact an essential turning point in human development.

The infantile neurosis, which will be discussed later on, can now be conceptualized as the final and most complex form of childhood disorder resting at the apex of the child's psychological development. It is preceded by a hierarchy of disturbances closely related to the ongoing maturational and developmental processes as they interact with each other and with the environmental pressures operating from without.

Since it is not feasible to present an exhaustive list of all possible developmental disturbances, the discussion will be organized around the various phases of development—oral, anal, and phallic. Typical problems and clinical examples will be examined to delineate the developmental tasks of each period and the type of problems manifested as the child attempts to cope with them. Emphasis will be placed on syndromes which might appear pathological unless their relationship to current development is understood. The more severe disorders such as psychosis, impulse disorder, retardation, and ego disturbances will not be discussed.

## Developmental Disturbances

### THE FIRST EIGHTEEN MONTHS—THE ORAL PERIOD

From the moment of birth on, the infant is subject to interferences which are often out of harmony with his own inclinations at the time. This is, of course, an unavoidable consequence of the immature status of the neonate's basic neurophysiologic rhythms, such as those governing sleep and vegetative autonomic functions. But even after some rhythms are established and as myelinization of the central nervous system progresses, interferences are still inevitable due to difficulties in mother-child communication. As noted by Anna Freud "where child management is not extremely sensitive [in infancy] this causes a number of disturbances, the earliest of which are usually centered around sleep, feeding, elimination and the wish for company" (8a).

One form of interference consists of inappropriate demands on the child or stimulation that is not compatible with the child's capacities. Such would be the attempt to impose a rigid four-hour feeding schedule no matter what, or an effort to effect toilet training in the first year of life. Many of these difficulties of the milder sort reflect the mother's anxiety and her vulnerability to being criticized as inadequate. In others, latent conflicts or problems a woman has had with her own mother, which are activated in the postpartum period, are played out between the mother and her own newborn child.

Case #1. A twenty-four-year-old mother of an eight-week-old daughter experienced severe anxiety attacks and an obsessive preoccupation that she was not able to gratify her child and make her comfortable. The baby was somewhat colicky and irritable at the bottle and it had been recommended that a pacifier be tried to provide extra sucking activity. What was so disturbing to this young woman was that it worked! She couldn't stand looking at her daughter giving occasional contented sucks on the pacifier in her sleep as infants do. She felt that if permitted and thus encouraged, the child would always want to suck and she envisaged her walking around at three, or four, or five with a pacifier constantly in her mouth—a prospect which upset her very much. She felt so revolted, she was unable to allow it; but, when the child became irritable, she would experience severe anxiety, feeling that she was an inadequate mother. In passing, she also indicated that she was so upset because of this situation that she had begun to smoke two packs a day—a marked increase over her usual two or three cigarettes a day. Also, she recalled that in her own childhood, she had been a thumbsucker, but was "cured" at around age four when she developed some kind of infection on her thumb. In addition, during consultation she presented herself in an infantile demanding way, impatient for immediate relief, and irritated at any attempt to get her to look into herself and explore further beyond the initial manifestation of the nature of her anxiety. At one point in discussing her plight in having a baby, she remarked, "Maybe I've bitten off more than I can chew."

It was evident that this young woman's own oral conflicts had been reactivated by the birth of her child. She defended against her own oral excitement by transformation into feelings of disgust, but the conflict reappeared in the form of excessive smoking that had the characteristic of a symptom, being both a direct gratification of oral drives and appeasing her superego by arousing fears of cancer as a consequence. When she deprived the child of the pacifier and reviled herself as an inadequate, defective mother, these self-reproaches represented angry feelings for her own mother by whom she felt she had been deprived of sucking or other oral pleasure.

Here, the birth of the child activated neurotic conflicts in the mother whose altered behavior could, in time, affect in a negative way this little girl's development. Commenting on the complexity of the interaction between mother and child, Waelder (23) noted "that the mother, as the earliest and foremost representative of the environment, has a selective influence upon constitutional endowment by stimulating and encouraging some things and discouraging others." Anna Freud (8) on the same subject elaborated this idea: "by rejecting and seducing, she [the mother] can influence, distort or determine development, but she cannot produce either a neurosis or psychosis. I believe we ought to view the influence of the mother in this respect against the background of the spontaneous developmental forces which are active in the child." Both authors agreed that the problem can best be approached in terms of the complemental series of internal and external factors.

Among the internal factors to be considered is constitutional predisposition. Work has been done on neonates which reveals a range of activity potential that appears to reflect an innate tendency of the infant's own neurophysiological apparatus (13). At one end of the continuum are infants who, from birth, are irritable, with increased muscle tone, active reflexes, and who show an increased responsiveness to the environment. Such infants are likely to be wakeful, irritable, and perhaps colicky. In case #1, the little girl seemed to be such a child. Her mother on the other hand, like many other anxious first mothers, might have had an easier time adjusting to her new role if the infant had been of a more placid, somewhat lethargic disposition—content to lie quietly sleeping long hours and feeding less frenetically. It is doubtful, though, that this particular mother would have been helped since her neurotic difficulties did not permit her to be comfortable vis-à-vis the infant no matter what the child did. The child here was being used for the externalization of the mother's own inner conflicts. Where maternal pathology is less severe, such happy combinations might lead to a reasonable mother-child relationship; for there are also women whose needs lie in the opposite direction—they are gratified by an infant's alert, hyperactive responsiveness and disturbed by placidity.

Therefore, in evaluating the complemental series of internal and external factors underlying these early disturbances, one must consider the factor of the infant's congenital activity type as well as other idiosyncrasies of his behavior and developmental pattern. Then, with this in mind, one must evaluate the extent and nature of the mother's own attitude toward the infant and herself.

These early disturbances are predominantly in the nature of external interferences by the mothering person. Though some schools of thought hold that complicated intrapsychic processes do take place even in the first weeks of life (School of Melanie Klein), internal conflicts in the child between the drives and the ego would not seem to be possible. By and large the control of the id is left to outside forces. The mother has control of what the child eats and can intrude her own wishes (or needs) even into the child's way of soothing himself to sleep. The conflicts between mother and child can be traced in their course from one period to another, as in the following example:

Case # 2. Marcia, a three-and-a-half-year-old girl, was seen in consultation after she had developed a fear of being bitten by a dog. It was easily surmised that this phobic symptom was related to the recent birth of her brother whom she had actually tried to bite on one occasion. In addition to the symptom, she had also become very clinging to the mother, objecting to even normal separations, such as for brief shopping trips. Also her usual bedtime difficulties were markedly increased, similarly related to anxiety over separating from her mother. For quite a while in treatment she required her mother's presence in the playroom where, in addition, she sought to be in actual physical contact with her.

The mother reported in the history that for some reason she found she had to interfere with the child's wish to fall asleep with the bottle at both nap and bedtime even when she became old enough to hold her own bottle and desired to do so. At bedtime there were troubled scenes with the mother trying to rock and hold the child who was cranky and irritable, unable to fall asleep. During the second year, mealtime became stormy with mother and daughter struggling over what she should eat and how much. The little girl had developed into a finicky child whose tastes seemed unpredictable and she also showed a tendency to become quite obstinate.

Thus the normally expected behavior related to sibling rivalry was intensified because of the unsettled relationship which Marcia still experienced with regard to her mother as a source of oral satisfaction. She was in conflict between her own desires for autonomy and independence which were age appropriate and feelings of having been deprived in oral terms. This special sensitivity to oral conflicts constituted a fixation point in her development which was now interfering with mastery of a subsequent developmental task, namely, sibling rivalry. In addition, there was heightened pre-oedipal ambivalence leading to clinging behavior interfering with the development of autonomous self-identity.

This brief clinical vignette illustrates the cumulative effect of developmental difficulties where achievements and structural changes in the psyche from one phase can contaminate and distort later phases. Developmental interferences in Marcia's oral period set the stage for later neurotic conflicts. (Marcia's phobia will be discussed in greater detail later on.) One might use the analogy of the construction of a building where weaknesses in the foundation can affect and compromise the structures that are placed on top of it. It also exemplifies the point that these early developmental difficulties do not cause neurosis but only form a matrix out of which later neurotic difficulties can emerge.

But the most serious disturbances are not those due to excessive stimulation or inappropriate demands for conformity by a neurotically anxious mother, but rather those which arise from deprivation of adequate mothering care.

Withdrawal of the mother with a severe postpartum depression, even though she may continue to go through the motions of caring for the child's physical needs, would represent one of the more common interferences of this variety. Anna Freud spoke of the child's becoming "infected," as it were, by the mother's mood. Children who are not handled sufficiently to give them adequate tactile stimulation and are otherwise deprived of mothering care develop a severe and often irreversible type of pathology with disturbance of physical growth as well as severe retardation in both emotional and intellectual capacities. These syndromes will be discussed elsewhere and are well described in the literature (20, 22).

Not all maternal influences are pathogenic or negative in their effect on the child. Though there is still much to be learned about the nature of communication between mother and infant, the mother's own interests can exert a selective influence in the course of the child's development as has been noted. For example, children whose mothers have a habit of cooing and talking to them while caring for them in some physical way talk earlier than those who don't (19). Exposure to parental preferences, such as music, must have an effect on the child's own tendencies in this direction. A strong reinforcement by parental encouragement and the exposure to the activity by significant adults can be said to libidinize this activity for the child and prepare the way for later more complicated processes of identification and paths of sublimation (8b).

*Stranger anxiety.* As part of his normal development the infant manifests an anxiety syndrome often referred to as stranger anxiety. It is seen somewhere between six and ten months, and consists of an avoidance behavior, crying, and other physical signs of distress when he is confronted with an unfamiliar person. Though such behavior is a source of embarrassment to parents since it can wound the sensitivity of an aunt or grandparent, it is a healthy sign of the infant's ego development. It signifies that his perceptual apparatus is now able to distinguish visually the mother's face from all others. Seeing the other face causes distress and means loss of the mother who the infant, by previous cumulative experiences, has come to associate with the gratification of his vital needs. Absence of such a reaction could indicate disturbance of the infant's perceptual capacity or may indicate a lack of a significant mothering figure with whom he has associated need satisfaction. It also indicates a beginning of awareness in the infant of the difference between self and external need satisfying object.

## TODDLER PHASE—EIGHTEEN MONTHS TO THREE YEARS

One of the critical developmental tasks of the toddler or anal sadistic phase is the development of the independent sense of self and thereby achievement of a degree of autonomy and independence. Motor independence is a maturational milestone. Development of walking and further motility skills arise as a result of many trial-and-error explorations like climbing or poking around the house or outdoors. Toddlers are bursting with energy and hard to hold down. Interference of any sort with this new-found freedom of movement is resisted. This is the age of "no," signifying, according to Spitz (21), an important step in psychological individuation and separation from the mother (16). These inner changes, both maturational and developmental, are accompanied by various signs of disturbance and anxiety that are inevitable and thus a normal sign of this phase.

There is a *normal behavior disturbance* with irritability, negativism, and unruliness. Because the child is engaged in an inner struggle to assert himself while at the same time he desires to please the mother to gain her love, the behavior often oscillates or is unpredictable. One minute you see a little man anxious to do what he's told, and the next you see a whining, irritable infant who must have his way. Such regression is normal as is the heightened ambivalence in object attitudes. Feeling of hate and love quickly alternate. Also because of this ambivalence, there is to a greater or lesser degree anxiety about being separated from the mother, expressed by clinging behavior. These phenomena are a normal part of this period insofar as they are seen only for short spans of time and insofar as they do not predominate in the child's life. They arise as a result of temporary disequilibria in the development of various aspects of the child's personality on the one hand, and conflict with the environment on the other.

One of the most significant achievements is that of sphincter control in relation to the process of toilet training. This is the area par excellence for the expression of a power struggle between mother and child. Often the training process only epitomizes the nature of the interaction between mother and child—the same struggles being waged over what is eaten or worn or the timing or nature of various activities throughout the day.

The following case illustrates such a power struggle between a disturbed mother and her eldest son that has gone beyond the normal bounds both in intensity and in time.

Case #3. An attractive and somewhat histrionic mother came for help with her eldest of two boys. At age four Carl was still not bowel trained. He would spend all morning in nursery school, come home and have a bowel movement in his pants. He often refused to sit on the toilet and acted as if he were afraid of it. Mealtimes were also the scene of frequent battles over what he would eat and how much. The mother was also beginning to be concerned that the younger boy, too, was starting to balk about training, and she feared he was emulating his older brother. The other major complaint was that, denied any request, he would have a tantrum till he got what he wanted. The mother was vulnerable to this sort of carrying on and would eventually give in in order to stop this behavior.

One year previous there was, in quick succession, hospitalization of the mother for a week, vacation by the parents alone in which the boys were left behind, and the death of the paternal grandfather with whom the boy was very close. In these troubled times, they were left with maids or whoever could be spared to look after them. The parents were not psychologically sensitive and made no effort to explain to the boy what was going on.

The mother was an actress prior to her marriage. She felt she had given up a successful career for her husband and regretted it. Also, since adolescence, she had suffered from morning depressions which sounded like micropsychotic episodes in which she would scream at anyone who disturbed her, making all sorts of threats of which she was later oblivious. For instance, she would scream at this boy when he came in in the morning, telling him to get out or she would kill him. She was taking Dexedrine every morning, claiming this was the only thing that helped her; she refused any attempts to try thyroid regulation, although studies had indicated her thyroid might be deficient. She was thus a very narcissistic woman with strong underlying feelings of dissatisfaction in her marriage and in her maternal role. Her own mother she described as cold and undemonstrative and not too involved with the children. Her husband disclaimed any problem with Carl and resisted the entire evaluation process, claiming that it was only with his mother that he was like this and that she was the problem. In nursery school they found Carl a charming, intelligent boy, but noted a tendency to play by himself rather than with a group. His vocabulary was well developed for his age, though his speech was infantile. In the playroom, phallic play interests dominated but were not exclusive.

The clinical picture, therefore, was characterized by severe conflicts between Carl and his mother, eating difficulties and behavior disorder, together with the vexing problem of stool retention. This problem seemed part of an ongoing pattern of the power struggle between the two. On the boy's side there was some evidence of previous oral fixation shown by his regression to a whining, demanding, thumb-sucking child who was a finicky eater. Also it might be suspected that the separations of the previous year (the mother's illness and the paternal grandfather's death, etc.) may have contributed to the stool retention as a symptom defending against the fear of object loss.

It was also noted that the mother complained of her husband's dullness in intellectual matters, and the lack of stimulation in the home. To compensate, she attempted to stimulate Carl intellectually, providing games and other activities far beyond his ability or age. She spoke unabashedly about his being a genius. She was evidently displacing much of her dissatisfaction with the marriage and her husband onto the child. He was to make up for what was missing both in her marriage and in herself. The burden of fulfilling such a function could not be borne by this youngster and he appeared to be recoiling from the excessive demands that she placed upon him (specifically that he produce, both mentally and anally) to please her.

Such a situation would not be just a developmental conflict; Carl, at four, was already suffering from neurotic conflicts fed by the pathological interaction with his mother. The existence of similar conflicts in the prior oral period and the persistence of these conflicts into the phallic phase of development signified that serious interference with the developmental process was taking place.

One good prognostic sign was that the stool retention still seemed to be focused mainly on the mother. During the evaluation process Carl went for a visit to the paternal grandmother while the parents had another vacation. There was no trouble with his bowels—no accidents—and no refusal to use the toilet. It might well be that as he moved further into the phallic phase, this particular symptom and perhaps some of the regressive whiny behavior might disappear, but the chances of his traversing the oedipal period without further and more serious difficulties was slim.

This case illustrates the complex interplay between normal developmental processes and maternal psychopathology on the one hand, and the possible influence of traumatic events (separation experiences) on particular developmental tasks on the other hand.

*Sleep disturbance.* Transient disturbance of sleep is often seen in the earlier part of the anal sadistic period (i.e. eighteen months to two years). As already indicated, there have been great strides and accomplishments. The toddler is busy developing his physical skills as well as expressing his own desire for independence. These changes, reflected in the growth and development of the ego, are a source of pride to the toddler.

At night the child fights sleep out of fear of losing this newly won control and ability. At this stage he is threatened by the normal ego regression which occurs at the onset of sleep. One specific fear is that sphincter control will be lost and the child will soil. Bornstein (1) treated a two-year-old child with severe sleep disturbance, causing her to sit bolt upright and stiff in bed lest she regress and soil. In the usual situation, the disturbance is not so severe, and after the pleasurable ego gains are consolidated, the fear of losing them in sleep will pass.

*Archaic fears.* In addition to this type of anxiety (the fear of ego regression) there are other fears which occur in a transitory way and without a pathological significance.

Losing the feces seen as a body part or prized possession can lead to fear of sitting on the toilet as in case #3. The content of the anxiety focuses often on the noise of the flushing and the latent fear is that of being flushed down along with the feces. Such fears often persist into the phallic phase with the anxiety then being displaced onto the fear of loss of penis. Other typical anxieties have to do with the unknown or new situations, such as going on elevators or new places in general; fears of loneliness; fears of the dark and loud noises (thunder, vacuum cleaners). Anna

Freud refers to these fears as archaic "since their origin cannot be traced to any previous frightening experience, it seems to be included in the innate disposition" (8c). But they are not phobias since they lack the complicated structure and are not based on an internal conflict with regression and displacement that comprises the dynamics of phobias. It is still an open question whether such proneness to anxiety in early years makes for a specific vulnerability to the development of phobias later on.

*Transient obsessional reactions.* At the height of the phase of anal sadism or shortly thereafter, there is often encountered behavior which looks like an obsessional neurosis with ritualistic behavior, particularly at bedtime, and excessive concern for orderliness and cleanliness. This is accounted for by an overshooting of the defenses of the ego in its attempts to control the drives of the anal period, particularly those related to bowel training. They represent reaction formations which, if not persistent and excessive, can form the basis of healthy character traits in the developing personality; i.e., they can become part of the autonomous ego (15). If for some reason, these reactions are reinforced and intensified, as with Carl, fixation at this level could be created, and the child might tend to regress to this level in the face of severe anxiety at a subsequent level of development. When this occurs, the conflicts that ensue and the symptoms that result represent true obsessive-compulsive pathology. This vulnerability is thus similar to the fixations of the earlier oral period and conflicts over food intake. Later manifestations of G.I. disturbance and neurotic disturbances of appetite are symptomatic expressions of regressive returns to the oral level.

*Stammering.* This is a transient disturbance often seen when difficulties are being encountered in the toilet training process. Frequently the symptom yields dramatically when parental demands ease off.

It should be noted that as development proceeds, the type of difficulty shifts from purely external interferences, such as maternal mismanagement in the neonate, to conflicts within the child. This progressive internalization proceeds *pari passu* with increasing maturation and structuralization of the personality. The conflict in the toddler over the wish to gratify his anal impulses at a time and place of his own choosing and the desire to please his mother is only possible with sufficient maturation in the ego and the laying down of superego precursors in the form of internalized controls. Similarly, the development of a symptom as a compromise formation, expressing in disguised and symbolic way some forbidden wish as well as satisfying the need for punishment, reflects a certain degree of sophistication in both ego and superego development.

## PHALLIC PHASE—THREE TO SEVEN YEARS

*Libidinal activities.* In the phallic phase, the genital area becomes the predominant source of erogenous stimulation in both boys and girls. Although phallic masturbation is seen earlier, even in the first year of life, it is not until this phase, which begins around age three, that the phallic zone is pre-eminent. It should be stressed that the succession of libidinal phases is a gradual one with much overlap (14). This fact underlies the ease of regression and the admixture of oral, anal, and phallic elements still seen from moment to moment in children prior to the onset of latency.

For example, the play pattern of a phallic child may start with guns and rescuing a female from a monster or "baddies." Drowning the monster may shade over into water play with the anal qualities of messing and cleaning up, so that the original phallic elements are lost. Though this is termed a regressive shift stimulated by anxiety and excitement created by the phallic theme, it is so highly reversible that such regressions are within normal limits. It is quite common also for phallic stimulation to lead to desire to urinate and such excursions to the bathroom can be used as useful guidelines to the libidinal activities of the child in the playroom. Such regressive overflow of genital excitement to the urethral zone, even if frequent, is, however, less ominous than shifts to the anal zone, interruptions of play being punctuated by the need to defecate. Anal fixation can be suspected, the older the child; by latency this behavior should certainly have passed, unless there is definite neurotic conflict present. For example, in case #3, Carl was engaged in a shooting theme between goodies and baddies. Suddenly he stopped and began to squeeze his buttocks together and his face paled a little. He agreed finally to go to the bathroom, but once there he would not sit on the toilet, but busied himself at the sink playing with the water. By his play pattern this four year old was showing phallic interest. The excitement that was created, however, was being expressed in a phase-inappropriate way through the anal zone.

*Sleep disturbance.* The phallic phase represents another period where sleep disturbance may become manifest. This time, in contrast to the early anal period, the difficulty in falling asleep is due to the presence of conflicts over phallic masturbation. The weakening of ego controls as sleep approaches, with relative quiet and darkness shutting out external stimulation, leaves the child more prey to his own fantasies and accompanying libidinal pressures. Tempted to masturbate, but fearful of the consequences, the child fights sleep. His behavior belies the anxiety with which he is coping and is misread by the parent as naughtiness in trying to break the rules by staying up later. The parent's anger in this context can reinforce the child's feeling of guilt, making the problem worse. Rather, a comforting but firm attitude will help break the vicious cycle. Intensification of attachment to soft toys or blankets has a significance during this period in protecting the child's anxieties and fears at the phallic level.

*Nightmares.* The ego's vulnerability to the thrust of the phallic oedipal drives is also revealed in the nightmares that are so regularly seen in this period. The manifest anxiety revolves around monsters, dinosaurs, kidnappers, witches, and the like, which are projections of the child's own hostile wishes. They also represent his fear of retaliatory punishment in the form of castration derivatives. A more severe form of nightmare, *pavor nocturnus*, if persistent, may connote a deeper disturbance in the child that is not just a developmental vicissitude. With *pavor nocturnus*, the child appears to be awake and may respond to questioning. He may be sitting up or walking around, but responding to frightening perceptions in the manner of a hallucinating patient. The next morning there is a characteristic amnesia for the whole episode. In the immediate situation, the parents can be of most help by definitely waking the child up. The cold tile of the bathroom floor, a drink of water, putting lights on and distracting the child with conversation can be useful in this respect. *Pavor nocturnus* should be investigated further.

*Behavior disturbance.* Pearson referred to this period—three to six—as a phase of normal behavior disturbance (18). The phallic child is faced with many crucial developmental tasks. He has to cope with and resolve the ambivalence of the oedipal triangle with attendant fears of punishment and intense rivalry and jealousy. He is noisily exhibitionistic to gain his mother's admiration and attention, but easily upset and crushed by failure, reverting quickly to the pre-oedipal whining, demanding role of the infant. Either way he can be exasperating—domineering and possessive on the one hand, or clinging or dependent on the other.

Similarly, he can be driven to reckless behavior to prove his masculinity but reduced to tears and hysterics by a slight bruise or cut. Whereas in the anal period, the major fear was that of loss of love of the object, now it is the fear of bodily damage, specifically injuries to the genitals which are so invested with meaning at this time. Anna Freud (7) termed the intense castration anxiety in phallic boys a realistic interference with the introspective process, constituting, therefore, a technical difficulty in the treatment of these youngsters.

*Transient phobias.* As part of the vulnerability to anxiety, phobias are seen as a form of defense and compromise with the libidinal drives that are so urgent at this time. Such complicated maneuvers for dealing with the drives were not possible previously due to immaturity of the ego apparatus. But adequate superego controls are not yet present to allow for smooth anxiety-free management of sexual and aggressive urges.

For example, in Mrs. Bornstein's case of Frankie (2), there was a period around age four and a half when he developed a fear that a wolf was under his bed which would bite his feet should he put them out of the covers. This occurred at a time when Frankie was struggling at night with his intense curiosity to go to the parents' bedroom to find out what they did in there. The phobia, then, could be seen as the ego's attempt to defend against Frankie's scoptophilic wishes at a time when his superego was not yet strong enough to maintain a prohibition against such temptations to satisfy his sexual curiosity.

The animal phobia, so typical as a transitory phenomenon in this period, is a result of such developmental conflicts related to sexual interests and anxieties. The passing away of such fears may signify important superego consolidations, so that such conflicts can now be more harmoniously handled without resort to compromise formations, such as phobias.

## LATENCY

The onset of latency is variously described in the literature as occurring anywhere between five and a half and seven. The reason for this spread is more a result of differences in the rate of development of children as they traverse this critical period of their lives than it is a theoretical difference among observers. More important than what age this so-called developmental "pause" or latency period occurs are the actual structural changes in the personality that accompany it. The solutions and the identifications which facilitate resolution of the "infantile neurosis" (the phallic-oedipal conflicts) lay the groundwork for the onset of latency. These psychic changes and developments set the basic form of the child's personality for the rest of his life. In later phases there are important additions and modifications, but the essential foundation has been laid at the time latency begins.

*Resolution of Oedipus in boys and girls.* The path followed by the boy and girl in psychosexual development divides at the phallic phase. For the boy, the threat of castration provides the impetus for his attempts to give up his erotic desires for his mother. They must be repressed and replaced by aim-inhibited tenderness devoid of sexuality. Identification with the father is an important mechanism in this process. It acts simultaneously to reinforce the boy's masculine identity and helps establish the superego. With this conflict properly resolved, the boy is now free both to like his father and to be like him. The former ambivalence of the oedipal phase is thus partly overcome by identification. (The father who is feared is now represented intrapsychically in the boy's superego.)

It is quite common to see oscillations between acting big and grown up and demanding to be treated as such (phallic exhibitionism) and fears of growing older in the early phases of latency. The more boasting and bragging, the more omnipotent the child behaves, the more he must also be suffering from inferiority feelings. Bornstein (3) described a case of a child who in his treatment hours claimed to be a brain surgeon secretly flown to the battlefield at night to operate on famous generals. Such excursions into this omnipotent fantasy were noted to occur following some slight or deflating experience particularly at school. The fantasy functioned as a defense against feelings of inferiority and hurt narcissism. Persistence of such grandiose tendencies with flight into fantasy beyond seven or eight is an indication of developmental failure in the area of self-image or self-esteem regulation. The child must not have been able to come to grips with feeling small and helpless. Something in the boy must have prevented a proper identification with and sharing of the father's phallic power and strength which enables him to look forward to the day when he too can be in fact as big as his father.

The little girl in the phallic phase at first behaves like a boy with sexual interest in the mother. But her awareness of the lack of a penis causes her to shift her love from the mother to the father. She then has to repress her masculine strivings and overcome feelings of inferiority due to penis envy. The Oedipus complex in girls does not begin till the awareness of her own "castrated" state occurs; in contrast, the threat of castration marks the beginning of the end of the Oedipus complex in the boy. A favorable outcome for the little girl requires her "ability to tolerate and strengthen her original passive drives and to channel her active masculine strivings into feminine sexuality" (4). If the masculine side is not repressed, the little girl remains in rivalry with the opposite sex and in latency presents the well-known picture of the "tomboy." In this situation the girl has not gotten over feeling inferior because of genital differences. She persists in trying to fool the world (and herself) that she is really a boy. Her femininity is denied and a pseudomasculine stance is adhered to defensively. Normally, in the girl, the Oedipus subsides slowly and the wish for the penis from the father hopefully becomes transformed into a mature wish for a child accompanied by a stable female sexual identification with adequate preparation for acceptance of the maternal role.

Resolution of the Oedipus complex thus involves shifts in libidinal interest and objects, changes in object relations, alterations in self-image brought about by identification, and important psychic structural developments, particularly in the superego. When the Oedipus complex is negotiated successfully, there is a general integration in the personality, with diminution of conflicts and lessening of inner turmoil. This whole consolidation process is facilitated by the apparent biological tapering of drive intensity as compared to the phallic period.

Rarely, however, does this process proceed smoothly and serenely. Developmental conflicts centered around phallic problems persist though their form may be altered. Early animal phobias are often replaced by renewal of separation anxiety signifying resurgence of ambivalence. This type of separation is structurally more like obsessional worrying for the safety of a love object because of repressed hatred or death wishes. The following vignette illustrates this point as well as many other typical conflicts in early latency.

Case #4. Natalie, an attractive seven-year-old, showed a combination of behavior disturbance and anxiety symptoms. She would fly into a rage over the slightest difficulty while doing her homework, venting her anger on her mother whom she had inveigled to come and help her. Nothing pleased her. She insisted on French horn lessons, finally overcoming her parents' objections, but then threw a fit when the instrument case was black instead of brown. During the day she was extremely hostile to both of her parents as they struggled in vain to please her to buy a few moments' peace. She would openly wish them dead and clamor for new parents. But at night Natalie was unable to go to sleep unless her mother put her to bed in a special way complying with various formulas and ritualistic arrangements. On the weekend she fought against the parents' going out, voicing anxiety about their encountering some danger. Occasionally she would reveal some worry about a car accident, especially if the weather were bad. She insisted on knowing what time they would be home. If they went out of town, mother had to promise to call at a certain time. Once when inadvertently this was not done, Natalie was inconsolable for hours.

As can be noted, Natalie's "separation anxiety" was like an obsessional symptom betraying death wishes toward the person whose safety was feared. But in the true obsessional symptom these death wishes would be repressed, i.e., unconscious. For Natalie, however, she could freely wish her mother dead in the daytime and mean it, only to have an anxiety attack in the evening when she experienced the wish as a fear.

Insomnia, partly warded off by obsessional mechanisms, occurs often as the extension of similar sleep difficulties (nightmares, etc.) of the phallic period when masturbation conflicts are heightened. Natalie manifested the typical obsessional rituals so frequently used to ward off these anxieties.

Natalie also had strong feelings of inadequacy and inferiority related to penis envy. Consciously she wished to be a boy and competed with them successfully in athletics, eschewing doll play and other more feminine pursuits. She couldn't wait to get home from school and change into shorts or slacks to go out and find the boys. Her outlook was that of a tomboy, not a reflection of heterosexual interest. She was struggling with and had not yet been able to repress her masculine strivings. Her interest in boys and her wish to be with them was based on identification, not object love. Thus, as with the death wishes which alternated with obsessional anxiety about her mother dying, Natalie could at times be very coquettish and seductively feminine. As she advanced into latency, the tomboy attitude dropped away. This particular expression of penis envy was overcome, then, spontaneously though other developmental interferences related to her castration complex persisted.

Mention has already been made of Natalie's use of mother as a scapegoat when homework proved difficult. Only by inference or very transitorily could it be seen how badly she must feel about herself in what she considered to be her academic inadequacy. Natalie approached any task with the preconceived notion that she would be unable to accomplish it. The slightest obstacle would appear to prove this contention that she was indeed no good. Natalie would then go to pieces. She would find some external source for the difficulties such as her mother or the teacher or attribute her difficulties to the distraction caused by ordinary activities in the household, e.g., her sister was talking too loudly, she could hear the TV downstairs. The whole family was forced to walk on eggs to try to avoid her carrying on in this way. This type of behavior represents an "intermediate stage of superego development" (6). The child is intolerant of any criticism from the outside. In the process of trying to internalize it, the child does not progress further than to an "identification with the aggressor." In the playroom, Natalie would subject the therapist to a tongue-lashing for minor infractions or shortcomings similar to the tirades she directed at her family. The guilt was projected onto the hapless scapegoat. The quality and intensity of her angry rebuke bespoke the harshness of her own budding superego. Unless such a superego is modified or mitigated, the child developmentally may remain fixated at that point. As adults these individuals have an infantile quality in their personalities. They take no responsibility. Everything is someone else's fault. Often they appear tied to a parent in a sort of *folie à deux* which replicates the early mother-child relationship. It is as if the superego was never fully formed. Responsibility for the consequences of what they do remain externalized.

Natalie, of course, was not experiencing merely developmental conflicts. She was well on the way to an obsessional neurosis, but to go into greater detail concerning the essentials of the rest of her case history would take us too far afield. She did present in an unusually clear and pathologically exaggerated way many of the "normal developmental conflicts" which are seen in early latency.

*Fear of castration and fear of death.* One other transformation which occurs in early latency is the change from open castration fear (fears of bodily injury or damage) to a fear of death. Although only five and a half, David (case #9), no doubt stimulated by the death of his grandmother, displayed more anxiety about death and all of its ramifications than he ever did about bodily injury. In the succeeding months after the funeral he brought home questions about death, heaven, and God. In more than one way he indicated a fear of his own death. He claimed he would never get married and then he would always stay in his present house. (That is, he would never grow up and die.) He toyed with what it would be like to be without parents and wondered who would take their places. This type of cosmological questioning about life after death is part and parcel of the educational process at the kindergarten or first-grade level. But the preoccupation with death betrays the fact that the child's interest is being fed as by an underground stream by his fears of death and continued, unresolved, ambivalent feelings toward those he loves.

*Peer relations.* Part of the latency process which follows the resolution of the oedipal conflicts is the displacement of interests from the oedipal objects to the peer group. Important activities in the child's life begin to take place outside of the home. Absence of such a transfer of libidinal interest or difficulties in adaptation to the group often reflect continued involvement with the oedipal objects. For example, an infantile neurosis has the effect of delaying latency and preventing these important extensions of the child's object relations from taking place. Such children are noted to suffer from lack of interest in peers, from school phobias, or from homesickness (8d).

*Family romance.* Along with the lessening of ties to the oedipal figures, the latency child shows evidence of disillusionment with the parents. They have lost their previous luster. This process is facilitated by the extent to which the child's own superego development enables him to cease having to rely unquestioningly on parental judgments.

A typical manifestation of this denigration of the parents is the so-called "family romance." The child fantasies that these are not his parents but rather poor substitutes for his real parents whom he imagines are very special or exalted figures from whom he has become separated. The myth of Oedipus contains such an idea though in modified form and similar themes are found in many fairy stories. Feeling adopted is another way the child expresses his dissatisfaction with his less-than-perfect parents. Anna Freud makes the point in this regard that reactions to adoption are more severe in latency due to this already phase-appropriate denial of the parents.

*Sublimation.* In early latency (up to age eight), the child may still be struggling with residual phallic conflicts and experiencing difficulty in consolidating his superego. By eight, things should have settled down, with the ego more firmly in control of the now lessened drives. Bornstein (3) finds it useful to divide latency into two stages—the first, five and a half to eight years, and the second, from eight to eleven—in order to deal with these developmental differences. Detached from the oedipal objects, the child is free to explore the world outside his family. He has the libido available for expanded object relations as well as for sublimated activities, such as hobbies. However, because these sublimations or attempts to discharge drive energy in an aim-inhibited way are not that far removed from the original aims, the latency child usually engages in enthusiasms rather than true hobbies. His interest, initially, is compelling and intense. But much to the parents' dismay after they have purchased the necessary equipment, the child drops the activity and goes on to something else. The path through latency into early adolescence is thus strewn with the discarded paraphernalia of lost enthusiasms.

*Learning problems.* One of the most important forms of sublimation is the learning process. Sexual curiosity is transformed into a thirst for knowledge, drawing its energies from previously sexually based desires to look, to probe, to find out how things work, where things come from, etc. Willingness to tackle the unknown, the ability to tolerate confusion, missteps, mistakes, failures, and the capacity to keep trying, all require a solid ego which can view these tasks in an unconflicted way. For a child who still experiences finding out how something works as the fulfillment of a forbidden sexual wish, learning continues to be an area of anxiety. Sexualization of learning constitutes the basic dynamics of neurotic learning difficulties in which sexual conflicts are carried over and contaminate this vital area of the child's life. Pressure on the one hand from his superego against his desire to learn, and on the other hand from the parents and teachers for academic performance, creates intolerable conditions for the child from which the only escape is often a withdrawal of interest in learning.

Problems related to the child's narcissism—the regulation of his self-esteem—also find exquisite means of expression in the learning process. That we learn best from our own mistakes and that practice makes perfect are two axioms the child with deep-rooted inferiority feelings cannot accept. To try something new and have it not come out right is to fail. The superego of such unhappy youngsters demands "instant" perfection. There is no allowance for trial and error.

Case #5. Ron, from the very beginning had difficulties in school. In treatment during latency it was learned that his frequent headaches followed experiences in class where he had made an error or had been unable to answer a question. Behind the headaches lay fears that his mother would not come for him after school. He would be thus abandoned by her because he was so stupid. His headache as a symptom expressed both an identification with the mother as a protection against losing her and a desire to arouse sympathy and interest in a regressive way.

In the playroom he showed other defenses against feelings of being a failure; he became grandiose in his claims of knowledge about abstruse matters in medicine or space technology, lecturing me in a condescending manner. Or he would play the part of the "teacher," concocting impossible arithmetic problems for me to do, slashing my work with big X's and sneering at my ineptitude. In the former omnipotence, there was a denial of reality and retreat into fantasy; in the latter situation, there is an excellent portrayal of the mechanism of "identification with the aggressor" and "projection of guilt."

The excesses of Ron's harsh, demanding superego were painful to behold. Whenever he was feeling particularly crushed, the slightest deviation or disappointment would throw him into a rage. If the ruler slipped when he was drawing a line, he would tear the paper to bits and throw the ruler across the room. The "offending" pencil would be broken to pieces. As our therapeutic work extended into this area of his narcissistic vulnerability, it emerged that Ron had the idea that only for him did these things not turn out right the first time. Other kids never had this trouble. For a long time he resisted learning to write cursively, but engaged instead in make-believe, scribbling "important" messages to the President and other leading figures. He responded well to the interpretation that he perhaps thought that other kids were somehow born knowing how to write, that only he, because he was born so dumb, had to learn.

Obviously, learning for this youngster did not just mean the fulfillment of a forbidden sexual wish to please his mother; it focused on deep-seated difficulties in his image of himself as hopelessly inferior and inadequate. The feelings of intense rage and depression stemmed from developmental conflicts earlier than those of the phallic-oedipal level.

The developmental task of learning presents itself full force for the first time in latency. Properly approached, it can provide a potent source of sublimation leading to acquisition of skills by the ego. Simultaneously these ego achievements can lead to great satisfaction for the child in terms of his self-image and the approbation and love of his parents.

It is a frequent occurrence in clinical practice to be consulted about children (usually boys) who only begin to show difficulty in school in the fourth and fifth grade. It is all the more puzzling since previous performance had led everyone to expect great things. Instead there is a downtrend at this stage of late latency. It is my impression that this difficulty stems from a shift in educational technique and style that occurs at this level of elementary education. It is no longer sufficient to be able to absorb information from the teacher in class; homework becomes a necessary supplement to the day's lesson. Chapters must be read and digested and the child must decide what is essential. He is called upon to do some independent thinking and organizing. Projects are assigned which require initiative and autonomy for their proper execution. The child is on his own. These children in the early grades have shown a capacity to attend passively, sopping up knowledge like a sponge, but the demands of fourth or fifth grade require the exercise of different ego capacities. These children then experience anxiety when called upon to be more active or assertive in pursuing an independent line of study. Conflicts over behaving in a masculine aggressive manner are stirred up in this new context of academic pursuits. It is a vexing diagnostic problem to distinguish those youngsters for whom the change in academic demands constitutes a temporary developmental disturbance from those whose real underlying difficulties are finding their way to the surface for the first time. One must rely on the panorama of the previous developmental patterns in making the decision for or against treatment at this time. The syndromes of learning disability in children will be examined in greater detail in another chapter.

## PREPUBERTY

During the transition from the oedipal period to latency, there is a regressive revival of pregenital trends. Anal and oral drive interests operate as a regressive defense against the anxiety-provoking oedipal material. Important character developments arise out of the reaction formations developed by the ego to deal with resurgent pregenitality. Traits such as orderliness, cleanliness, and regard for time are useful adaptations that ensue. There is a similar regressive movement of the libido toward the end of latency in what has been termed prepuberty. Unlike the previous period, more seems lost than gained by way of character developments. Many of the child's previous achievements and social adaptations appear to dissolve. He seems less mature than before. Delinquent trends can appear for the first time (8e). Unless properly understood, this breakdown in behavior and control can be alarming.

For example, homosexual behavior can occur as isolated episodes even into early adolescence. Normal object relations during latency are "homosexual" as an indication not of incipient perversion, but as an expression of the narcissistic basis of object choice. Boys like other boys with whom they can identify. The aberration of the "tomboy" has been referred to already as a young girl who persists in maintaining a phallic identification. She is "really" a boy and therefore wants to be with those of "her kind."

Real concern should arise about the eventual sexual identity of a latency boy who prefers the company of girls. While the revival of pregenital trends, including passive longings, can be instrumental in fostering homosexual behavior, the ultimate outcome depends on many factors among which is the age of the partners. There is less danger of homosexuality where the ages are the same and there is no element of coercion. (For a more complete discussion see Anna Freud, 8e.)

*Motor activity.* In prepuberty the child also reacts to his passive wishes by a flight into physical activity to reinforce his feeling of being in control. Any situation which arouses passive dependent desires and which restricts physical expression can be very anxiety-provoking. In child therapy such repetitive actions as coin-flipping, playing with paper clips, or foot-tapping can serve as discharge outlets. The child at this age is too old to play and too young to free associate. Educators and camp counselors sensitive to this phenomenon learn to punctuate sedentary activities with some periods where motility can be expressed and restlessness drained off.

Patterns of activity have been subject to study as they reflect the ebb and flow of resistance in treatment (5), e.g., tossing paper airplanes back and forth in the playroom serving as a means of keeping distance from the therapist.

The increased restlessness and need for motor outlets may also reflect prepubertal stirrings of libido. During latency, sexual pressures are either lessened or can be drained off in the many sublimated activities (learning for sexual curiosity, physical skills for phallic exhibitionism, etc.). Resurgence of more intense genital sensations in boys can lead to renewed conflicts over masturbation. The passive experience of tumescence to which boys are so subject can also be a source of great anxiety. Fears of helplessness and loss of control or fears of the pressure of drives can form a potent stimulus to the increased motor activity of this period. Being in control of one's body can serve an important defensive function while simultaneously restoring the narcissistic equilibrium threatened by such irruptions from the id. In pathological cases masturbation conflicts can lead to a need to carry out physical activity to the point of exhaustion unconsciously equivalent to detumescence.

In addition to the normal recourse to motor activity as a defense against experiencing his own inner feelings, particularly passive trends, the older latency child uses reality as a means of avoiding contact with his fantasies. For this reason he is unable to free associate in therapy, and other means must be employed to gain information about unconscious processes. This push toward reality expresses itself in the child's concern for real knowledge of the world in terms of facts and figures. The younger child uses numbers in the service of fantasy. To him a zillion and a thousand represent equally immense, unfathomable quantities. The prepuberty child wants to know how many million make a billion and tries to figure how long it takes light to travel to the moon and back. He already knows the velocity of light. In the girl these same interests may appear as sublimated activities in following recipes or in learning fundamentals of baby care on younger siblings or on baby-sitting chores in the neighborhood.

Such is the picture of the child as he rounds the corner of latency on his way to adolescence: developmentally complete in many respects, but yet to face the final integration of his personality after the sexual maturation of adolescence. The foregoing picture, however, can be but an overview focusing on particular vulnerable areas subject to disturbance which may or may not have lasting significance. Emphasis has been placed on the developmental tasks of each period and on reactions which might appear to be pathological but which only represent some temporary disharmony. Only careful scrutiny of the entire developmental process will suffice to distinguish transient from more serious interferences, such as neurotic conflicts and full-blown neurosis.

## Separation—Object Loss As a Developmental Interference

In a developmental framework, it can be easily seen how the same event occurring at one point in the child's life can have a different meaning and impact than when it occurs in another phase of development. The longitudinal axis in the study of the evolution of psychic structure or other vital functions comprises a line of development (10) in which the specific function can be studied from phase to phase. As an example of such a developmental line the reaction to object loss will be discussed at various ages.

Object loss is a critical event whenever it occurs, but in different ways. During the early years, the loss of an object can be catastrophic since there is real physical as well as psychological dependence. Important components of ego development will be distorted or lacking in the complete absence of, or with deficient mothering.

Case #6. Perry lost his mother from a fulminating leukemia when he was six weeks old. He was cared for by a succession of mother substitutes hired by his father. Some lasted a few months or less, others as long as a year. None was considered satisfactory by his father, but he tried as best he could to provide a home for his only child. When Perry was seen in consultation at four, he presented a severe problem of stool retention, sometimes going for days without a movement even though in obvious abdominal discomfort due to cramps and fullness. He was otherwise in good physical health and appeared as a charming though somewhat soft youngster. He was brought by a foreign woman who was his current caretaker and it was noted that he left her without any trace of difficulty whatever. His language was peculiar. At times he would chirp unintelligibly as if to himself, whereas he could name such objects in the playroom as "microscope." He had to interrupt his play often to concentrate on holding back his stool, which was evidently accomplished only with great effort and concentration. Both in theme and quality, his play was more like that of a two-year-old. Dump trucks and blocks were his favorite items. In one dramatic session, he constructed a series of barriers which had to be negotiated one after the other to allow passage of a small car. Following this he went to the bathroom to attempt a movement for the first time during a play session. However, he showed no sign of concern about leaving or arriving nor any particular warmth or hostility. He seemed, in effect, indifferent to the examiner as an object.

Although there are many other complex and intricate facets to this case, it is used here to illustrate the severe disturbance in object relations stemming from long-standing deprivation of consistent maternal care. Language development as well as cognitive ego functions were also impaired; psychosexual progression semed to have halted at the anal phase with a persistent severe symptom of retention for which an organic basis had been ruled out by pediatric examination. The damage occurring early was diffuse; the long-range outlook was bleak.

Such disruptions in maternal care occurring in the earliest months of life lead to severe ego disturbances, childhood psychoses, or severe developmental retardations.

In the toddler or anal sadistic phase (one and a half to three) there is normally a heightened ambivalence in the child's attitude toward significant objects, such as the mother. Re-emergence of earlier clingingness and anxiety over separation from the mother are often vexing but phase-appropriate manifestations. There is fear of abandonment coupled with the belief in the omnipotence of his own angry thoughts toward the mother. At this level in the child's mind, the wish and the deed are considered synonymous.

Fixations in this area can arise due to acts of fate such as illness or death of a parent or hospitalization of the child. Regardless of the reality, children in the anal phase regularly view such events as rejection by the parents and attempt closure psychologically by fantasizing reasons for which they should be abandoned. In this period, the major fear is a fear of loss of love.

Separation problems encountered in the beginning of nursery school at three or three and a half indicate that this developmental hurdle has not yet been overcome. Later anxieties about going off to school and actual school refusal can represent regression in object relations to this stage of pre-oedipal ambivalence. Here the child's anxiety is due to his belief that the parents' safety can only be counted on while they are in sight or close by. There are always, of course, related fears of abandonment should any-thing happen to the parent. School refusal in these instances is actually a fear of leaving home rather than a fear or wish for avoidance of school as a phobic situation.

In examining children during this age and even up to age five, it is not uncommon for them to be unable at first to come to the playroom alone; characteristically the child reaches for the mother's hand and pulls her along. Therefore it was an abnormal sign for Perry to react with such indif-ference on his first visit to the office. Marcia (case #2) needed her mother in the playroom for the first several months, which was pathological in significance despite her age (three and a half) because of both the inten-sity and the persistence.

In the phallic phase separations are perceived within the rubric of the oedipal conflicts and masturbatory guilt.

Case #7. Jimmy at seven and a half was being seen because of phobias and anxiety attacks which threatened to keep him from school. Quite early in treat-ment he began fabricating reasons to go to the waiting room to see his mother (he wanted to show her a picture he made, etc.). After this was observed a number of times it was noted that it occurred following play activity with strong oedipal flavoring, such as rescuing mothers or other females from dan-ger. He was asked about any worries he might be having about his mother in the waiting room. Gradually he revealed that he would get the thought of someone attacking her as she sat out there and then he would want to go and check to reassure himself. These fantasies turned out to be similar to others which expressed in a disguised way Jimmy's own erotic wishes toward his mother. The sexual nature was submerged behind the sadomasochistic idea of an attack (the mechanism by which these unacceptable wishes were trans-formed into a symptom of anxiety hysteria is discussed elsewhere in this chapter).

Here, the point to be made is that Jimmy's "separation anxiety" was a symptom of his neurosis—an expression of this latency boy's unresolved oedipal conflicts. Jimmy's fear of abandonment and his preoccupation with death represented punishments for his oedipal desires.

Separation due to death makes for difficulty particularly in the phallic phase when the child's lack of awareness and understanding work against an easy resolution. For, in addition to the cognitive problem of understand-ing death as a reality, the child is also coping with his death wishes connected with his oedipal feelings.

Case #8. Linda, a four-year-old, saw her mother deliver a stillborn eight-month fetus at home. The mother was hospitalized for almost a week. After her return the child began to display a variety of symptoms and behavior changes related to her attempt to cope with what had happened. She regressed in a dramatic but reversible way with crawling and baby-talk and wanting a bottle. She also initiated a game on her block with her playmates called "dead baby" in which she always pressed for the lead role. Also she began at night to complain of abdominal pains and asserted she had blood in her b.m., which could not be confirmed. This was connected with her observing the mother's labor pains and afterwards with the blood secondary to the delivery; but also much earlier, at two, Linda had witnessed the mother having attacks of colitis with bloody diarrhea. Identification thus played a prominent part in Linda's attempt to cope with both losses—the mother and the fetus as a prospective sibling.

Over the course of treatment, which was brief but intense, it emerged how the events she had witnessed had been understood by Linda in terms of her own sexual conflicts over masturbation and oedipal guilt. At the time of the trauma, she had been suffering from persistent urethritis. It had, in fact, developed at almost the same time she learned of the mother's pregnancy. In her play and fantasies, Linda showed how she equated this urethritis with her mother's bleeding during the stillbirth and a laceration she had observed on her mother's knee previously. Also it emerged that the burning sensation of the urethritis was associated with an accident of a neighbor who burned her hand on the stove and had to go to the same hospital as her mother. Burning was due to touching with the hands, and this led to ideas of danger about touching with the hands when they were not clean. This theme developed into expressions of her own feelings of guilt about touching herself in masturbation as being the cause of the urethritis.

Burning also brought up bee stings and mosquito bites which she had suffered. These unconsciously related to her ideas of impregnation—the doctor gives mother an injection. Further dissection revealed her own wishes to have a baby in this way. Her wish to take the mother's place and have a baby was part of her ambivalence to her mother's hospitalization since she was left at home with father during that time.

Without going into all the further intricacies, suffice it to say that the traumatic event and separation from her mother was taken up by Linda's ego in terms of what, in a phase-appropriate way, was occurring and being worked out in her psychosexual and ego development at the time. Prior to the stillbirth there was no indication for psychiatric treatment; her pediatrician recognized the possible relationship to masturbation and he also was sensitive to the possible psychological effects of vigorous manipulations in treatment of the urethritis. (Interventions such as cystoscopy could in themselves act as developmental interferences and lead to fixations and distortions in the child's subsequent sexual development.) The aim of treatment was prophylactic, i.e., to prevent permanent distortion in Linda's own concept of herself sexually so as to enable this little girl to achieve a full feminine identity and unambivalent acceptance of the maternal role in later life. In other words, treatment was undertaken to prevent fixation due to this particular trauma.

Death as a real separation is always a problem in the young child. Not the least of the difficulties is the irrational, anxiety-laden attitude of adults who cannot be of real help to the child because of their own need to deny. By emphasizing life-after-death concepts such as heaven, or worse, by resorting to subterfuges, such as telling the child that the dead person went on a long trip, they unwittingly foster and reinforce denial in the child. This prevents his coping with death and acquiring the means to cope with future losses more adequately. Often enough, the child has sufficient difficulty with his own need to deny death, as in the following case:

Case #9. David, a five-year-old boy, developed tic-like gasping symptoms following the death of his maternal grandmother with whom he was very close. They were first noticed on the day of the funeral while he was at the grandmother's house waiting for everyone to return from the cemetery.

Over the next several weeks the symptoms continued and efforts were made to help him talk about what had happened. David explained that this gasping was his "new way of breathing," and behind this there seemed to be a fear that unless he did this he might "forget" to breathe altogether and die. For some time before, as with most children today, David was exposed to educational efforts against smoking and had often chided his grandmother to stop because she would develop cancer. She did die of cancer which, however, was unrelated to smoking.

One day, several weeks after the funeral, he was with his family passing a cemetery in the car. He volunteered that headstones were put over a grave if you loved the person who died very much; and if you loved them very, very much you also put flowers. He then complained about not being able to go to the funeral. It was explained that young children didn't usually go to funerals, but the promise was made to take him to the cemetery if he wanted. He then asked what would happen if a person were buried and was not really dead. Encouraged to explain further, he said he thought that the person might wake up and be unable to get out of the coffin because of all that dirt on top. Then they wouldn't be able to breathe. He made a play of words about the similarity between "cough" and "coffin." The symptom was seen briefly during this discussion and then disappeared entirely.

In subsequent weeks, however, the subject of death frequently made its appearance, showing that David was continuing to work through the problem in all its facets, now unimpeded by the symptom. For, as with Linda, he had attempted at first to cope with the loss by identification with his grandmother. This took the form of her still being alive in the coffin and through his symptom he was making her breathe—he was breathing for her. His symptom then reinforced the denial which stood in the way of any realistic resolution of the loss. When this fantasy became verbalized he could then begin to work through the idea of her being permanently dead; in addition, any guilt about her death was assuaged by the earlier comments about loving someone who died by supplying a headstone and flowers to prove it.

Separation has been discussed here as a prototype of an external interference which affects a child's development. It has been seen how early object loss, like early trauma in embryological development, produces serious and diffuse impairment of vital ego functions. Perry (case #6) at age four had severe disturbance in such ego functions as speech; his libidinal development was arrested and his object relations blunted.

In the toddler, separation anxiety occurs as a "normal" expression of ambivalence in object relations. Overcoming this ambivalence is a phase-appropriate developmental task. Marcia (case #2), whose relationship with her mother was already poor, stumbled at this hurdle when it was made more difficult by the arrival of her brother. A transient neurotic symptom was the result. It looked as though Jimmy (case #7), although in latency, had regressed back to the pre-oedipal ambivalence of the anal phase. But closer examination revealed his need to go to his mother from the playroom to reassure himself that she had not been attacked as he fantasized. Contact with his mother was sought for relief from anxiety brought on by a dangerous sexual fantasy in which his own repressed erotic interest in his mother had been projected onto an imaginary attacker.

David's response to death and the loss of his grandmother (case #9) was a transient tic-like symptom which showed minimal involvement with his current psychosexual life. Encouragement to verbalize was all that was needed to facilitate the working through. But for Linda (case #8) the tragic stillbirth and separation from her mother threatened to intensify the oedipal conflicts which the mother's pregnancy had already stirred up, creating the vexing physical symptom of urethritis. Her symptoms were more profuse and extensive. Separation was only one thread in the fabric of the developmental conflicts with which Linda was faced at the time.

One wonders if the term "separation anxiety" has not been used too loosely to retain any usefulness. Its meaning as a phase in the development of object relations during the anal period has been blurred by the practice of describing any anxiety related to need for contact with an object as "separation anxiety." Such anxieties can really only be understood against the background of the child's developmental status and past history.

## Childhood Neurosis

Anxiety hysteria, conversion hysteria, and obsessive-compulsive neurosis are seen in almost the same manifest form in children as in adults with similar symptomatology and underlying dynamics. However, as has already been pointed out, sufficient structuralization of the personality to enable such a neurosis to be formed occurs only when the child has achieved latency. The most significant structure in this respect is the superego, which doesn't develop sufficiently or begin to consolidate till the Oedipus complex is resolved. Another prerequisite for a neurosis is an intact ego whose defenses can oppose the drives sufficiently, particularly those drives which are objectionable to the superego. And the latency period is the first period of development in which the ego has achieved that kind of organization and strength. Prior to this, neurotic conflicts of various kinds can be observed even in very intense and damaging forms. But they exist as fragmented reactions in relation to specific conflicts, both external and internal in origin; and they are not organized together as a psychopathological unit.

THE NEUROTIC PROCESS

Essential to the understanding of the formation of a neurosis are two interlocking concepts: intrapsychic conflict and signal anxiety. One of the most important functions that the ego as the executive agency of the mind has to perform is perception and reaction to a danger situation. The ego's method of registering the existence of such a danger is termed signal anxiety. This subjective apprehension of danger appears not only when some objective external situation threatens, but also when conflict between the drives and the ego occurs. Such conflicts are occasioned by the stimulation of an unacceptable aggressive or sexual wish which threatens disruption of the psyche by violating prohibitions laid down by the superego, the internalized repository of external prohibitions. To such "danger situations" the ego brings to bear its defensive apparatus by which the offending impulses can be prevented any access to consciousness. If this process is complete, then repression has been successful. When repression alone is not sufficient, further defensive maneuvers have to be undertaken to render the drive innocuous.

The train of events envisaged thus far begins with the emergence of an unacceptable drive (sexual or aggressive), signal anxiety produced by the ego because of the danger situation, followed by various defensive maneuvers by the ego whose task it is to find a solution for the conflict. If the drive cannot be blocked by repression alone, the ego can try to find alternative means of expression for the drive while at the same time satisfying the superego's requirement for punishment. Such compromise formation is understood to be the underlying process in development of a symptom.

For example, Sal, a five-year-old boy, became very jealous and angry about the new baby which he was allowed to feel growing in his mother's stomach. His wishes that the baby would stay in there and never come out were opposed in that form by the defensive apparatus of his ego. Instead Sal developed a symptom of painful constipation. This initial aggressive wish against the new baby came into conflict with the boy's love for his mother and his fear of punishment for wanting to hurt the baby. The wish became transformed into a painful somatic reaction—the constipation. Here by the defensive process in the ego the conflict was "solved" by the use of the mechanism of conversion. The unacceptable impulse thus achieved some partial discharge somatically, though in an altered and symbolic way, and the superego requirement for punishment was accomplished via the suffering of the symptom.

If the balance of forces had been different and Sal's ego had been unable to withstand the wish to harm the baby or prevent its birth, the boy might have actually hit the mother's stomach. Here the ego and id would have acted in concert and the resulting pathology would be an aggressive act exposing the child to the external danger of parental punishment. The fact that this impulse would be given direct access to motility indicates the presence of a compliant or weak ego. Such a situation is normal for a much younger child and thus the significance of such behavior would vary according to the age of the child. But a child of five, like Sal, should be able to have control of such impulses without requiring prompting or admonition via an external authority. His own superego should be developed enough to fulfill that function. Thus the presence, as in the first instance, of a symptom is of great diagnostic significance concerning the processes of ego and superego development. Since Sal's mother did not have to oppose his wish, it is clear that the prohibition was internalized and there was thus an intrapsychic conflict with the resulting symptom, constipation, as a compromise formation.

The presence of intrapsychic conflict is then an important indicator for the process of development. Similarly the signal function of the ego is a sign of ego advancement. The lack of appropriate reaction to such impulses, which could lead to reprisals from the environment, would indicate a failure in ego development or an ego deviation. Such reactions would comprise non-neurotic pathology of the kind referred to previously as uncontrolled expressions of sexual or aggressive drives. By contrast, neurotic reactions represent quite advanced and sophisticated responses by an intact ego against drives which are opposed by a superego made up of internalized parental prohibitions. The conflict which ensues is thus an internal one fought out by the drives and the superego, in which the ego must mediate and find a solution satisfactory to both parties. It has already been noted that such reactions can occur on a transient basis, indicating a developmental hurdle that for some reason cannot be smoothly negotiated.

### REGRESSION: THE UNCONSCIOUS, FIXATION

In addition to repression, the ego has other mechanisms of defense at its disposal. Among the other major defensive maneuvers employed by the ego is regression. Like an army retreating from recently won positions to more secure ground, the child faced with intolerable anxiety occasioned by phallic-oedipal drives can give up this advanced level of libidinal interest and return to earlier fixation points previously passed through. As with the army this retreat does not solve the problem, but merely changes the ground on which the battles are to be fought. Regression of the libido to pregenital levels (oral, anal) still leaves the child faced with the fantasies, anxieties, and guilt at that level.

In the example of Sal, the little boy jealous of the new baby on the way, the eventual manifest level of difficulty, constipation, did not refer at all to having babies or being jealous of a rival to his mother's love. The oedipal position was first abandoned by the regressive movement of his libido back to the anal level, and there emerged in terms of his wish to hold on to or destroy his own feces. The ego still opposed this expression of the anal sadistic impulses and the feces are painfully retained instead of being expelled.

Two further aspects must be stressed. First the entire process occurs without the child's awareness; that is, it is in the *unconscious*. Both the original thoughts and wishes as well as the ego's reaction to them proceed silently. The emerging symptom appears, then, to the naïve observer as only a fortuitous happenstance. Many such symptomatic expressions occur in childhood without their significance being appreciated. Second, despite the anal quality evident in the form of the little boy's symptom, his problem is still an oedipal one. This is so even though the mode of expression of the conflict has been defensively degraded from the phallic to the anal sadistic level by the process of libidinal regression. In a different child (e.g., case #2—Marcia) the same problem of anger toward a sibling eventuated in a fear of being bitten, indicating that for this youngster the main fixation point in her development occurred at the earlier oral level. In Marcia's case it was a particular vulnerability in her mother for the area of feeding which made this phase very anxiety-laden for both mother and child. This created a special sensitivity to and proclivity for conflict at the oral level. This is what is meant by *fixation point*.

Had there been no regression at all, this same conflict could have led to an anxiety attack in the little boy where he might have become afraid that he would be hurt in some way or perhaps kidnapped by strangers (as he might have unconsciously wished to be done to his soon-to-be rival). This symptomatic configuration would produce the clinical picture of anxiety hysteria or phobia where the manifest symptomatology and content of the anxiety retain strong phallic oedipal tones.

From the above it is seen that only by careful examination of the clinical manifestations, understood in the context of the child's developmental level, can the true nature of the conflicts be understood. The level of conflict cannot be read from the surface content of the symptom any more than a dream can be understood by simple inspection of its manifest elements. It should be further noted that the hallmark of a neurotic conflict is that regression occurs with regard to the drives. The ego stands more firm, directing its efforts (defenses) against the drives associated with the fixation points to which regression has occurred. Should the ego regress also and tolerate either the messy, soiling behavior or the sadistic outbursts of the anal child, there is, then, an easygoing relationship between the ego and the drive, and internal conflict no longer exists. The difficulties encountered by such a child would be external in origin due to opposition from the environment. Such a state of affairs is normal in early childhood where regulation of the id is left to the outside world, but persistence of such patterns or return to such behavior indicates a potential for a type of pathology which is non-neurotic in nature. Such is the situation with certain types of character disorders, impulsive character, and what is descriptively termed immaturity.

For a more complete discussion of the neurotic process and the basic concepts such as signal anxiety, intrapsychic conflict, the unconscious, repression, regression, and other mechanisms of defense, the reader should consult the writings of Anna Freud, Berta Bornstein, Gerald Pearson, and others whose works have been referred to so far.

## ANXIETY HYSTERIA

There are children who develop complex and fixed phobias with attendant great anxiety as the predominant feature of their pathology. There are others who appear to somatize their conflicts and present various physical symptoms similar to the conversion phenomena of later ages. Others show marked diffuse anxieties without focal conversion reactions or phobias much like the adult anxiety states. As with adults, there is never a pure culture of one type or another. These three entities (anxiety states, phobias, and conversion hysteria) share one common feature: The phallic-oedipal level organization has been consolidated and maintained despite the threat of severe castration anxiety.

The manifest anxieties show a close connection with castration and/or themes of punishment for oedipal wishes. For example, an eight-year-old boy, Peter, fears a robber will come and steal all of his father's money. Here the boy's own disguised wish to steal his father's power and source of strength is attributed to the fantasy figure of the robber. There is some anal regression also, since the boy's unconscious wish is really to castrate the father and acquire his genital capacity and not take his money.

Injuries and wounds involving loss of body parts as unconscious symbols of the genitals also abound. The agent of this destruction is often some monster or other figure drawn from current television programming, horror films, comic book villains, or other current fantasies. Those who condemn such media as being the cause of these anxieties are led to the simplistic notion that prevention can be achieved by eliminating such influences from the child's life. Such an approach completely overlooks (or denies the fact) that these anxieties basically derive from the child's own hostile and aggressive wishes to inflict some harm on others which he is defending himself against by projecting these feelings onto some suitable external object. First, there is repression of the idea, that is, the child is unaware that he has it. If this does not suffice, the wish is attributed to an external agent who will carry out the prohibited deeds. The superego demand for punishment is usually met via the allied fear that some form of harm will befall the patient either by the robber or through an associated anxiety of bodily damage. For example, Peter had a dream in which the manifest content was the same as his robber fear, but, in addition, he dreamed that he broke his leg while jumping from the house which the robber had set afire.

It must be stressed that such knowledge is not gained from simple inspection of the patient's accounts of his fears of such anxiety dreams, but rather is derived after much painstaking work over a long period of time and only after exploring many such fantasies, dreams, and play sequences. The therapeutic task is to reconstruct the salient features of the patient's conflicts and associated fantasies, utilizing the tendency to repetition and stereotypy which characterizes neurotically determined behavior.

In the less complicated anxiety states one sees the mechanisms of *repression* and *projection*. In the formation of a true phobia, the process becomes more complex, but the oedipal flavoring is still there. As has been noted, some relatively simple forms of phobia occur in the prelatent period. For descriptive purposes, they are easier to dissect in order to illustrate the basic mechanism involved.

For example, a three-and-a-half-year-old girl (case #2—Marcia) had been upset at the arrival in the household of a baby brother. Her initial reaction of hostility and annoyance at this new rival for her mother's affection was met with great disapproval by her parents. She then became more diffident, if not accepting of his presence, but simultaneously developed a terror of dogs, even those from the neighborhood with which she had been on friendly terms. She avoided the park or tried to, since dogs often ran loose there, and she spoke in anxious terms about a fear that they would bite her. Dissection of this simple phobia revealed that the little girl experienced her anger toward the baby in oral terms—her resentment focused on the feeding attention being given by the mother. Her past history, particularly in her oral period, was characterized by a struggle with the mother who tried to wean her very early from the bottle, and was intolerant of thumb-sucking; in addition, she would not let the child fall asleep with a night bottle. This latter circumstance led to a difficulty in falling asleep that was still present. Also, she was a fussy eater, and there were frequent power struggles at mealtimes between mother and daughter. It was revealed that shortly prior to the outbreak of the phobia of dogs, she had been severely reprimanded by her mother for actually trying to bite the baby.

Marcia experienced the wish to bite the baby and harm it; rather than her wish being opposed by her superego, which was not yet sufficiently developed, it was the mother who threatened punishment and the loss of her love for such behavior. This external opposition to her wish by a loved object created a conflict which was "solved" temporarily by the banishment of the wish (repression) shown by the surface change in her attitude toward the baby. But repression failed; the wish re-emerged and was then projected outwardly. It was not she who wished to do some biting, but rather someone else who wished to bite her. Instead of being the aggressor, by the mechanisms of *projection* and *reversal*, the child became the victim. A further step removed the connection with the brother entirely. The source of the biting was displaced onto a symbolic substitute for the brother—the phobic object—in this case, a dog. With Little Hans (the famous case reported by Sigmund Freud) there was a phobia of horses. His fear of being bitten by the horse represented Little Hans's own wish to hurt his father. Freud noted the great value that this process of symbolic displacement had for the child; it enabled him to live comfortably in the same house with the original object, his father. The price he paid for this was a restriction of his ability to go outdoors because of his fear of being bitten by the numerous horses that abounded in the streets in those days.

The completed process in the phobia then, involved:

1. Repression of the unacceptable wish.
2. Projection onto the outside world as the source.
3. Reversal in which the patient becomes the victim rather than the perpetrator.
4. Displacement of the source of danger onto a symbolic substitute for the original object.
5. Avoidance maneuvers to prevent anxiety occasioned by contact with the phobic object.

There is a basic difference between these early phobias in the prelatent period, many of which are concerned with animals, and the later phobias of the fully developed anxiety hysteria. Notice that the conflict of the little girl was not a fully internalized one. Opposition to her biting wishes had to come from her mother. In an older child these same orally tinged aggressive impulses would have been opposed by the child's own superego as the internalized representative of parental prohibition. The truly neurotic conflict is fully internalized, existing between the superego and the offending impulses (id); the ego has the task of mediating the conflict and finding a solution sometimes in the form of a compromise formation termed a symptom.

CONVERSION

Monty, an eight-year-old adopted boy, was doing poorly in school. When faced with new work or any task that he did not understand, he would often burst into tears. He began complaining of headaches and stomachaches, and asked frequently to go to the school nurse. It got so bad that the other children would begin to laugh as soon as he raised his hand. He was a very fearful boy who avoided roughhousing or contact sports on the playground because of fears that he might get hurt. This surface picture seemed to depict a boy lacking in the usual masculine boisterousness and aggressiveness one would expect at his age. Analytic investigation revealed that these somatic complaints and many others were conversion reactions. Most of his phallic assertiveness had been repressed and instead he unconsciously identified with his mother. Specifically he had identified with her as being the victim of a sadistic sexual assault by his father. This was his interpretation of events when he witnessed the parents having intercourse at an earlier age. As is often the case in witnessing the primal scene, it had a traumatic effect, distorting subsequent development in the boy due to both the exciting and terrifying nature of what he had seen. It made him fearful of his own masculine aggressive wishes, which made identification with his father more difficult.

In the learning situation at school, knowing the right answer had the connotation for Monty of being like his father; he retreated from this position out of fear of reprisal for daring to compete with his father. At eight, then, this youngster had begun to live out his neurotic conflicts in crucial areas of his life, such as learning, which became a vehicle for the expression of his difficulties in growing up and being masculine. His passive feminine identification also came out in his repeated desire to wrestle with his father. It is interesting to note in this connection that when Monty walked in on the parents having intercourse and asked what was going on, he was told by his father that mommy and daddy were wrestling.

In conversion hysteria the ideas are repressed, but they can be uncovered via analysis of the physical symptoms that have emerged as a substitute formation. In the case of this little boy the symptoms represented an identification with the mother who in Monty's unconscious mind was seen as the victim of the father's assault.

Of course there were many important facets of his neurosis that were connected with the fact of his adoption. The material presented here was selected only to illustrate the process of conversion.

## OBSESSIVE-COMPULSIVE NEUROSIS

In this group of disorders the phallic-oedipal strivings have been lost by regression. The libido has given up the advance position and returned to the anal sadistic level. The ego then has to cope with conflicts revived around the fixation points established when this phase was first traversed. Often the history will reveal an initial period of anxiety with some fears and/or somatic reactions. This is past by the time the child is seen and the obsessional picture predominates, with rituals, compulsive acts, magical formulas, and the like. This can be clearly seen in the following clinical vignette in which the disturbance focuses on sleep.

Case #10. Len, an eight-year-old, had several disturbing nightmares; he began to balk at going to bed at night, expressing fear of "more bad dreams." He began to avoid his usual fare of television cartoon shows because of the prevalence of monsters and demons that were showing up in his dreams. He demanded to have his door open to the hall and the light kept on. If it were dark as he went upstairs, he would run as if for his life to the switch at the top of the stairs. Once his mother heard him say with great relief, "Made it!" Going to bed became more and more prolonged. He would call out frequently to his parents in an almost patent effort to see that they were available. After about a week he began to develop a "system" on going to bed. There was a routine check of the closet and great attention was paid to having doors ajar several inches. His bedspread had to be folded just so, his shoes had to be lined up by his bed, and certain exercises had to be performed with an old stuffed toy that had been abandoned but which suddenly was taken off the shelf and began to spend the night in a special position on top of the bedspread.

By the time he was seen, other obsessive-compulsive rituals and thought patterns complicated many of his ordinary activities, such as eating and dressing. The earlier phobic anxieties had given way to a compulsive neurosis. However, the essential underlying conflicts were still those related to his masturbation and accompanying sexual fantasies. The former was given up, however, and the latter repressed. Instead, Len was preoccupied with keeping things even, straight, or at exact right angles. He was involved with touching rituals, so many times with the left hand, so many with the right hand; but then he would not be sure and would have to repeat. He worried about such matters as parallel lines meeting.

Both in manifest symptomatology and in the underlying dynamics the obsessional neurosis which emerged during latency in this boy was similar to that seen in the adult. In his developmental history evidence could be found for fixations at the anal sadistic phase to account for the use by his ego of particular defenses characteristic of the obsessional state closely related developmentally to the anal sadistic level. Toilet training was complicated by a traumatic observation of parental intercourse which Len understood as an attack. Also during the training period, around two years of age, he developed a penile infection for which circumcision was required. He was frequently admonished not to touch the bandage and concerns about cleanliness were heightened due to the realistic fear of infection and sloughing off of the sutures. Close connections between circumcision and the problems around toilet training no doubt acted as a forerunner to the intense castration anxiety that he experienced in the subsequent phallic phase when Len's investment in his penis was at its height. Complications caused by traumatic incidents or even severe developmental conflicts often can have future effects in distorting subsequent phases of development leading to new developmental conflicts, or, as in this case, being partly responsible for the outbreak of neurosis.

The defenses typical of the obsessional neurotic were clearly shown by Len. *Reaction-formations* to dirt and aggression were revealed in many of his symptoms which had to do with fears of contamination and germs. He used some thought patterns for the control of impulses and attempted through the magic of rituals to ward off or neutralize danger. Delay in carrying out activities that had been drawn into his conflicts represented the *defense of isolation*. Heightened *ambivalence* revealed itself in his object relations. There was a return of some of the sadistic cruel behavior that he had displayed during the period of the later anal phase following the circumcision and the primal scene observation. This same ambivalence lay behind the doubting thoughts and the endless doing and undoing maneuvers of the symptoms themselves.

Also as part of the regression of the drives away from the phallic level, the type of conflicts one sees in obsessional neurosis have more to do with activity versus passivity rather than the sexual dichotomy of masculine and feminine. The obsessional child wishes to do "bad things" to others, but fears having things done to him. During the anal stage in the child's life, his behavior actually oscillates between these two modes. He is at times cruel or mean, hostile to others, provoking or teasing, which gives the impression of the wish for punishment (a normal behavior disturbance of this period, as spoken of above). In the later neurotic manifestations of this type of conflict in object relations, the now more mature ego takes stronger measures in such outbursts. The child is very polite, even obsequious, overconcerned with doing harm to others, quick to deny any angry feelings. The torturing sadistic behavior, as seen in Len's case, is confined to pets and other animals with occasional outbursts toward younger children. In the symptoms, however, these aggressive impulses are expressed in a cloaked way, as in the fear that some harm has been done (representing the underlying wish), followed by some expiatory or undoing gesture.

Pearson has stated (18) that there might be two etiologies for obsessional neurosis. One, as described by Freud, related to the sexual conflicts of the repressed Oedipus and another, more severe, related to the chronic problems with aggression and the fear of loving based on patterns of early parental rejection.

This latter type of obsessional state, with severe, long-standing, and persistent pathology, may be a forerunner in childhood not of a later adult obsessional neurosis, but rather may presage a more malignant schizoid or psychotic development. Anna Freud (8) referred to cases like this as indicative of deep splits in the personality only temporarily held together, as it were, by a neurotic solution.

For example, Ricky was eight and a half when first seen in consultation. At two he had severe anxiety dreams about being bitten by a dog. At three there were severe phobic reactions not only to dogs but chickens and other birds. During the later oedipal period, four to six, he became fearful of needles, concerned about dirt and germs and infections, developing great scrupulosity about cleanliness. There were also nocturnal rituals to enable him to sleep. He went from anxiety states to phobias to a severe obsessional state prior to latency. He was seen at eight and a half with severe anxiety about going to school. But it very quickly emerged that Ricky felt that he was being persecuted by his classmates, that some poison had been put on a needle on his seat. He began to experience similar fears from strangers on the street, and gradually he was unable to leave his house at all, preferring to hide under his bed. This boy was already having a full-blown paranoid psychosis in latency.

Ricky's sad case illustrates the unreliability of predicting the form of later pathology from the character of the childhood disorder. Here there were severe developmental conflicts and an obsessional neurosis fairly well developed prior to latency. It has similarly been found that children with phobic reactions in prelatency do not necessarily develop anxiety hysteria as their choice of neurosis; more often in latency they manifest an obsessional type of picture.

There is thus much more fluidity in childhood allowing for variety of psychopathology prior to the consolidation and fixity of later years. This factor is especially important with reference to character development.

## NEUROTIC CHARACTER DISORDERS

In adult nosology we are used to evaluating the more enduring and repetitive traits in the patient's personality—his style, as some have referred to it —in terms of character structure. A neurotic character is an individual whose pathology is revealed in the way he lives his life, his attitude to objects, his sexual life, his way of working, his values, his way of thinking. Close relationship can be seen to exist between these character traits and the type of symptom neuroses which develop. The patient with phobic symptoms reveals in his character exaggerated cautiousness, tentativeness, approaching new situations with trepidation. The obsessional character with stinginess, punctiliousness, concern for details, lives a tight, orderly, but somewhat drab existence because no room is left to chance.

However, this close correlation between character structure and symptom was not found as expected in children. The situation is much too fluid in childhood to find such descriptive labels helpful in organizing one's thoughts about a child patient.

Certain character traits, particularly the reaction-formations developed in the anal period, such as cleanliness, punctuality, concern for others, etc., can form the basis of a stable, adaptive personality provided they can remain free of conflict; i.e., they become part of the autonomous ego described by Hartmann (15). But a characterological diagnosis alone in childhood is not very useful, since it implies a permanence or stability not yet achieved developmentally. The child with hand-washing compulsion and nocturnal rituals may also be messy and sloppy in his personal habits with seemingly no sense of time. A child with many phobias and anxieties or conversion symptoms, on the other hand, may be strongly "obsessional" in his character, i.e., orderly, fussy about details, concerned about neatness, cleanliness, punctuality, etc.

One can be concerned about the child whose developing personality lacks fluidity and is perhaps hemmed in by inhibitions and restrictions.

Treatment may be warranted in the absence of symptoms with the hope of restoring a more fluid relationship between the drives, the ego, and the emerging superego. Anna Freud (9) has referred to these premature closures in the personality as calcifications to convey the type of deleterious effect on development that ensues. Character traits themselves, in keeping with the chemical metaphor, were described as precipitations in the ego of previous conflict situations.

# 3

## Ego Disturbances in Children

WILLIAM STENNIS, M.D.

## Introduction

Serious disturbances of the major ego functions (perception, memory, synthesis, object relationships, control of motility, speech, defense, and reality testing) form a rather large group in the psychopathological disorders of children. Although not classified as such in the current diagnostic and statistical manual of the American Psychiatric Association (1), this group of disorders may be considered together for the purpose of understanding etiology, psychodynamics, and treatment approach. It includes those disorders more often diagnosed as mental deficiency, organic brain syndromes, the various childhood psychoses, and the "certain severe disturbances of the ego in children" of Dr. Anna Marie Weil (17).

As a group, these children are set apart from others because of outstanding deficiencies, difference, or strangeness in one or more of their ego functions. Where there is clear evidence of "lower than normal" IQ on a congenital or hereditary basis, perception, memory, and synthetic functions of the ego suffer most seriously. Without smooth functioning of these aspects of the ego, reality testing is inefficient. Although speech, defense, control of motility, and object relationships may also be deficient, it is the first three mentioned functions that are most regularly and seriously affected. All of the psyche is built on an organic substratum and the functions of the ego are unusually sensitive to damages or malfunctioning in that substratum. However, the presence of damage, even serious damage to the central nervous system, does not necessarily mean that the psychological adaptation of the individual will be impaired. This is especially true where the damage is primarily to the motor area of the cortex. When the damage has been in an area that is concerned with perception, memory, or synthesis, it is more probable that the other ego functions will also suffer. Children with "ego disturbances" (Weil) or one of the various forms of childhood psychosis have more severe disturbances in their object relationships or in the nature of their defensive structure, although even this is likely to be closely related to disturbances of the primary ego functions of perception, memory, and synthesis.

## Structure and Functions of the Ego

The ego itself is basically a theoretically constructed model concerned with mediating between internal drives and external reality. In 1895 Freud "regarded the ego as a group of neurons with special characteristics" (2). But in his 1938 outline of psychoanalysis, Freud gave his most precise definition of the ego as he had constructed it.

*Here are the principal characteristics of the ego.* In consequence of the pre-established connection between sense perception and muscular action, the ego has voluntary movement at its command. It has the task of self-preservation. As regards *external* events, it performs that task by becoming aware of stimuli, by storing up experiences about them (in the memory), by avoiding excessively strong stimuli (through flight), by dealing with moderate stimuli (through adaptation) and finally by learning to bring about expedient changes in the external world to its own advantage (through activity). As regards *internal* events, in relation to the id, it performs that task by gaining control over the demands of the instincts, by deciding whether they are to be allowed satisfaction, by postponing that satisfaction to times and circumstances favourable in the external world or by suppressing their excitations entirely. It is guided in its activity by consideration of the tensions produced by stimuli, whether these tensions are present in it or introduced into it. The raising of these tensions is in general felt as *unpleasure* and their lowering as *pleasure* (5).

If we take this latter definition of the ego as that of an adaptive agency, it is currently possible to talk about the functions of the ego in neurophysiological terms. For example, the reticular activating system is an alerting system. The hypothalamus controls autonomic activity. The limbic system integrates primarily internal sensations, deeply related to self-preservation and cortical evaluation of these sensations. The cortex gives fine perception of the outside world, stores memories of previous experiences, and makes fine discriminative judgments while constantly checking, in a sense, with the limbic system.

But in more traditional terms the ego functions are as follows:

1. Perception.
2. Memory.
3. Synthesis.
4. Control of motility.
5. Defense (the concept of defense is implied by Freud: "avoid excessive stimuli").
6. Reality testing.

In more recent years, the functions of

7. Speech.
8. Object relations.

PERCEPTION

Perception may be defined as "the receiving of an impression through the senses." Perception probably begins with a physical, chemical, or electrical change in a sense organ, roughly analagous to the change which occurs when light strikes a photo-sensitive cell. If, however, we attempt to deduce that something has happened on a cellular level, we must go to all sorts of rather complicated lengths to establish that a change has taken place, for example, in the rods or cones of the eye. Chemical or physical changes may occur but they do not signify perception. If we connect our photo-electric cell to a simple galvanometer, we can see that a change has taken place. The needle is deflected, current has passed through the wires, the magnetic field has been created and a needle moved. When light strikes the eye, a physiochemical change takes place in the retina and a "current" flows along the nerve to the cortex in a similar fashion.

A cell in the cortex is stimulated and we can measure this in an EEG, but has perception taken place? I think not. Let us carry things a bit further. There is a device known as a voice-actuated relay. It is an electrical device whereby when one speaks into a microphone a current flows, closing a switch that may control the starting of, for example, a tape recorder. It is roughly similar to the photoelectric cell. Current is created by the pressure of the sound waves; physical energy is converted into electrical energy which closes the switch. This is an interesting device in that its sensitivity may be changed. For example, it can be made to pick up the softest of sounds. Whether or not it responds can be changed. One might say that it can be "turned on" by a pressure of oral activity, just as certain young ladies might be "turned on" by a pressure of another type of oral activity. We can even change how long it stays turned on after the sounds— or oral activity if you wish—stop. Quite a machine! We might even say that this machine may be adjusted to "hear" footsteps coming down the hall, or the sound of a lover's voice. But has perception taken place? Again, I fear our machine must fail. But perhaps we haven't given it enough of a chance. If we rewind the tape we find that it has made a record of what has been said. Does it then have a memory? Does the fact that it has moved indicate that it has control over its motility? Has an impression been made on it? Do the little iron filings, magnetically rearranged, constitute an impression? A mold?

What a silly experiment and what an inadequate thing our language is. Of course the machine does not perceive. Perception is all the things we have mentioned, but much more. Perception involves not just the passive reception of stimuli but an active examination of sensations from the sense organs, and even a screening out of impressions made on the senses which we do not wish to become consciously aware of. The blemishes on our lover vanish when we are in love, although our senses must record them.

But when love turns sour, those same blemishes take on a much broader significance. Mentally defective children seem to have an impairment of the process of perception, although their vision or hearing may be intact. The impressions they receive are fleeting and of little usefulness to them. Sometimes children who are organically damaged seem overly distracted by sensations. Like the tape recorder, they seem to respond to even the slightest sounds. They may be distracted, for example, by the hum from air conditioning or fluorescent lighting, sounds that most of us do not even hear.

Psychotic children may be unable to perceive anything, so withdrawn are they, or a small cut may be perceived by them as something that signals complete fragmentation.

Perception is a fascinating subject as a function of the ego. In psychoanalytic terms, it has most meaning to us when we are able to correctly perceive our primary love object. Perception matures only in terms of the success of our object relationships.

## MEMORY

Memory must be preceded by perception, that is, if we discount the earthworm experiments in which earthworms "learned" certain tasks, were subsequently ground up and fed to other earthworms. It seems that the well-fed earthworms "learned" the new tasks much faster than a control group. At our present level of understanding of memory, it is difficult to know how to evaluate the findings of these studies. Memory is probably one of the most easy of the ego functions to define. It is simply a storage of information with capacity for recall. As has been shown by hypnosis and the experiments with subliminal stimulation, both perception and memory can take place out of conscious awareness. Memory has been linked to the RNA in the glial cells, and to other chemical shifts. Others have postulated the storage of memory through particular synaptic processes. In ego disturbed children, memory may be hypertrophied as in the so-called idiot savants, absent as in the autistic child who cannot recognize his mother, distorted as in the child who recalls fantasy as reality.

Like perception, memory serves its most important function when it helps the individual to recognize the primary love object and to seek from that love object the affection and care that is necessary for survival.

## SYNTHESIS

In his *Principles of Psychoanalysis,* Dr. Herman Nunberg discusses very adequately the synthetic function of the ego. He compares the synthetic function of the ego to the sexual striving of the id, that is, "to join other objects with the aim of creating a new unit." In the ego this same tendency "finds expression in the faculty of binding, unifying, creating."

He continues,

the ego then *creates*—out of the infinite number of perceptions, impressions, feelings, emotions pertaining to the psychic representation of the objects—a new, and under certain conditions, independent formation called the superego. This new psychic agency is thus formed through assimilation and integration of quite a number of traces left in the ego by external and internal stimuli. . . . The synthetic function of the ego thus manifests itself in the assimilation of internal and external elements, in reconciling conflicting ideas, in uniting contrasts, and in activating mental creativity.

Nunberg feels that the need for causality, which has an "instinct's compelling force," is a manifestation of the synthetic function of the ego. There seems to be a need to connect two facts so the second seems determined by the first. The synthetic function also includes a tendency for simplification, generalization, interpretation, and finally understanding. Nunberg concludes that the synthetic function "represents a principle of the highest order of mental life. . . . Synthesis thus brings about not only unity of the whole person, but also simplification and economy in the ego's mode of operation" (13).

Piaget has shown in his delightful experiments that true causality in the child begins at about eighteen months, when the child can understand that there is a cause and effect relationship between an external object acted on by another person. He regards the associational "connection" between the face of the mother and the relief of tension prior to that time as being perceived by the child in a kind of continuum that does not allow for the separation of two events, but certainly the perception of the significance of the mother to the child as a preserver of his existence is an important early precursor of the function of synthesis. If the child does not understand that he will lose the mother's love if he does not control his impulses, the synthetic function is operating quite deficiently (14).

The breakdown of the synthetic function as seen on the Rorschach is one of the most reliable evidences of disturbed functioning of the ego. If, as the test progresses, we see the child's ability to unify and synthesize progressively deteriorate, a major disturbance of the function of synthesis is present.

## CONTROL OF MOTILITY

This term is rather confusing since its semantics apparently suggest a kind of cellular or neurophysiological governor or dampener which I don't believe is correct. Hyperactivity in children with organic brain syndromes has been a classical sign of this disorder. Studies have indicated that children with organic syndromes have no more or less motor activity than other children, even though clinically they do give this impression. But children with organic syndromes are distractible (disorder of perception) and shift their interest, often creating the impression of hyperactivity. Instead of completing one task, they scurry off to begin another. Is this not more readily seen as a disorder of synthesis where the urge to bind and unify an experience is deficient? When we speak of control of motility, I believe we speak of purposeful control of motility. The disorders associated with the motor cortex which produce abnormal movements do not refer to the psychological function of control of motility. In certain circumstances (i.e., hypnosis or automatic behavior), the direction or control of the motor behavior has been surrendered to another ego, whether it be that of the hypnotist or the unconscious of the patient.

If we view control of motility purely from the conscious standpoint, there are several important developmental things we can say about it. An infant whose major needs are fulfilled has less of a "need" to move about in an effort to attract attention or "do something" about his state of distress. A maternal-child relationship, then, in which the child is "reasonably" well satisfied and with less of a need to move about probably marks the beginning of the psychological ability to control motility. When the child can change his position in space, the maternal figure physically restrains him when he places himself in danger. Later her verbal "No" does the same thing. The earlier physical restraint, added to the verbal "No" and internalized in the context of the oedipal situation, form the basis for true control of motility. As we progress along the developmental scheme one can see that a single ego function such as control of motility blends into more global models that we may begin to call "ego" or "superego" as it becomes interwoven into the fabric of the total personality. The influence of the father in this final synthesis or precipitation or internalization of controls has perhaps been underemphasized. It is his "No" stated verbally and nonverbally to all pregenital impulses that aids in the final synthesis. It is his task to balance the mother's "Yes" with an appropriate "No" that enables the "ego" to "precipitate" at the end of the oedipal phase.

## DEFENSE

Freud's concept that the organism avoids "excessive stimuli" has been carefully elucidated by Anna Freud in her book *The Ego and the Mechanisms of Defense* (3). While the concept of defense against unconscious impulses is among the more important contributions of psychoanalysis to our understanding of human behavior, its usefulness in recent years has been poorly understood. It is not uncommon for a patient to exhibit in any one segment of behavior numerous mechanisms of defense, and this is characteristic of human beings who have been exposed through their parents and ego ideals to a number of ways of protecting themselves from excessive stimuli, whether they come from within or without. However the number of defense mechanisms that any one individual uses regularly, and especially in situations where basic core conflicts come to the fore, generally is not more than two or three. The fact that one uses a method to ward off the recognition of internal difficulties is probably infinitely more important than what specific mechanism is used. The unconscious impulse warded off is the important issue.

That mechanisms of defense are used in the growth or humanization process is also an important concept that has been insufficiently stressed, probably because it has been insufficiently studied and not well understood. For example, in the second six months of life when the infant has some recognition of the significance of the mother in terms of his understanding that she is necessary for his survival psychologically, there is objective evidence that he begins to imitate her behavior, so that more and more specific and human behavior occurs. The behavior seems to reflect the statement, "If I cannot have my mother with me always to protect me from the fear of losing her forever, I can at least keep part of her with me —her behavior." Although it is difficult if not impossible to verify this, we see retrospective evidence that this operates in older patients. Dr. Anna Marie Weil in her paper on ego disturbances remarks that in these children "identification becomes a substitute for object relationships" (17). And we have observed many adult patients who in a stressful situation can even observe that their behavior duplicates behavior they have observed in their own parents. This concept of duplicating behavior of someone who seems more secure or more in control than the patient has been confused by the use of several terms that purport to describe different mechanisms. Residents in training frequently have difficulty differentiating imitation, introjection, and identification. What difference does such hair-splitting really make in the ultimate understanding of patients and in dealing with them psychotherapeutically?

During my own residency in child psychiatry, the resident in the office next to mine had to be away. He was treating a psychotic child who was able to come to his office from the in-patient unit. Somehow the boy had not received word that his doctor would be away. I heard noises coming from the office and on investigation found the patient lying on the couch, rolling from side to side, thumb in his mouth saying, "Dr. Michaels is here, Dr. Michaels is here!" This complete inability to allow one's self to be aware of a terribly painful affect is necessary and frequently used to ward off many kinds of anxiety, from the case of this child to that of a neurotic man in analysis. This particular adult patient was unable to see, despite overwhelming evidence, that his wife was repeatedly unfaithful to him. It is fair to ask, "Was he repressing this, denying it, or rationalizing it?" What difference does it make except to help us and then him if he is unable to admit to consciousness a fact that would cause him extreme pain either in the form of anxiety or depression? The necessity of denying impending death in many terminal illnesses is frequently recognized.

When a three-year-old child shifts the blame for a broken ashtray to a younger sibling, or a guilty parent of an ego disturbed child blames doctors and teachers for not making her child better for the purpose of un-loading her very large and unmanageable burden of guilt, thus reducing her pain, are not similar things happening psychologically? People reduce their anxiety by shifting the blame.

How many experienced clinicians can differentiate between ego restric-tion and ego inhibition? Ego restriction has been carefully defined as representing the warding off of disagreeable external impressions in the present because they might result in the revival of similar disagreeable external impressions from the past. Ego inhibition is said to be operating when an individual is defending himself against the translation into action of some prohibited instinctual impulse, that is, against the liberation of pain through some internal danger. Why is it helpful clinically to differ-entiate these two mechanisms, since the end result is that the patient is cautious, shy, and reluctant to extend himself?

The mechanisms of defense need to be restudied, redefined, and re-duced in number. The concept is too useful to remain in the confused state that now exists. In studying children with ego disturbances, defense mechanisms are often transparent and rigid. The child often seems to be a distortion of the most inefficient and unyielding mechanisms of defense of his parents. One must constantly recall that these children exist in a state of very high anxiety, that their defenses must be tenaciously grasped lest the personality of the child fragment and a state of psychological nonbeing ensue. The anxieties of loss of the love object, loss of the object's love, and the fragmentation that might ensue should either of these first two anxie-ties occur are the things most severely defended against in these children. This is perhaps more important to understand than just how they do it.

## REALITY TESTING

Testing of reality requires an intact perception, memory, synthesis, matura-tion, and a warm, human relationship designed to lead the child in testing the environment. There are aspects of the environment that can be taught, but other aspects that must be learned through experience. The parent must allow the child to test reality within bounds he can assimilate. If the parent shields the child from all of his efforts to test reality, his tools (perception, memory, synthesis) will atrophy. If reality situations beyond the child's ability to master are repeatedly presented to him, the child will eventually balk at the repeated failure, giving rise to negativism and eventually perseveration, evoking high levels of anger in a parent because the child does not take as large a step as the parent wishes. The develop-ment of an adequate ability to test reality depends upon intact primary ego functions and a sensitive human relationship that takes the time and effort to break down the steps required to learn how to test reality into dimensions that the child can understand and assimilate.

In the previous discussion of "control of motility" the role of the father was mentioned. In no other function does the father play a more important role than he does in "reality testing." In the family structure it is the role of the mother to supply the child's needs—to say "Yes," to be indulgent, a "pushover," to lend spice and joy and fullness to life. Within the family, but more important within the world, it is the task of the father to say with deep emotion, "Yes, all of those things are marvelous—but if you are to survive against the overwhelming forces of nature, you must be able to test reality (the outside world) and recognize that you must deny yourself some things that you now feel that you must have. You will find that you can do without many infantile things that have become dear to you. As a matter of fact, in leaving behind childish things a new world will open for you that contains new pleasures that you haven't even glimpsed before." This is summed up so beautifully by the Apostle Paul in his first letter to the Church at Corinth, "When I was a child I talked and felt and thought like a little child. Now that I am a man my childish speech and feeling, and thought have no further significance for me" (12). There is much evidence that this attitude of the father within the context of the oedipal situation enables the child to make the important synthesis so necessary for an adult personality. His denial of the mother to the boy and his refusal to become involved with his daughter says "No" not only to the genital impulses so paramount at that time, but as well to *all* pregenital impulses as well. Childish (i.e., oral, anal, oedipal) speech, feeling, and thought must be given up, abandoned, sublimated, repressed. When this does not happen because the father has not been able to convey this to the child or because the neurological substratum is defective, not only is reality testing impaired, but the child also is flooded with feelings and thoughts that belong to an earlier time and that may seriously hamper his abilities in many areas of ego function. These inner or "childish" fantasies are often so compelling that the child simply cannot direct his energies to the testing of reality.

### SPEECH

Speech begins with global words or phrases that signal a need. Its precursors in the form of crying or babbling testify to the empathy that humans have for the helplessness of their young. Speech does not reach major importance as an ego function until the acquisition of the semantic "No," which signals that the child has learned to say "No" to himself as his parents have said "No" to him. This indicates that speech now has a function of delaying action with respect to impulses. When man first hurled an invective instead of a spear, said Freud, civilization began. The use of speech as a method of delaying action has been underemphasized, but its importance to the humanization of any new being cannot be underestimated (16).

OBJECT RELATIONS

All of the above functions of the ego must take place in the context of an evolving relationship with other human beings through a continuum. We begin life in an autistic state; that is, we feel that everything that happens to us happens simply because we will it to happen. There is no inner and outer life, no me and others, simply me. Were it not for our maternal figures we could not survive such an "unrealistic" attitude. But with their care we do and, with growth, begin to recognize that it is not ourselves who are responsible for our existence but those who care for us. We "see" them first only in part: breasts that nourish us, hands that cover and hold us, and finally as whole objects rather than part objects. As they care for us we lend a new dimension to their lives and give it new meaning. They give to us and care for us, but our existence gives something to them that simply did not exist before we existed. Our relationships are intermeshed, interwoven, symbiotic. When we first recognize the extent of our need for them, we feel terror when they leave us, but as our memory and experiences grow, we can hold a constant image of them in our minds even when they are absent. This enables us to separate from them for brief periods of time without fear of disintegration. We first imitate them and then identify with the prohibitions they place on us. We compete with one of them in the oedipal triangle; and as we lose, we finally gain independence of our childhood. Let us look in detail at the evolution of the ego as it passes through these stages: autistic, part object, whole object, symbiosis, object constancy, separation, identification with the prohibitor, competition, and finally true independence of the primary incestuous love objects.

## Evolution of Ego Functions

The assets and liabilities of the finished personality are based on the characteristics of the particular individual's central nervous system, its maturational progression, and its relationship with the environment. This relationship with the environment involves chiefly its relationship with other human beings. The functioning efficiency of the ego is determined by two things: (a) the characteristics of the central nervous system as reflected in its passage through maturational stages; and (b) the quality and evolving character of the object relations through the stages of psychosexual development.

An objective observer in a nursery can see easily that infants respond quite differently from the very beginning. Some are quiet and placid; others are irritable. The irritable infants have difficulty becoming settled or achieving homeostasis in the outside world. Although there is a range of activity and ability to achieve the kind of balance that we regard as normal, there are many who fall outside this range and function in a sub-standard way from the beginning of life. When motor development is slow or shows evidence of paralysis, objective evidence of this can often be collected early. However, when perceptual capacity is impaired, much more difficulty is encountered in delineating the problem. For example, the diagnosis of deafness in a newborn infant, particularly when it is not complete or when it involves a distorted reception of sounds, is difficult. We have virtually no method of testing the infant's capacity for memory or synthetic functions. When the organic defect of the child is purely on the motor end, he may be able to receive stimuli accurately and to integrate them properly and develop reasonably well. The reverse is not true. A child limited in the functions of perception, memory, and synthesis has a major handicap. This is a major handicap because it does not enable the developing infant to evolve object relations in the same way that the child who has a normally functioning central nervous system can. His perception of the object and its functions, as well as his ability to classify and integrate the stimuli from the object, is impaired or confused, hampering his capacity for imitation, introjection, and identification.

The organically deficient child frequently has a maturational timetable that is either slow or uneven. This unevenness often throws the mother of the child off guard. For example, she may expect the child to smile between one and two months of age. If he does not, she may give up trying to make him. If his negativism comes out at three and a half instead of two, she may be completely bewildered. Both of these factors change the quality or rhythm of her relationship with him. This maturational timetable is more crucial in the first year of life than in later years, but if this maturational progression does not coincide with the mother's expectations, ego development is likely to be impaired. The mother's expectations are, of course, derived from her own experiences with her own mother. If these have been rigid or deficient, her ability to perceive variations from the normal and to react adaptively may itself be impaired.

There is another side to this as well. A child may begin life with a reasonably intact central nervous system, but when he is ready to smile, the mother may be too depressed to stimulate him or lead him forward as a reward for smiling, or there may be no mother around if he is in a poor home or in an unstimulating agency. When a child is ready for a particular maturational step and the environment does not help him make it, the receptivity of his central nervous system for change and growth may begin to decline. If the required response never comes, the resulting damage to the ego or to its organic substratum has the style of an organic change in the central nervous system and in time this may be irreversible. The developing infant is most susceptible to this damage and the damage is most permanent in the first year of life, although it may continue through other stages of development.

The ego, if viewed as an adaptive agency, is influenced chiefly by its organic characteristics and the quality of its object relationships. At one end of the continuum might be a child with a severe organic deficit and reasonably normal parents. On the other end would be a child with little or nothing initially wrong with his central nervous system, but whose primary objects are unable to supply the stimulation and leading so necessary for proper development. In between is a mixture of both types and to varying degrees. But the end result is an individual who has a reduced capacity for adaptation (15).

Dr. William Goldfarb has studied a group of psychotic children intensively. Each child was examined neurologically, psychologically, and psychiatrically. In addition, a psychosocial and psychiatric study was made of the child's family. Dr. Goldfarb discovered that the children who had the most positive neurological signs had the least disturbed families and those families who were most disturbed had fewer positive neurological signs (7).

Numerous studies of the results of adequate physical care, but gross emotional deprivation, show that not only was the development of the central nervous system impaired by this kind of deprivation, but physical growth in general was long delayed. Harlow's studies show that infant monkeys who were deprived of mothers strikingly resemble autistic children (8).

The clinical picture that we refer to as ego disturbance involves the consideration of two etiological factors, the functioning efficiency of the central nervous system and the quality and evolving character of object relationships. It is extremely difficult for a child to develop proper mechanisms of defense, rewarding speech patterns, adequate reality testing, or control of motility without a warm human relationship and intact perception, memory, and synthetic functioning of the ego.

## Disturbances of the Ego in Children

The major types of ego disturbances in children are mental deficiency with as yet an unknown or uncertain etiology, organic brain syndromes, childhood psychoses, and ego disturbances (Weil). The problem of mental deficiency will not be considered here.

### ORGANIC BRAIN SYNDROME

Classically the brain-damaged child is distractible, impulsive, has a short attention span, is emotionally labile, hyperactive, and restless. His frustration tolerance is low and his anger explosive. Although occasionally children with this clinical picture may be mentally retarded, they need not necessarily be so. In fact, in my own clinical experience, they more often show symptomatology of a developmental arrest than they do of mental retardation. A few have superior intellectual capacities, but where the organic syndrome is signficant most have disturbances of major functions of the ego. Perception, memory, and synthesis are almost always involved.

Their ability to learn, to adapt smoothly to social situations, and to use appropriate judgment is often absent.

Where the organic brain syndrome produces moderate, severe, or profound mental retardation, the organic causative agent is usually more easily identifiable and the child will show rather severe and generalized impairment of all of the major ego functions. This category includes most of those classified under the clinical subtypes of mental retardation.

### CLINICAL ILLUSTRATION
### ORGANIC BRAIN SYNDROME

The family constellation consists of

1. The primary patient—Polly, age ten and a half at the time of the evaluation.
2. Kathy, age fourteen, her older sister.
3. Father, age forty-five.
4. Mother, age thirty-eight.

Polly was brought for evaluation because of "immature behavior." Her parents were concerned about her "slow emotional development" as chiefly manifested in her temper fits and in her inability to take "No" for an answer. Her mother said, "Every command she fights, it's a battle a day." Somewhat apologetically the mother said that perhaps they were expecting too much of her, or "maybe she didn't have enough therapy."

They explained that Polly was taken to see a psychiatrist at the age of four because of "horrible nightmares." The parents recalled that Polly used to wake up screaming, running around the room or sitting rigidly on the bed or floor. Although her eyes were open, she seemed terrified and could not be roused from this state immediately. Two and one-half years later the parents took Polly to a clinic when she was six because she was unable to take "No" for an answer and had severe temper fits.

In describing Polly currently the parents say that she is like an exaggeration: "When she's happy she's all smiles, when mad she's very mad. She's always restless and constantly in physical motion." She prefers muscular activity and loves to play with boys. For the six months prior to the evaluation she has played with some girls but seems to prefer baseball to dolls and always has. She has shown some feminine interests in her clothes more recently, however. "When she's a girl, she's a girl. When she's a boy, she's a boy!" Most of the things she does she does quickly and with great intensity. The father expressed the apprehension that Polly speaks very loudly at home but in school they report that she speaks almost in a whisper.

They feel she needs a tremendous amount of attention. Recently she wanted her father to help her fix a baseball glove to make a pocket with soap. When he was unable to help her immediately, she flew into a rage, called him "cheapskate, mean father, selfish, you don't love your kid." The father is somewhat bewildered by this behavior because he feels he gives her much love and affection.

Both parents report that Polly loves men and loves to sit on their laps. She is more cool toward women but she seems to have to be physically in contact with men.

Though her gross motor coordination is good, her fine motor coordination is poor. There has been some improvement lately in her drawings. She does well in school in the fifth grade in spite of the fact that she never does homework, getting primarily B's and A's. She works quickly and her work is often sloppy. When she is told to do it over again, which is quite frequently, she has a temper fit, yelling and screaming to the point where "you just can't get through to her."

With her friends she is popular and has lots of sleep-over invitations. She is outgoing, though a bit aggressive and sometimes overbearing. Her teachers report that she has tremendous enthusiasm for new things but very little follow through. The parents also report that she has flighty interests. As they began to describe her many good qualities, the mother concluded, "I wonder why we're here. I hate to say it but she's a charming child . . . if it just weren't for those daily upheavals . . ."

*Developmental history.* The parents were married three years before the first pregnancy. It was a planned child, the mother's health was good. There was considerable bleeding during delivery but the baby was healthy, weighing six pounds. Kathy is now fourteen and making a good adjustment.

Though the parents felt they could live with one child, Polly was planned as a companion for Kathy. The father had no sex preference but the mother and her family wanted a boy. They were not disappointed with a girl, however, and the mother said, "It's good for a girl to have a sister." During the pregnancy the mother's health was reasonably good. She had considerable nausea and vomiting and took Bonamine for the first six weeks. Between the second and third month she had some staining and may have received some hormonal injections. The labor was quite short. The mother felt the doctor had to go to a flower show, so that the water bag was broken and a single injection of Pitocin was given to induce labor. Birth records indicated that the mother had Demerol, nitrous oxide, ether, cyclopropane, and a pudendal block. The birth weight was six pounds and the baby was healthy. The mother and child went home from the hospital in four days. Polly was an active baby in utero, but essentially fairly quiet. She was an average sucker, a thumb-sucker which continues to the present time at sleeptime. She was named after the paternal grandfather and the maternal grandmother.

Polly was bottle fed by choice and was said to be a good eater. At the age of ten days she rather suddenly began to have diarrhea. She quickly became dehydrated and was admitted to the hospital with a rather severe

Salmonella infection. She was hospitalized for ten days, had cut downs, a fungal mouth infection, and was treated with Chloromycetin. After she returned home she required much work from the mother, having to be fed every two hours, stool specimens had to be taken to the public health department regularly, diapers soaked in Lysol, and the mother recalls that they were concerned over any loose bowel movements for the first two years of her life. Because she was on Chloromycetin, it was necessary to do rather frequent blood counts. Though it was later established that the infection probably came from the hospital nursery where she was delivered, the father was later discovered to be a carrier and has had the feeling that he may have given the infection to Polly. Throughout this period of time Polly was a pleasant, tranquil child. She was responsive and seemingly alert. Exact age of sitting alone was unknown, but she was felt to be slower than her sister. She walked at fourteen months, also later than her sister. Talking was also slightly delayed. She took to solid foods rather easily and without difficulty.

Toilet training was begun near the end of the first year. She was seated on a toilet seat for ten to fifteen minutes after meals. Her mother read to her. There was little pressure and no complaints from Polly. By fifteen months she was trained for bowels with no accidents or smearing episodes. She was enuretic until the age of nine and a half. At eighteen months she was weaned from the bottle slowly with fruit juices given in a cup. She was very attached to furry toys and still takes a panda to bed with her.

At the age of two and a half, Polly had the sudden onset of a strangulated inguinal hernia. She became quite irritable and fussy one evening. She bothered her parents so much with this "bad behavior" that she was given a spanking by her father. Following this she went into shock and had to be hospitalized. The mother did not stay with her following the emergency surgery although the surgeon recommended it. When discharged from the hospital several days later, Polly said that the Gray Lady fed her oatmeal and she thought that the Gray Ladies were going to be her mother. The most upsetting thing about this hospitalization to her were the rectal temperatures. To this day she has a conscious memory of this, has never allowed it again, and on another occasion when a medication was prescribed by suppository she absolutely refused. Surgery was in the left inguinal region. Following this she was "proud" of the scar. The doctor who did the surgery told the parents that it might be a weather indicator and for several years whenever it rained Polly would complain, "My hernia hurts." After she came home from the hospital she wanted to be carried around for a few days but then began to walk without difficulty. When they returned to the surgeon for removal of the stiches she was quite fearful that he would hurt her but the mother was able to reassure her. An examination of clinical records indicated something a bit different. The parents reported then that Polly cried each time she looked at the scar. Although it is not exactly clear from the records, there is some indication that following the surgery the nightmares may have begun. She awakened at least once a night screaming. She did not recognize her mother or father, and when her mother would try to hold and comfort her, she would thrust her away. In spite of their severity the nightmares seemed to subside for a period of time. Just before her fourth birthday she began nursery school at the synagogue in the morning. Her mother was there one morning a week. She was cooperative and seemed to enjoy herself. There were no separation difficulties or other problems. Several months later she began a new nursery school in the afternoon and to this she also adjusted well.

It was in the first half of the fourth year that the *pavor nocturnis* began. After these had gone on for a period of several months the parents sought psychiatric help.

At the age of five the parents consulted their pediatrician with respect to her bed wetting. He suggested an alarm device. Polly objected to this strongly. Whenever she wet the bed she would wake up and wake her mother, who would then change her and the sheets. Finally the parents began to insist that she take care of these things herself. This was followed by a few temper fits but the parents were consistent and Polly gradually took over the task of changing her own pajamas and bed.

It was in December, just after her sixth birthday, that she was taken to the Child Development Clinic. The temper fits had apparently become much worse and the mother said that she was desperate. They were also concerned with the continuation of the bed wetting. The nightly ritual would go something like this. Polly would wet the bed and get up, insisting that the parents change it for her. When they refused, she would throw a temper fit. She yelled and screamed, said she was a slave to them. The alarm device frightened her. Her father said that he always knew when Polly wet the bed because she would let out a sigh of relief that he could hear from their bedroom.

The parents were also concerned about her flirtatiousness with older men in the neighborhood. They said she did not play well with older children and tended to seek out younger children. She was often extremely stubborn and refused to obey. In school she was described as shy and obedient. She liked boyish games and was extremely restless. "While reading her a story you are constantly aware of the writhing body beside you," said the mother. Mealtimes were especially hectic. There was much confusion with many things being knocked over. Polly had extreme temper fits at times, throwing herself to the floor, yelling, hitting her mother or her sister. Bedtimes were absolutely terrible. She usually threw the first fit when she was told to go to bed, saying her sister was favored and demanding that she had the right to stay up as long as her parents. She used to insist that her mother tuck her in, that the mother read or sing to her. When the mother left, she was out of bed with requests for water, trips to the toilet, etc. When the parents finally put a stop to this, there was another temper fit. She was finally forcibly put to bed and threatened with a spanking. Usually she got a spanking and eventually fell asleep sucking her thumb and whimpering.

In the middle of the night the mother was frequently awakened by Polly's crying which grew louder. She would find her half asleep and would usually escort her to the bathroom. In the morning she was difficult to awaken, fretful, moody, and cried when the mother finally got her awake. There were frequent arguments about clothes. She would rip them off, throw them to the floor, and refuse to wear what her mother had selected.

At the time of the interviews the parents reported that Polly played mostly with a friend David. Although they played sports most of the time, they also liked to dress up. In this play David was always the female and Polly was the Indian, the father, or some other male. Of sexual differences she said to her mother, "You know, David has it neat with his penis, and all. He doesn't have to sit down." And the mother observed, "She's always had an interest in the penis." The past summer at the shore she came in while her father was dressing and asked to see "that little sack that mom was telling me about." Her father demonstrated his scrotum to her.

The father at the end of the history-gathering interviews confessed his concerns about his daughter's sexual identification. Though he is somewhat encouraged about recent feminine traits, he is especially worried about the rectal thermometer business. "I hope this doesn't make her frigid someday," he says. The mother has gone through a book on pregnancy with Polly and says, "She knows when I get my period I'm not pregnant." She frequently asks her mother if she has had her period and if the mother says, "Yes," she says, "Well, no baby this month."

Kathy wants another child but not Polly. The house is, as one might expect, quite open to nudity: "For a long time we've not tried to hide anything." The parents don't know about sex play with David. Masturbation has been noted both at school and at home since the second grade. When asked what she was doing, Polly said, "It itches and I scratch."

*Clinical interviews.* Polly was seen for three diagnostic interviews, a summary of which follows. At the first interview she was quite anxious, showing much undirected restlessness and complaining mildly that her sister was able to go swimming this afternoon while she had to come for an appointment. When asked why she came she said that she had temper fits whenever she was punished. She yelled and screamed at her parents. She gave as an example that she and her girl friend had been punished for waking her older sister. She said that the tantrums had been going on for about a year. When I asked whether or not anything upsetting had happened during the past year, she spoke of the death of her grandfather whom she remembered as a kind man who used to play with her a great deal. He used to cut her hair. He died suddenly. When she was a little girl her favorite game was riding horsey on his knee. The night after he died she had a nightmare that he died because she was riding his knee. The nightmare woke her and she had difficulty going back to sleep. I asked her whether anything had really happened in her life when she felt responsible for hurting someone. She denied this but then proceeded to tell me of her friend David falling from a high diving board and having a mild concussion and cut finger. This upset her very much, she confessed. That night she had a dream that she was able to fly through the air like Superman and rescue David. David is her playmate in many muscular games. She has had other nightmares about a vaporizer in her room that seemed to turn into a witch. Then she asked me what psychiatrists really do. I told her I was aware that she had been in treatment before and wondered what had happened there and what she thought psychiatrists did. She said that she did nothing but play in her previous treatment and concluded, "He didn't get anything out of me." I told her that I wasn't even trying to get anything out of her and look how much she had told me about all of the many problems she had. She said that she should have been consulted about coming here and I agreed, saying that sometimes parents don't realize how much kids want to know about that sort of thing. She also agreed and told me that she didn't know until she was seven that she had had Salmonella when she was an infant. She was interested in some Indian dolls in my office, where I was going on vacation, and a number of other personal questions.

The second interview was held one week later. She was restless, explored the office, and said she had been everywhere in my office and that she was quite impressed with the things I had there. She told me that her sister's birthday was today and that she had had an argument with her mother over wearing a particular sweater. On the way home from school she and her friends pretended that they were escaping from a German concentration camp and that the school principal was really the commandant of the camp. After a period of silence she was distressed that I had no questions to ask her. On exploring the toys she began to play with a gun, shooting it at me. At the end of the interview when we were scheduling a time for her third appointment, there was much disagreement over the time and she almost threw a temper fit in my office during the discussion of this with her mother. I patiently arranged a time that was acceptable to her one month later.

At the time of this third interview she was less restless and said that things were going well. She was at a day camp but hoped to go to overnight camp next year. She began to pace the floor and wondered how long a pace was, how long my office was, how long her foot was, and wanted to sit in my chair. Again she admired the Indian dolls and told me of being tried in "court" at day camp for being too rough with some of her fellow campers. She said that her biggest problem is still her temper. She was told about the psychological testing and the EEG, as well as the fact that after the studies were completed I would meet with her again to explain the findings to her.

*Psychological testing.* Polly was seen for testing in August of her eleventh year. The psychologist noted that there was a slight tomboyish quality in both her appearance and manner. Near the end of the first testing session, she was tired, became restless and slightly hyperactive. She obtained a Verbal IQ of 121, a Performance of 114, and a Full Scale of 120. There was a significant variation in her verbal functioning. She was only approximately average in arithmetic and very superior in verbal conceptualizing and vocabular ability. In the visual motor subtest she was only at a low average range in synthesizing parts of concrete objects to a whole.

Weak ego controls and anxiety appeared to be interfering with the utilization of her general cognitive and intellectual abilities in both verbal and visual motor tasks. She had a periodic difficulty in finding the right word or phrase and seemed to block easily or become rigid in motor or conceptual thinking in situations where she was being timed or in situations that were emotionally loaded such as in the Rorschach.

The psychologist felt that she was a girl with some ego weakness and regressive features presently precipitated by anxiety due to concerns about her hostility, the latter interwoven in several ways with a variety of oedipal problems. In spite of this, reality testing was essentially grossly adequate.

An electroencephalogram was reported as follows: "'This is a maximally abnormal record marked by a fairly discrete left temporal spike focus which occasionally fires bilaterally. The spike activity becomes more frequent with sleep and drowsiness. These abnormalities would be compatible with a chronic epileptic focus in the left temporal region."

Polly was diagnosed as a brain-damaged youngster and her parents counseled about handling her in a more structured fashion. The use of medication was recommended and the parents cautioned about the need for intensive psychotherapy to undo some of the more maladaptive behavior patterns Polly had developed over the years, especially with her peers.

On the recommendation of the neurologist she was begun on phenobarbital but she experienced a paradoxical reaction with increased irritability and hyperactivity. Next she was tried on Valium with an immediate dramatic improvement. She was begun on 1 mg. daily with a gradual increase to 6 mg. daily. About a month after beginning the medication she decided she no longer wanted to take it. Her parents had been forewarned that this might happen and had been counseled to have her check with her doctor. In spite of my efforts to persuade her not to stop taking it, she was insistent and was allowed to do so. Within a week she suggested that we begin again. Over the next nine months she was seen once monthly. There was steady improvement in her relationships with her family and the temper fits virtually disappeared. In spite of this improvement, Polly seemed increasingly unhappy. It appeared that she had so isolated herself from her peers by her previous behavior that she would need psychotherapy to aid her progressive development.

Over the next three years Polly was seen twice weekly in psychoanalytic psychotherapy. Both mother and father were seen weekly for almost two of these years. Serial electroencephalograms were obtained every six months. These were discussed in detail with Polly. She knew the reason for them as well as the reason for the use of the medication. Gradually the spike focus disappeared, and by the time she was fourteen the EEG was completely normal. Polly was withdrawn from the medication and improvement was sustained. Her circle of friends gradually widened. She began to enjoy being a girl. Her school performance gradually came closer to her intellectual endowment. Neurological maturation, medication, and psychotherapy had all contributed to her progressive growth and development.

## PSYCHOSIS

There are several types of psychotic children. They generally have a disturbed relationship with people.

The first type is *early infantile autism* (as described by Kanner) (10), which begins in the first year of life and is characterized by an unresponsive child who, as he later develops, remains in a world of his own. He is unresponsive to his parents and frequently the parent gives up making an effort to encourage him to be responsive.

CLINICAL ILLUSTRATION

EARLY INFANTILE

AUTISM

A young couple called for an appointment because of their concern about their four-year-old adopted daughter Carol who had made a very poor adjustment at nursery school. She was described as "aggressive, strong-willed, and negativistic." Because of this, she had been asked to leave nursery school just a month earlier. Carol had been previously seen by a group of psychologists who had told the parents that she was an "autistic-like" child. The parents were so distressed by the possibility of this diagnosis that they wanted another opinion. She had also been seen by a neurologist who found no neurological abnormalities and a normal EEG. He was impressed with her inability to relate to animate objects.

In my history-gathering sessions with Carol's parents they complained about her in several dimensions but many of the elements of her early history were obscure. They saw her essentially as an angry and aggressive child who was disruptive of the family situation. The mother said that Carol was not happy, had never been happy, and that she didn't know how to make her happy. They reported that "from the beginning" Carol was more fascinated with objects and animals than with people. She at times laughs inappropriately, which is distressing to both parents.

Both parents were not without problems of their own. The mother was the oldest in a reasonably stable family of four and had an essentially happy childhood. She was successful but not popular in high school and married her husband when she was twenty-three. Their courtship was long and stormy, as their marriage has been. Most of their disagreements have been over finances. Although her husband has assets of half a million dollars, the cash flow through the family has been small, necessitating many hardships that somehow seem inappropriate. Because of his outspoken nature she says that her husband has many enemies. He has a mildly hypomanic air about him and does not create a very trusting impression. He is the only child of schoolteacher parents. Apparently indulged by his mother, he began to have difficulty when he went away to college. He was in several colleges with an erratic academic record. He was frequently in arguments with professors, and as a result of his refusal to budge on what he considered to be a "moral point," never received his diploma. He was vague in describing his current business, which seemed to have something to do with advertising and real estate.

Carol was adopted from a private agency two years after they had adopted their son Tim from the same agency. They had made an effort to have children of their own but could not because the husband had a reduced sperm count. Carol was adopted at the age of two and a half weeks. A pediatrician who observed her for those first two weeks described her in the following way:

Rather irritable and willful baby. Hates her bath and screams all through it. Is inclined to hold her breath when crying and face turns purple. Fusses when put to bed after feeding and does not stop until she has rolled from side to stomach and crawled up to top of crib digging her face into the corner.

When the parents got home with Carol she continued to scream. Nothing seemed to comfort her. The adoption agency reported that the pregnancy was uncomplicated but added that the mother had received gamma globulin because of exposure to measles. This was the mother's first pregnancy but she was noted to be Rh negative. Mid-forceps were used during the delivery. The baby weighed five pounds, thirteen ounces, but breathing was slow and extremities were blue. The Apgar was seven. Otherwise she was considered a normal child. Her mother said of Carol, "She was like a china doll, beautiful but cold and unresponsive." They could not recall when or even if she ever smiled at them. For the first three to six months of her life there was a real question in their minds over whether or not they could keep her. Of Carol's screaming her mother once said to her husband, "'I don't know how long I can stand this." At the age of two they enrolled her in nursery school, primarily, I believe, to give her mother some rest.

After seven months she was removed because the teacher threatened to quit if Carol was not taken out of school. Toilet training was begun in the spring prior to her entry into nursery school, was a prolonged struggle, but was eventually completed before she began nursery school.

Carol was seen for three diagnostic interviews. During the first interview she made only fleeting eye contact and talked in the third person, referring to herself as Carol. She kept with her a plastic bath toy which she related to more closely than she did to me. She was able to identify a few toys which I pointed to on the shelf as well as name their colors, but when presented with some very simple puzzles she was unable to approach them at all, even when M & M candies were offered as a reward. During this interview I hid myself from her within the office but where I could still observe her. She did not notice my absence for a good ten minutes. She was infinitely more absorbed in relating to the toys than she was in relating to me. Much of her speech was repetitive and referred to two of the toys that she was playing with. Finally, in an effort to force a relationship with me, I removed all of the toys in the office as well as the plastic bath toy which she had brought with her. This precipitated whiny noises which evolved into shrieks and then Carol began to bite her hand, hit the couch, and finally lay on the floor in a severe temper fit. After several minutes the temper fit subsided and she said, "Want fish, Dr. Stennis," referring to her bath toy. I told her I would give her the fish if she would look into my eyes and tell me that she wanted it and this she was able to do. By the third interview I had been able to evolve a kind of relationship with Carol and was able to teach her some of the simple geometric puzzles. The success was obviously pleasing to her. I refused to do any of the things that she asked me to do without her first making eye contact and frequently rewarded her with praise and candy. By the end of these three interviews, it was my impression that she was primarily an autistic child, but that the prognosis was reasonably hopeful in view of the fact that she was able to evolve some kind of relationship with me when forced. I was concerned, however, over how much the parents had to give in the considerable work this child would require over the next several years. In a final interview with the parents I confirmed the diagnosis but emphasized the hopeful signs. I outlined a program of work with both parents and the child involving the teaching of object relations and minor perceptual and integrative skills. They were eager to get her back into a nursery school, which I counseled against for the time being.

Although I had suggested frequent visits I did not hear from them for several months. When I next saw Carol she had indeed improved. Her mother had worked very hard with her but was obviously exhausted. Strains had begun to appear in the relationship of the parents, primarily because of the father's lack of support of his wife and continuing strange financial stresses. In spite of a lack of cash the father had bought a cabin site in the mountains with the excuse that the return to nature would be good for

Carol. The appointment to meet again with both parents was broken. I had a request several months later from a local clinic for her records and later heard that the parents were again unable to follow through with recommendations and were considering having the child institutionalized.

The second type, the child with a *symbiotic* psychosis (as described by Mahler) (11), develops fairly well until some traumatic event, such as the birth of a sibling, causes him to go into a marked regression. He may alternate between severe autistic withdrawal and a frightened clinging to an adult. He is often fearful of many things. In both of these types of children defensive structure, reality testing, speech, and object relationships are severely impaired.

At this point it would probably be useful to differentiate clinically between autistic and symbiotic psychoses. The most usable differentiation can be made on the basis of the child's relationship to animate and inanimate objects. The diagnosis takes on more validity, of course, when historical factors complement the clinical picture.

Primarily autistic children simply don't care about people. They generally separate easily from their parents, make little if any eye contact with the examiner, and will not seek him out if he hides himself in a closet or behind a chair, curtain, or screen. Young autistic children rarely speak, and when they do their speech is primarily descriptive and often mechanical. When restrained from a pleasureful activity, they withdraw into a corner and either suck their thumb or rock or both. They will generally choose one toy or object (if they have not already brought one with them) and devote their entire attention to it. They may smell it, taste it, twirl it, or caress it, but this thing, whatever it may be, receives all their attention and love. Although they may be stimulated to laughter by tickling or being lifted high into the air, they avoid being cuddled or physically loved.

Although they show many similarities, children with a symbiotic psychosis do show some clinical differences. One should bear in mind that there is a developmental continuum in all the ego disturbances.

Symbiotic children seem to have reached a stage of some knowledge as to the significance of a maternal figure. They have more difficulty separating from the mother, who may have to be allowed to accompany them into the playroom. Even then they want to cling to her. I have noted that when held these children tend to prefer a "primate-like" clinging behavior where all four extremities try to bind them to the maternal figure where some form of facial juxtaposition is possible. I have found it diagnostically useful to have the mother try to hold the child with his back to her abdomen. I have yet to see it successfully done. While these children also prefer inanimate objects, they can be "seduced" away from them. When their play is directly interfered with, as when a favorite toy is withdrawn, a howl of protest is raised. Occasionally they will hit the hand of the interfering examiner. Crying, throwing a temper fit, hitting out, or seeking the maternal figure are more usual defenses than complete withdrawal. These children can be more easily "reached" in human terms than can those with an autistic psychosis. Speech remains primitive with descriptive nouns, perhaps a few simple verbs, and rarely any personal pronouns.

Dr. Elizabeth Geleerd has described a group of *latency age psychotics*. She stated that these children have no friends among their contemporaries but are demandingly possessive toward one adult. They are not completely out of contact, but have a low frustration tolerance and react with severe temper fits or dangerous destruction. They have phobias, compulsions, tics, and nightmares. They lack control over their drives. Dr. Geleerd felt that these children are arrested at the stage in which the inability to control the mother completely is countered with negativism, temper fits, and fears. One can see in examining Dr. Geleerd's description that these children have disturbances in object relationships, defensive structure, control of motility, and reality testing.

CLINICAL ILLUSTRATION

LATENCY AGE PSYCHOSIS

I evaluated Peter at the request of his previous psychiatrist with whom he had been in treatment for the past two years. Recent psychological testing indicated the presence of much psychotic thinking. He was not quite ten when his father first consulted me. The historical information was obtained from the father and a maiden aunt who was acting as a maternal figure. Peter's father was now divorced from his wife. They were both from extremely wealthy and successful families. After five years of marriage with no children they decided to adopt. They got Peter from a private adoption agency quickly arranged because they were in "something of a hurry." Peter was eight weeks old at the time of the adoption. Although his wife was at first quite enthusiastic, she soon complained that the child was overactive and cried too much. As her enthusiasm waned his own increased. He said that he felt his wife really wanted children only because it was the social thing to do. He recalled that she was not exactly overworked with the child because they had a nurse from the very beginning. The nurse was described as cold, meticulous, and "always in a dither over the nursing equipment." She had the primary responsibility for Peter's care until he was three years old. There were no specific feeding difficulties, "all he wanted was more," and no sleeping problems. He was a large, muscular, active baby. He crawled at eight months, walked at thirteen months, and began to talk in short sentences at thirty-one months. When he was one and a half, his sister Kristin was adopted from the same agency. The details of toilet training were obscure though it was thought that it took place between the ages of two and three. Peter had rather frequent temper fits. He wet the bed until the age of six and sucked his thumb until the age of eight. At three years of age his first nurse was replaced with a very proper but cold English nanny who was rigid, compulsive, and restrictive. He seemed closer to an Irish maid than to anyone else around this time.

At four he began private kindergarten. From the beginning he had a problem with his peers. He was antagonistic, had frequent fights, and was often rebellious.

In his sixth year he transferred to an exclusive private school and there too was a discipline problem. He also began to have difficulty learning. During this time marital stress between the parents became more acute. After consulting a psychiatrist they decided to secure a divorce. Before it became final the mother became quite ill with pneumonia and was in bed for several months. She fired Peter's nurse because she felt she was showing favoritism toward Peter and not his sister. Although Peter had little reaction to his nurse's leaving or to his mother's illness, his difficulties in school increased to the point where he was asked to leave school. Peter was seen at this time by a psychologist and a neurologist. The neurologist found an EEG pattern that showed "questionable" functioning. The psychologist considered his problems "primarily neurogenic" and recommended that he see a child psychiatrist. This was not done at that time. He was placed first in a local public school where he could not be contained and then in another private school for children with "mild" problems. The divorce became final when Peter was eight. Although the father wanted both children, they went to live with the mother who remarried shortly after the divorce. Peter did not last long there and eventually returned to live with his father whose sister came to live in and help manage the household. Repeat psychological testing revealed a Verbal IQ of 121, Performance of 125, and a Full Scale of 125. The tests also revealed constriction of emotional and intellectual responses to his environment and strong feelings of insecurity. Peter was accordingly begun in psychotherapy. At nine he had to change schools again because it was becoming apparent that he also had a rather severe learning disturbance. The new school reported him to be hyperactive, grandiose, demanding, and seeking the total attention of all of the teachers. He continued to get along poorly with his peers. Because progress in treatment was slow, repeat psychological testing was done which indicated he was close to being psychotic. This precipitated the referral to me. His previous therapist indicated that he wished to terminate his relationship with Peter and his family.

Peter was seen for three diagnostic interviews. He was a very large boy for his not quite ten years of age, with an expression that only partially obscured his very high level of anxiety. He was able to tell me that he had come to see me today because his father and his doctor did not seem to know how to help him. When I wondered why, he said that he had problems learning at school and that the teachers did not give him enough attention. After only a few minutes he said, "I like you." When I wondered how he could come to know that he liked me so quickly, he told me that my head was the same shape as his. Then he began to talk about experiments he had read about where they make test-tube babies and he began to fantasize himself as a great scientist who would make babies to order.

The more he talked, the more bizarre the fantasies became and the higher his anxiety level rose. He seemed most grateful when I suggested that the thoughts sounded as if they were pretty scary and maybe he would like for me to help him talk about something else for a while. I structured the rest of the interview with questions about his school and family and friends. I learned that he was a pretty lonely boy with really only one friend at school. In subsequent interviews whenever the fantasies became too grandiose I stepped in with more structure and was able to learn about his interest in "noises and explosions" which he demonstrated for me. He also told me about his teddy bear and his toy snake which he pretends is a boa constrictor trying to squeeze him to death. By the third interview he was able to play with some of the toys and involve me in a competitive situation although he insisted on doing things exactly his way.

His father was told that he was indeed on the verge of a serious emotional breakdown and that intensive therapy was recommended. Peter was seen in intensive psychotherapy over a period of eight years. It was stormy indeed. There were times when I had to simply cancel a full day of patients to help him pull himself back together. A teacher would mildly reprimand him for something and he would run away from school. His father would forbid some wish of his and he would run away from home. Many evenings he ended up at my front door. We would have some popcorn, talk it over, watch a little TV, and I would take him home. Almost everyone in his family at one time or another actively tried to destroy the treatment situation. They tried to send him away to school several times but he simply refused to go and I refused to support their wish to send him away. He finally made it through high school, and although still very self-centered, demanding, and a bit impulsive, was not actively psychotic.

## ARRESTED EGO DEVELOPMENT

Dr. Anna Marie Weil described another group of children who show "severe ego disturbances of a non-neurotic type characterized by a lack of progression." Although Dr. Weil recognized these children within a special group, she considers them as a further extension of the cases described by Kanner, Mahler, and Geleerd along a continuum. Historically, they show family histories that are tainted with "a complementary series of constitutional factors interacting with damages in early life." These children show a marked delay, unevenness, and resulting distortion in ego development. They are most frequently recognized in latency when they stand out because they are not as reasonable, controlled, or integrated as their peers. They may be highly intelligent or talented, but they have an excess of infantile behavior. Whereas the normal latency age child may show quick regressions and quick recoveries from these regressions, these children are likely to regress easier and remain in a state of regression longer. They have a serious disturbance in object relationships that results in a retained feeling of omnipotence, persistence of magical thinking, inability to accept the reality principle, poor reality testing, poor synthetic or integrative functions of the ego, and inability to use age-adequate defense mechanisms, and an abundance of diffuse or bound anxiety. They show poor social, emotional adaptation, severe problems around manageability, and multiple "neurotic-like" symptoms (17).

CLINICAL ILLUSTRATION

ARRESTED EGO DEVELOPMENT

Mark's parents consulted me when he was seven years, nine months old. His mother saw him as too demanding. His father was annoyed at how much Mark upset his mother. He had virtually no friends at school or in the neighborhood. His parents had nothing good to say about him. A typical incident would begin when he would refuse to leave the television set for supper, saying that he was not hungry. When his parents insisted, he would sit at the table and suck his thumb. In order to make him stop sucking his thumb, they had whipped him, bandaged it, and covered it with bitter herbs, all to no avail. His mother expressed a conscious wish to kill him.

Mark's mother's history is tragic. Her own mother died a suspicious woman who thought family and neighbors said unkind things about her and plotted to make a fool of her. She was disdainful toward her husband, a rather passive man, and during the last few years of her life made him sleep in the attic. He showed his preference for his oldest daughter by taking long walks in the woods with her and by constantly berating Mark's mother, whom he said had "not a brain in her head." She was a lonely, unhappy child. Dolls and later horses became her best friends. She worked as a clerk and secretary after graduation from high school. At twenty-six she married. The marital discord was so great in the early months of her marriage and her depression so deep that she saw and talked to a "little green man." After the birth of her second child and a severe conflict with Mark, she ran away. This eventually brought her into psychiatric treatment.

Mark's father's childhood was also unhappy. He was born with only three fingers on his left hand. He compensated for this by doing well academically. He now is a successful consulting engineer who is working on an advanced degree.

Mark's mother did not become pregnant with him until two and a half years after her marriage. She was Rh negative and her husband Rh positive. The pregnancy was uneventful but she described the eighteen-hour labor as "very hard." The baby had slight initial breathing difficulty and a hematoma over the left side of his skull. Breast feeding was discontinued several days after delivery because of insufficient milk. When Mark was four days old, his maternal grandmother suddenly died. His mother's father came to the hospital and accused her of causing his wife's death. She became severely depressed. Mark was a "lazy baby," difficult to feed and frequently vomiting following feedings. The rest of the time he was merely apathetic. During the early weeks of his life, his father had to be away frequently. His mother felt frightened and helpless. She was "bedeviled" by her father who visited her frequently for the sole purpose of blaming her for his wife's death. She knew little about children, complaining when Mark sucked his thumb at two months. She weaned him abruptly at ten months. He did not walk until the age of two years. Poorly coordinated, he fell frequently. His mother had a miscarriage in his second year and again became very depressed. Toilet training was begun at two and a half and was not difficult, but Mark was enuretic until the age of six and continued to soil periodically. He began to talk at three, and almost immediately spoke of the content of his frequent screaming nightmares where he yelled at a green monster with a red hat who was after him. He had an elective tonsillectomy at three and a half and was frightened and depressed following that period. At four he wandered into a large chicken house and began to yell at the chickens. In the resulting excitement, 100 chickens were killed. He told his parents that he did it because he wanted to see them die. In kindergarten at five he was restless, strong-willed, and uncooperative. His mother was pregnant at this time with his brother John and became quite depressed over her ability to care for a second child. Mark's behavior was impossible for her to cope with.

Mark was in the second grade when he was initially evaluated, and although he was doing passing work, he was a behavior problem and isolated completely from the other children. He sometimes pleaded for children to come and play with him. At Christmas he announced to the class that whoever gave him a gift should select one he liked or he would throw it away. He played only at war or with models of prehistoric monsters and would only watch television shows that were violent.

In clinical interview Mark was a strange-looking child. He had buck teeth, a small head, with low-set prominent ears. His long extremities and short body gave him a somewhat simian appearance. His gross and fine motor movements lacked smoothness. Predominant affects during the interview were anxiety and/or excitement. Language and thought were age appropriate, and intelligence was about average. He easily told me that his problems were that he was frightened and shy. He said that his mother threw dishes at him when she was angry and that he once killed a dozen chickens. He said he frequently had nightmares of monsters and dinosaurs chasing him. He complained that he was lonely because he had no one to play with. His play involved only the guns and toy dinosaurs who fought with and ate each other up. His play became so violent that it seemed to frighten even him.

Mark had many positive subtle neurological signs; his gait was awkward, his finger-thumb opposition was clumsy, there was asymmetrical positioning of his outstretched fingers and involuntary movement and tremors. The neurologist who saw him considered delayed maturation, mild brain injury, or a more severe congenital malformation of the deeper structures of the brain.

On psychological testing, his Full Scale IQ was 119 with a Verbal of 113 and a Performance of 122. He was troubled by the psychologist's long fingernails and worried about what she had hidden in her mouth. He had more difficulty with the unstructured material. Poor problem solving and integrative functions were evident. The projective tests showed much fear of abandonment and special anger at the mother for not having supplied needs. The classical geometric tests for organicity were not abnormal, but the general impression was of an ego disturbed youngster.

Mark's parents rejected any suggestions for a special summer camp for him as well as for psychotherapy. A year later they returned asking for treatment. Only one thing could distract Mark from violent play—deep interest and involvement in his daily life. We drew pictures together, collected stones together, built models together, and talked of his loneliness, his struggles with his mother, and his frequently absent father. He learned about my interests and hobbies, traveled over maps with me prior to my vacations, exchanged Christmas presents with me, and gratefully received birthday presents from me. For two years he took on prescription from me 4 mg. of Stelazine daily and knew that it kept him under control. I taught him the art of making and keeping friends and the style of getting along with adults. I persuaded his mother that no devils lived within him and his father that Mark needed only a little time and interest. In four years he grew into adolescence and junior high school. Although no scholar, he passed with average grades, and he has friends who now share his interests as he shares theirs. As treatment ended his mother showed me his school pictures over the years. Remarkably the fear and tension of the second grade gave way to happiness and success in the seventh. Once yearly a letter comes from Mark and from his mother telling of his continuing progress.

## Principles of Treatment

Treatment of children with severe disturbances of their ego functions begins with the moment of first contact with the child's parents. The diagnostic evaluation must be extremely thorough. It must include a meticulously detailed history of the child's development, his current environment, and the parents' backgrounds. Several clinical interviews with the child at intervals of not less than one week are necessary. Neurological and psychological examinations likewise must be done, as well as any other specialized testing that will establish wherever possible the specific factors involved in the etiology of the ego disturbance and the relative weight to be applied to each factor. This detailed and unhurried examination allows both parents and child to develop an important relationship with the physician that simply cannot be developed in a short period of time.

The children who present rather severe disturbances of multiple functions of the ego, such as is seen in children with mental deficiency, severe organic brain syndromes, and the psychoses of early childhood, are best managed by strengthening the parents' and teachers' functions as auxiliary egos for the child. When I am asked to evaluate a young child, I encourage the parents, if their anxiety level is high, to be an intimate part of the examination—to see how much difficulty the child has with simple puzzles—to allow them to help him with his many diagnostic tests as they wish, and to do as thorough an examination as I can, sharing with them as many findings as they can possibly assimilate. If I see a very limited potential evident, I urge them to work actively with the child until progress ceases so that we both arrive at a conclusion about the extent of the child's limitations simultaneously. By that time, we have usually become old friends and they are infinitely more ready to accept the child's limitations from me than they might have been previously.

With these severely handicapped children, I return to Itard and an "education of the senses" (9), with the primary purpose of enriching object relationships. It is through the child's contact with significant human beings that he will learn more how to use whatever potential he may have to find a more satisfying relationship with people and with the world. Before a child can use his eyes for seeing, he must be able to see his mother's or his teacher's eyes and face. Before he can use his hearing, he must hear her voice above all other sounds. Before he can explore the outside world, he must explore her face. Before he can know that he is a human being, he must know and have control over his own body. These initial steps must be on a one-to-one basis. If the child is young, his mother can often be taught these techniques. If a teacher is involved, for a time a one-to-one ratio is essential until object relationships have been established.

Eye contact can be fostered by gently cupping the hands underneath the child's chin or on the side of his face and by reducing distracting backgrounds. Hearing can be enhanced with a set of earphones to feed only the mother's or the teacher's voice to the child, thus screening out background noises. The sense of touch is heightened by much close physical contact with the child and encouragement to explore the teacher's facial features. Body image may be fostered by working with the child in front of a mirror, and even if he does not yet have speech, he can be taught to compare his facial features with those of his teacher, i.e., her eye with his eye, her mouth with his mouth, and so forth. Motility control is often helped by the use of medication, but sometimes it will require just twenty minutes of sitting on the floor with arms and legs wrapped firmly but gently around the child, who has become temporarily psychotic in a temper fit until this has subsided. In effect, you are saying to him, "Don't worry, if you cannot control your impulses, I can help you do so. I will not allow you to hurt yourself or others!" The teaching of speech should begin with words that are invested with a high degree of interest— usually those which signal a need—then proceeding to significant human objects such as mommy, daddy, followed by body parts, eyes, mouth, nose, hands, feet, and then more familiar household nouns.

In addition to these basic perceptual skills we must help the child to master one further essential ingredient—what we call the synthetic function of the ego, the ability to put things together, to seek cause-and-effect relationships. This we do most effectively by frequently putting things into juxtaposition that have an important relationship. We give repetitive structure to the child's world, and when we require of him a sequential task, we make the steps small enough so that he can have the success that gives immunity from our educational enemy, perseveration. Constantly we must encourage, praise, support, and radiate a sense of hope.

All of the while we must involve the parents in what we are doing. To bind their guilt we must give them something to do. Parents of severely handicapped children must be given an opportunity to work off some of their guilt. In my experience, giving them a task to accomplish is infinitely more helpful than simply having them talk it out. In most food gathering cultures, seriously handicapped children were killed or abandoned. The food gathering cultures saw these children as a real threat to the life of the tribe because it was often a task to gather enough food to keep yourself going. In each of us, there is a recognition from the beginning that handicapped children require more from us, and we frequently have an unconscious anger at the extra help that the child needs. Prolonged anger frequently provokes guilt which becomes so severe that it must be projected to others, such as teachers and doctors who have responsibility for the care of the child. This guilt also shows itself as overprotectiveness. This guilt can be handled most effectively through having the parents become actively involved in helping the child.

The treatment of children with less severe ego disturbances, most of whom fall into the years of latency when we first see them, has a slightly different emphasis. One must be prepared to form a corrective objective relationship with them. By becoming a real person, hopefully the child will more closely identify with the therapist and borrow some of the style of the therapist's ego's functioning. The major conflict areas that are approached in an effort to develop insight center around fear of loss of the love object and/or fear of loss of the love object's love. These should be dealt with in terms of current object relationships and as a current conflict. One refers to the remote past with caution. In the treatment room, one needs to remain very adaptable, providing limits of stimulation, structure, or lack of structure over a wide range. In some instances, the therapist must become a need-gratifying object before the child can progress beyond this stage. Uncovering is strictly avoided although unconscious material on any level (oral, anal, phallic) may have to be dealt with when it surges to the surface. In these children "phallic" or "oedipal" or "neurotic" conflicts often show through quite openly. How one deals with them depends on the state of the child's ego functioning at that point in time in areas other than therapy. If ego control is tenuous in the outside world, caution should be exercised in dealing with or "analyzing" this material. The child frequently may react to exploring sexual material as seduction and more rather than less anxiety is released, which often complicates adjustment in the outside world. The educational aspects of teaching delay and sublimation also form an important part of therapy with these children. Occasionally the use of drugs is helpful, but only with the cooperation and understanding of the child. A structured environment and specialized teaching program may also be of considerable aid.

Work with parents of the ego disturbed child has a unique style as well. The parents should be helped educationally to see that the child may see things differently and be concerned about things which are not of concern to them. If one helps them to see how their child functions, often they can more readily empathize with him. Parents play a major role in helping the child to gain control of his impulses and in teaching him appropriate defenses. The purpose of the therapist is to help them, through education, to act as more efficient auxiliary egos for the child.

## Summary

Children classified as ego disturbed manifest a strangeness, difference, or deficiency that sets them apart from the majority of other children of their age. They have a major defect in one or more of the ego functions of perception, memory, synthesis, control of motility, speech, object relations, defense, and reality testing.

They have a history of probable organic insult which impairs the functioning efficiency of their central nervous systems. Multiple failures at adaptation at various stages of development are characteristic as well as multiple and often shifting difficulties. The regressive pull seems to be winning over the progressive thrust. Object relationships are frequently poor.

In a series of clinical interviews, these are often frightening children who will ask for part of your soul. They show much anxiety and distress over their difficulties, although they may not be able to verbalize or communicate this distress. Thought content often shows too much primary process. Their thinking, choice of words, and manner show marked deficiency or signs of disorganization. The fear of loss of the love object predominates.

On psychological testing, most of these children show organic signs. Oral, anal, phallic, and oedipal material is abundant and tangled in a disorganized fashion. Anxiety level is very high and defenses often disintegrate in testing, especially on the Rorschach. Thinking is often disorganized and shows major deficiencies in the function of synthesis and integration.

Most of these children fail a significant number of the soft or subtle neurological signs and frequently show a hard, or localizing, sign.

Treatment is often long and difficult. The therapist must actively reach out to the child, either in the form of setting limits or stimulating him. The interviews vary in structure with the needs of the child, but often reach both extremes. The first step is to become a significant need-gratifying object for the child. Hopefully, through identification the child borrows the healthy defenses and desirable personality traits of the therapist. The therapist also teaches adaptational skills. In order to emulate him, the child must have considerable information about and involvement with the therapist. The child is often treated as a close friend and/or family member. Work with the parents involves much education, active help, and extensive emotional support, designed to help the parents grow into more adequate auxiliary egos for the child.

More so than with any other group of emotional disorders in childhood, Freud's statement in his paper on "Analysis Terminable and Interminable" is appropriate: "The liberation of a human being from his symptoms and inhibitions and abnormalities of character is a lengthy business. . . ." (4).

# 4

## *Vicissitudes of Adolescence*

STANLEY H. SHAPIRO, M.D.

### Introduction

As a phase in personality growth, adolescence is of critical importance. Due to the thrust of biological maturity, upheavals in psychic equilibrium occur which provide another chance, as it were, to resolve basic personality conflicts held temporarily in abeyance by the defenses and ego organization achieved in latency. The upsurge of libido that is the psychic correlate of physiological maturity is the catalyst and, to some extent, modulator of all of the characteristics of the adolescent process. New identifications with alteration in the ego ideal, self-image, and the whole system of self-esteem regulation comprise some of the critical transformations of the ego and superego under the impetus of increased drive intensity. These changes are also reflected in the object relations of the adolescent who must traverse the perilous terrain from the security and comfort of dependence on the parents, only partially breached in latency, to the full independent functioning of the young adult.

Much of the visible adolescent turmoil takes place in the arena of his growing peer relations and is accompanied by the diminishing importance of the parents and their values. This very crucial phenomenon of adolescent rebellion must be understood as a psychologically necessary disruption of which the social aspects, in terms of behavior and group action, are secondary consequences. While the dynamics of group processes in adolescence are an important area of study in their own right, the internal stresses and strains of the individual cannot be ascertained by a sociological approach.

The most fruitful method of study is that of psychoanalytic developmental psychology viewing the personality structure as emerging according to inborn sequential unfolding (maturational pressure) combined with the impact of the particular environmental forces encountered by the individual. This process viewed longitudinally comprises personality development. Any significant area of the personality or of its functioning which can be singled out for separate longitudinal study comprises a developmental line with regard to that function (5). Within this framework both conscious and unconscious mental activity can be subsumed. One can trace the vicissitudes of development of the structure of the personality with regard to such functions as the defenses, the superego, or various autonomous ego activities. This point of view provides a baseline for the assessment of behavior as being appropriate to a given developmental phase. Difficulties or conflicts which are appropriate to an age can be understood as arising from the demands of development. These demands create disharmony or disequilibrium in the personality manifested as developmental conflicts which initiate a search for solutions. In the course of reactions to these developmental disharmonies both progressive and regressive movements may be noted. Struggle for a solution to a given developmental task can be deemed successful if the outcome leads to further growth in the personality upon which new developments can be based as maturation proceeds. Development is thus a cumulative process. An understanding of pathological vicissitudes of behavior can be achieved by assessing the pathology in terms of its interference with ongoing development. As previously described in the chapter on the infantile neurosis, some conflicts are phase appropriate whereas others are holdovers from previous phases; still others represent impingements from the outside which comprise developmental interferences (9).

Both pathological and normal behavior can therefore be viewed as vicissitudes within a general framework of development. Freed of commitments to a nosological scheme, but connected to a maturational organization, some of the internal processes of adolescence can be discussed using terms and ideas which can be applied to an understanding of both normal and abnormal phenomena. It will thus be possible to stress vicissitudes which signalize normal developmental crises but which may otherwise be considered and appear quite alarming. More malignant psychotic developments and asocial behavior patterns will be discussed elsewhere.

Adolescent development may be conceived as a combination of two related tasks: one, to master the changes in the body and its functions which are the consequences of physical, particularly sexual, maturation; and two, to master changes in the sense of self with the dual quest for independence and a stable sense of identity, both sexual and otherwise. Many developmental (phase-appropriate) conflicts can be traced to the impact on personality processes of the biological upsurge of the sexual drive. Not only sexual activity itself and sexual identity formation but also many other related areas of ego development (body image, intellectual development, sublimations) derive from the onset of physiological puberty. The first signs of these internal shifts and changes occur roughly during the chronological period of eleven to thirteen. These pre-adolescent developments constitute the interface between latency and puberty. In order to comprehend the upheaval of early adolescence the stage must be set in latency.

### PRE-ADOLESCENT DEVELOPMENT

After successfully overcoming the throes of the phallic oedipal struggle, the child enters latency. Though sexual interests remain active they are more or less covert as the child becomes absorbed in the mastery of reality beyond his own body and his own immediate family. Latency is a period of intellectual and physical growth and consolidation. Blos (3) summarizes the fruits of latency as the mastery of reality and the mastery of the drives (i.e., sublimation). The child who does not successfully resolve his oedipal conflict and who therefore develops a neurosis will not enter latency. Similarly normal adolescent processes will not unfold unless preceded by a successful passage through latency. Thus each stage in personality maturation becomes the base upon which the next phase unfolds and each phase thus exercises an important and at times decisive influence on the succeeding one.

Yet, as paradoxical as it may seem, the hard-won stability, the character structure established during latency, is not suitable for the quantitative and qualitative upsurge of drive activity and the subsequent adaptive demands of adolescence. The situation may be likened to the molting process seen in crustaceans, such as lobsters and crayfish, whose external skeleton or shell must periodically be shed in order for the animal to grow. The upheavals which are so characteristic of adolescence indicate that this "molting process" is taking place. But as Anna Freud (4) has pointed out, "The people in the child's family and school, who assess his state on the basis of behavior, may deplore the adolescent upset which, to them, spells the loss of valuable qualities, of character stability, and of social adaptation."

## DELAYED ADOLESCENCE

One of the first developmental vicissitudes to be encountered is the delay of adolescent onset. This is signified by a continuation into the early teens of latency behavior with no sign of the expected turbulence.

Case #1. Stephen at fifteen was slight of build and had not as yet experienced any secondary sexual changes, such as body hair development, voice change, and the like. Always a good student, his application to his studies was far in excess of what was required and bordered on obsessional perfectionism. Indeed he had many features of the obsessive compulsive in his character structure, which had developed and continued from latency. He was punctilious, tidy, compliant, and fearful of authority. His strict regard for the rules to which he adhered with almost a legalistic fanaticism made him a questionable asset in games with his peers. As would be expected, he veered away from athletic pursuits and found success and pleasure in such activities as the debating team. All his aggressiveness and competitiveness focused on verbal, intellectual pursuits and he delighted in fault-finding and one-upping both peers and teachers. But at home he let his guard down, as it were, and was given to temper outbursts, demanding, whining behavior, and fierce rivalry with his brother, four years younger. This behavior was also of long duration and had undergone little change over the years. Stephen was thus still a latency child at fifteen, with no apparent heterosexual interests; his sexuality was limited to the crude locker room vulgarity more characteristic of the eleven-year-old.

In Stephen's favor was the parallel delay in sexual maturation which had not yet assailed the latency structure from within. Those children whose defenses against drive activity are so excessive as to be able to contain the libidinal thrust of puberty are in serious circumstances. The previously adaptive "taming" of the drive now can prevent normal maturational processes in the psyche from taking place. When maturation does occur there is greater danger of a complete overthrow of the ego, producing the disorganized decompensation of psychosis. Such an eventuality is to be considered when strong reaction-formations and other signs of an obsessive compulsive character structure persist unchanged into early adolescence despite the physiological maturation.

In contrast to Stephen's delay in entering puberty, many ten- and eleven-year-olds appear precocious and their behavior resembles a charade of adolescence, with exchanges of ID bracelets, talk of going steady, etc. This façade is unfortunately often misread by parents whose need to relive their youth makes them impatient for their child to grow up. Much unnecessary pain and discomfort can ensue from the premature boy-girl parties sponsored by such parents who do not distinguish the intense *verbal* interest from a desire for an actual relationship.

Case #2. Patti, age eleven, reported to her therapist that she was very embarrassed in school. Playing softball she hit the ball very well but it was caught by Robert. Now everyone will think that Robert likes her. She went on to indicate that she and Kathy both like Robert and they spend a good deal of their spare time discussing him, keeping tabs on his whereabouts. Neither would dream of talking to Robert for that would cause everyone to know that they liked him; so that there is virtually no contact in fact. That this love interest "from afar" is something less than even puppy love is given away by the total lack of jealousy between the girls. As a matter of fact almost all of the girls are in love with Robert, who is "the most popular."

There is as much homosexual libido involved as heterosexual, since the common fantasy of "being in love" binds the two girls together as confidantes with whom each can share (and learn to verbalize) intimate feelings and attitudes in the supporting presence of a trusted sounding board. The capacity to form such friendships is a good prognostic sign indicating a potential ability to separate from the mother who is the original confidante.

ADOLESCENT UPHEAVAL

Some of the typical anxieties in early adolescence focus on the physical growth and change related to the development of the secondary sex characteristics. In both boys and girls there is often anxious covert competition. Girls show an ambivalent concern for the menarche. Those who haven't experience doubts and fears around the question, "Will I develop?" The intensity and fixity of these fears is a function of how much guilt and how many unresolved problems related to infantile sexual activity might remain. Boys likewise keep score on who has and who hasn't gotten his sperm yet. Behind this interest always lurks the fear that maybe something is wrong and it isn't going to happen ever.

Case #3. Tony was the kind of eleven-year-old who was taken as mascot by older boys because his social precocity made it possible for him to be tolerated. But for Tony this posed an extra burden; he always had to keep up and appear to know what was going on, even if he didn't. One day during a treatment session Tony blurted out, "How do you masturbate?" He had been trying to masturbate and was confused because nothing was happening. His real question was, "How do you know when you are having an orgasm?" It was clear that Tony was not yet developed enough for ejaculation to occur and was beset by doubts. These doubts were enhanced by the fact that the older boys were way ahead of him in development and were talking freely about their sexual activities. To compensate for this defect Tony was first to volunteer when some marijuana was obtained. Likewise he went out of his way to be insolent with his teachers, not seeming to mind the punishments it brought. In his book the gain in prestige as a "no-nonsense tough guy" with his peers was well worth it. For Tony, anxiety over his lack of sexual development led to behavior designed to supply a substitute expression as proof of his masculinity.

Adolescent onset is a vulnerable time for the child with previous difficulties. Old conflicts are rekindled by the renewal of libidinal interests and old anxieties are re-experienced.

Case #4. Alice at eleven was tortured by the fear that she would never develop physically as had several of her "early bird" girl friends. These fears were easily traceable to residual guilt over sexual explorations and masturbatory behavior from her oedipal years when she was seen in therapy. But as great as her fear of not developing was the dual anxiety about being sexually mature. Alice was obsessed with the idea that her period would come as a kind of flood leading both to serious medical consequences as well as embarrassment. Knowing that menarche signified that she was capable of having a baby, she had fantasies of getting pregnant on a date without knowing it. These ideas were not shared outside the therapy except in greatly diluted form.

Like a magnet she was attracted to stories and television shows which dealt with illegitimacy and accidents, which in turn disrupted her sleep with nightmares. These florid anxieties and recrudescent neurotic symptoms appeared suddenly and lasted five months. During this time Alice was seen again in therapy. The symptoms subsided after sufficient connections were made with the conflicts and problems that had re-emerged and were well known from her earlier period of treatment, which was at the height of her oedipal struggles.

Treatment was able to be discontinued when her ability to function in school returned and she was anxiety free the rest of the day, signifying that her development could now continue unimpeded.

## MASTURBATION CONFLICTS

When menarche occurs and spermatogenesis makes its appearance in nocturnal emissions, despite the relief that everything is in working order, new anxieties arise. Now the problem is that of being in the grip of an internal process over which one has no control. The feeling of being controlled from within by his own drives and urges stands parallel to the sensitivity displayed by the adolescent to being controlled from without. There are avenues available for expression of the struggle against the external adversary or authority as the ubiquity and intensity of adolescent rebellion attests. However, it is much more difficult to cope with the internal enemy whose power is directly perceived and from whom there seems no escape. The young adolescent boy's concern about his own body and its functions often borders on the hypochondriacal as a result. Whether it be muscular size or strength, acne, hair, weight, the same general pattern of anxiety prevails. Is it working right? Is it normal? Can I control it? These patterns are most often clearly delineated in the young adolescent's struggles with masturbation.

Case #5. Both of this fourteen-year-old boy's parents were big, tall people, as was everyone in his family; yet he worried about whether he would ever be tall. Though he appeared like a reed, he spoke of dieting because of a "pot belly." Jack also planned exercise programs to build up his muscles. These anxieties were fed by constant comparison in the locker room with others of his age mates, some of whom naturally were more advanced physically, since this aspect of physiological maturation is subject to individual variation. To compound the difficulty Jack found himself admiring those of his peers whose genitals had already begun to develop and enlarge. He had great difficulty revealing this in treatment because he interpreted his competitive interest in penis size as evidence that he must be a homosexual.

Jack masturbated but had trouble admitting it even though he was well read enough to know the medical facts. The act was performed in a driven way as a means of relieving a variety of tensions and anxieties and hardly seemed a pleasurable pursuit at all. Particularly for Jack it relieved tension over the feeling of being controlled. Just the fact of having spontaneous erections was a source of great distress. He worried about it happening at inopportune times, particularly at parties or when he was going to be in the presence of girls. He utilized masturbation to dissipate temporarily this fear of being controlled by his own body. But as part of a vicious cycle the anxiety over being controlled then gave way to guilt feelings which expressed themselves as anxiety that he had now damaged himself and perhaps would no longer be able to have an ejaculation. He tortured himself with thoughts that he would never be able to marry and have children. Mirroring Mark Twain, who is quoted as saying that stopping smoking was quite easy because he had done it hundreds of times, Jack was perennially swearing off masturbation only to become prey to the fear of the unwanted erection and the intrusion of the disturbing sexual fantasies. And for this there was only one "cure"—masturbation. Thus the cycle would start again.

Normal development is uneven, marked by forward bursts of growth, regressive movements, and occasional plateaus of consolidation and relative calm. Regressive shifts both in libidinal interest as well as level of functioning are common in adolescents. "Dirty talk" with strong anal components is a typical expression of libidinal regression in early adolescence. Some of the hypochondriacal concerns about body functioning and the diet fads which go along as projected solutions to overcome weakness or acne, etc., can be understood also as regressive forms of anxiety expressed in oral or anal terms. This regression takes on more serious significance with the revival of old conflicts and anxieties which re-invade other areas of functioning so that a transitory neurosis is re-established.

As Stephen's (case #1) voice began to change and he shot up in height, the previous outward façade of intellectual superiority and aloofness from his peers started to crumble. Difficulty concentrating on his studies was traced to the intrusion of thinly veiled sexual fantasies in which he depicted himself in the role of a great athletic hero performing under the admiring gaze of a beautiful movie star.

Stephen flirted with being discovered masturbating by being careless in disposing of the Kleenex, and had fantasies of mother walking in on him, catching him in the act. He both feared being caught but wanted her to know he was a man. He consciously assailed himself for his weakness in giving in to masturbating and worried about damaging himself in some way, even though he had read enough to know otherwise. His previous perfectionism gave way to a recklessness about his work, particularly about handing it in on time. Stephen delighted in being able to write themes at the eleventh hour, handing in the original draft and getting an A. He frequently was late for appointments because of missing his train by a minute's miscalculation. Vague plans and "long-distance" interest in girls appeared for the first time. Stephen displayed the same "fight against time" by trying to masturbate to a point just short of ejaculation, paralleling the way he handed in his work at the last minute, and tried to time his arrival at the office down to the last second. But it must be stressed that all of these vicissitudes occurred internally. All Stephen's parents noted was that he appeared more moody, which they attributed to his "growing up."

Like Jack (case #5), his masturbation conflicts were expressed in anal terms and obsessional defenses of isolation and undoing predominated. Being controlled by either his own body or by others reflected Stephen's concern over passivity. Behind his anxiety over time was the need for mastery and control. If he came early for an appointment, he was under the therapist's control; if he came late he was also not in control vis-à-vis train schedules, elevator service, etc. Perfection could be achieved only by arriving in the waiting room just as the door was opened. Stephen viewed his sperm anally as a valuable product to be conserved; in masturbating he struggled to retain the sperm, trying to masturbate just short of orgasm but still obtaining relief from sexual tension which was producing the unwanted erections and the disturbing sexual fantasies.

In this boy the libidinal thrust of puberty had rekindled old conflicts related to masturbation and phallic exhibitionism which had been handled mainly by regression to anality and the use of obsessional defenses. His difficulties focused on the polarity of control (activity) and helplessness (passivity). Doing his schoolwork took on the characteristics of the desired but conflict-laden sexual activity which he tried to handle with the same maneuvers of control and perfectionism with which he masturbated. This is what is meant by the sexualization of function—where an autonomous activity (academic learning) becomes invaded by, and the vehicle for, the expression of sexual conflicts.

The overall organization of these conflicts in symptomatic behavior and in character traits revealed the presence of an obsessional neurosis erupting through the bulwark of Stephen's latency obsessional character structure. This character structure was too rigid to accommodate the adolescent stirring of libido when it made its belated appearance. Stephen presented the picture of a classical obsessional neurosis in adolescence, which was seriously jeopardizing his development.

Physical maturity and the re-emergence of the sexual drive combine to pose tremendous problems for the adolescent. These problems revolve around the adjustment to the physical and physiological changes of sexual maturation and the psychological concomitants of such changes which amount to the need for an overthrow of the stable personality patterns achieved in latency.

Anxieties have been noted in relation to the actual functioning of the genitals (menstruation and spermatogenesis) which is often displaced onto other parts of the body and regressively experienced in oral and anal terms. What the adolescent really thinks about these processes is shrouded in secrecy, shared only with intimates. Anxiety, shame, and the universal fear that they are the only ones to feel this way combine to make this information hard to reveal to any adult. The derivative expressions, such as hypochondriacal concerns, compulsive exercise rituals, food fadism, etc., are the usual visible manifestations of this turbulence along with the more rapid mood fluctuations and inconsistency of behavior. To the ordinary observer these processes do not reveal themselves as indicative of sexual conflicts which are appropriate to the age. Rather, they appear to be part of the general behavior pattern of adolescence and reflections of group or social activities.

While the true nature of these concerns generally remains very private, other aspects of adolescence operate much more visibly. The social scene of adolescence is a highly charged arena where many developmental problems are played out. From the point of view of the individual adolescent, the wider sphere available to him outside the home and away from the parents provides an opportunity to pursue the quest for independence and the establishment of a sense of identity which comprises the second major developmental task in adolescence.

## SEXUAL IDENTITY

In addition to the need to accommodate to an altered body image and the maturing of the sexual functions, the adolescent must forge a sexual identity which transcends physical and physiological fact. The development of a stable self-concept is anchored largely in terms of sexual identity. This key area is naturally most vulnerable, bearing as it does both on highly charged libidinal functions and on narcissistic concerns related to self-image and self-esteem.

Some reference has already been made as to the anxiety shown by boys about the adequacy of their physical functions. The anxiety is clustered around conflicts over masturbation as residual interferences from the infantile period. The developmental task of achieving genital primacy is crucial for the adolescent. It means organizing libidinal strivings in relation to heterosexual aims focused on achieving discharge via the genitals. Clinically, one can often see how difficulties in this area are reflected in other areas in ego functioning. The boy who does not feel his genitals are adequate will also demonstrate feelings of inferiority in intellectual functioning. Spiegel (10) indicates that it is an open question whether there is a cause and effect relationship between the achievement of genital primacy and ego synthesis and intellectual achievement during adolescence.

Case #6. Charles at eighteen described his difficulty with girls as due to his inability to pursue them despite great interest. He needed continuous reinforcement and reassurance that the girl was amenable; each new escalation of intimacy had to be clearly signaled as acceptable by the girl. Charles openly envied girls their prerogative for being passive and receptive. His fantasy was that the girl should come to him and in a sense be the pursuer, while he could assume the more feminine role. In trying to understand his inhibition, he verbalized both a fear of humiliation should his overture be rejected (narcissistic injury) and, more deeply hidden, fear of his own capacity to be aggressive which he equated with any show of masculine assertiveness. His anxieties crystallized in a fear of impotence—the ultimate humiliation. His unconscious wish to be a girl was revealed in dreams and during drug-induced "highs" in which he had the illusion that the lower half of his body was that of his sister.

His own concept of cure was to "prove" his masculinity by performing successful intercourse. This he attempted with a prostitute under sordid conditions and with a great deal of anxiety which he attempted to assuage by alcohol. The results were predictable—a self-fulfilling prophecy of impotence precipitating a severe anxiety state and a conviction that he was a homosexual.

While the stumbling block for boys lies still in the area of their castration anxiety, which prevents adequate masculine assertion, girls experience difficulty from another direction. For the girl, proof of femininity derives from external sources—being loved by a boy. This need to be loved subserves both narcissistic and libidinal aims. Heterosexual strivings are reinforced in a direction away from the father onto a substitute object. Identification with the mother as a sexual woman occurs simultaneously and this can absorb the pre-oedipal attachment (homosexual libido) as well as alleviate the oedipal rivalry. "I can be loved by someone *like* my father and therefore be *like* my mother." This replaces "I want father to love me, not mother" (oedipal); and "I want father to love me rather than be loved by mother" (pre-oedipal—homosexual). The more complicated oedipal strivings and conflicts of the girl are played out over a long period of time extending into adolescence. The end point with boys, by contrast, is sharp and definitive in order for them even to enter latency. The girl's need to be loved as proof of femininity places her under great moral pressure. Society to some extent urges and rewards the pursuit of masculinity; but with girls there are strong currents against proving herself sexually (double standard).

In the more liberalized youth culture of today, with the advent of the pill, the situation is much worse. Social change has made it harder and harder to say no.

Case #7. Audrey, a nineteen-year-old art student, reported that she was getting involved with a boy, passing from the platonic level at which she found herself comfortable, to the "making out level" in which her "hang ups" were coming to light. She told how they've been "making out" in his apartment, but no intercourse as yet. She suspects it's in the offing from the way he has been talking. She doesn't know what to do and is beset with doubts focusing on whether he is finished with his old girl friend who has just left town for several months. Suppose she "does a thing" with him and then he goes back with the girl friend upon her return. She knows she'll feel terrible and like a fool, but what can she do? She thinks of avoiding him in order to forestall his wanting to sleep with her. Yet she wants to sleep with him, feeling that she likes him very much. She chided herself on her inability to accept having sexual relations on a friendly basis. Why should she make such a fuss about it, about separating love and sex? She tries to convince herself that there is something abnormal or sick about her not being able to "do a thing" and let it go at that, even if the old girl friend does come back. It is humiliating for her to think that she will be jealous if he left her for the old girl friend; but she can't help it. Maybe if she were away at some "straight" college going with some "straight" boy this would be okay, but she is not. All her friends espouse this free love philosophy. She is ashamed of her "hang ups" in doing so. She spoke admiringly of a "great" girl "who slept with a lot of guys—even with one guy just because he hadn't done it before—just to help him out. Then she got married and is very happy."

Audrey is caught in a typical bind, feeling ashamed of very feminine (albeit not unneurotically tinged) feelings about sexual relationships and love. She is trying to put down these feelings in favor of the Bohemian free love philosophy espoused by her peer group at art school. Her only defense is to effect a painful withdrawal from the situation and thus lose the boy altogether if she gets found out. She could see no justification for asking him where he stands with the old girl friend and where she stands with him. That's too square. The cards are stacked in favor of the boy who has the backing of the group. She is made to feel that there is something wrong with her in making such a big deal "about going to bed with a guy." Under such circumstances who can draw the line between proving one's self and promiscuity? Sexual relations become degraded into a mechanical act devoid of emotional connotation. Many adolescent girls are thus pressured into sexual relations which are inevitably self-depreciating and/or dehumanizing.

## ADOLESCENT REBELLION

Independence has many ramifications, most of which revolve around the adolescent's needs to detach himself from the parents and their protection and guidance. The beginnings of this detachment process or "object removal" are seen in early adolescence (7). The deterioration of behavior and habits that so often characterizes the youngster on the threshold of puberty clearly has a rebellious connotation. Personal habits of cleanliness and tidiness are replaced by an insouciance to dirt and disorder reminiscent of the two-year-old. The carefully nurtured and often hard-won work habits of the latency period appear to dissolve.

This is also reflected in the academic slump often seen in the sixth or seventh grade, especially in boys whose previous high performance makes this turn of events quite a striking phenomenon. Also in boys, the decorum of sorts that they are able to muster in the classroom becomes harder to maintain as they seem to become infected by a restless, noisy boisterousness. Pressure for self-assertion stems from within as the adolescent boy seeks an adequate outlet for the increased libidinal energy with which he is assailed. This need for immediate discharge through action is fed also by the narcissistic pressure to prove himself to his peers. Academic rewards alone cannot provide the sustenance for these narcissistic and drive pressures. In addition, school is a natural substitute arena for acting out resentments to parental authority.

Case #8. Kurt at twelve was an interesting and charming youngster who strove for the unusual, the picaresque, and even the bizarre in both his ideas and his appearance. He had a definite need to be different which at times was refreshing and stimulating for his teachers. Among his peers he was a pacesetter. His hair was longest and his dress was always at the thin edge of what was acceptable at his school. Both his parents were hard-working successful people who ran a "tight ship" at home with parental authority unquestioned. But, in addition to these winsome aspects of his adolescent rebellion, there were also self-defeating side effects. Kurt's need to stand out required him to be the one to raise his hand in class as the teacher, exasperated at their behavior, berated the class rhetorically, "Who wants to go and sit in second grade?" Kurt would also fail to produce the contrite expression of regret for his behavior and the obligatory tears when called down to the principal. He simply would not work for a teacher he disliked, despite the consequences which, several years in a row, amounted to spending his summers in school.

This behavior and parallel plummeting of his schoolwork began on the threshold of puberty in sixth grade. Previously, Kurt had been studious and well behaved (even overly so). Personality difficulties were revealed only in some phobic manifestations and sleep disturbance.

One can get some measure of the intensity of drive pressure and the struggle for narcissistic gratification from the often observed fact that "making the team" or just "being one of the guys" can override any considerations about schoolwork which previously were so important. The return is not immediate enough or definitive enough to satisfy the adolescent boy's pressing need for recognition and acceptance.

This early form or prodrome of the "adolescent rebellion" represents in part the need to throw off the yoke of parental control and authority. It is brought about by the resurgence of the drives with the reawakening of the libidinal interests of the Oedipus complex. This reawakening of sexual interest in the parents is now made more threatening by the onset of biological maturity. But it is not only girls having to distance themselves from their fathers because of renascent sexual interest and boys being frightened by their recognition of mothers as sexual objects. The accession of the libido is bisexual. The noisy activity of boys protects them against their passive homosexual wishes. Girls find fault with their mothers and are openly provocative by their criticism of the mother's values and ways; and behind this façade of continual bickering one can detect the operation of defenses against attachment to the mother. The continued need for a mothering figure is often detectable in the apparent paradoxical attitude toward the mothers of one's girl friends. One's own mother is viewed with contempt, "But if only I had so and so for a mother. She's so understanding and nice." This need for "object removal" also impels greater interest in other adults as objects for identification. Teachers particularly can fill this role in a constructive and meaningful way for the young adolescent. For the disturbed adolescent, the therapist can provide a model for identification removed from incestuous dangers. The downgrading of the parents receives group support and reinforcement, while at the same time it fosters great dependence on and interest in peers. But seen only from the outside one can mistakenly perceive the individual youngster's behavior as a reflection of group process and therefore a socially induced phenomenon. This view captures only the last steps of a complicated internally driven process which creates the need for the group action.

Dissolution of apparently well-established work and study discipline also comprises part of the first phase of adolescent rebellion. When maintained within limits that are not self-defeating, the rebellion can be viewed as part of a normal development fostering the necessary and at times painful task of setting one's self off as an independent person. Many of the former needs met by the parents are now sought from peers— advice, encouragement, solace, information—all come from the peer group whose importance increases as the parents are devalued. It is thus a serious clinical sign to learn from a mother that her teen-age daughter tells her everything, including the details of her sexual activity on her dates. For the adolescent, having a "secret life" is not only a right and a privilege, it is a developmental necessity. Though this point has validity for the whole of childhood, it is particularly crucial for the adolescent for whom distrust of adults is developmentally appropriate. For this reason some of the most difficult patients to treat are the children of professionals in the field or children who have been raised "by the book," i.e., by parents who continually interpret to the child the hidden meaning of his behavior which they have gleaned from some psychological text. These children have had to develop strong defenses against being understood and are often "allergic" to attempts to interpret their behavior.

Thus adolescent behavior is paradoxical. Sloppy, messy, disorganized activity, which indeed is regressive, at the same time provides a defensive distancing from the parents and their values; and, further, it serves constructive movement in the early adolescent years, helping to focus interest and attention on the peer group and on other less threatening adults who are accessible.

## SEPARATION AND INDIVIDUATION

Letting go of the parents and finding one's self as an equal in the company of peers may sound easy, but the transition is anything but smooth and harmonious. To keep the parents at arm's length entails at best a continuous background noise of tension punctuated by frequent explosions over such trivial matters as coming to meals on time and fulfilling household chores. This situation has been described as that of having a sullen, dissatisfied boarder in the house instead of a child. But these external battles only reflect an internal struggle as the adolescent tries to put down his own wishes to be cared for and watched over as in the past.

These urges reawakened with the other drives and libidinal interests are strongly condemned as regards the parents, but regularly appear displaced onto the peer group.

Case #9. Nora's melodramatic battles with her mother merited a wider audience than was available at family dinner table, for this fourteen-year-old girl's tirades were a ludicrous parody of a television soap opera. The slightest comment by her mother—even a question—would initiate a barrage of invective. She also criticized her mother's docility and lack of independent opinions. She voiced contempt for her mother's values and her way of life, decrying her mother's enslavement to the home and her lack of interest and accomplishment in the outside world. On the other hand, a cold dinner due to mother's being at a meeting brought snide remarks about meeting one's responsibilities and obligations. At fourteen Nora was attractive, but as yet she did not date. Her closest friend was Denny with whom she spent most of her free time. She patterned her behavior and ideas in line with Denny. Nora could not tolerate disagreements and was unbearable to be around until things were patched up with Denny. Each new development or new piece of information about her peer group was processed through Denny. It was a common joke that Nora should have an open telephone line to Denny's house. What to wear to a party and post-mortems the day after required long conversations. When Denny spent any time with another girl, Nora could only be described as jealous. Nora was only at peace with herself when she had established a consensus with Denny on all matters of importance. Denny thus replaced Nora's mother in this important function of stabilizing and modulating Nora's own view of the world and her current position in it. If Nora's contemptuous attitude toward her mother were not strident enough alone to warrant suspicion, then her slavish dependence on Denny whom she used as an alter ego should suffice to reveal the strain on Nora as she tried to break her passive dependent attachment to her mother.

Throwing over the values of the parents the adolescent simultaneously disrupts whatever internal harmony has been achieved between the ego and superego—the latter agency, of course, deriving from an internalization of parental mores in the first place. In addition, the whole balance of self-esteem regulation painstakingly built up during the latency period is threatened. The latency child should have begun to replace the need for parental reassurance by a self-contained narcissistic balance "derived from achievements and mastery which earn objective social approbation" (3a). But this process is imperfect and incomplete. Some external sources of approval are still necessary.

Such twosomes as Nora and Denny, each reinforcing the other in the struggle against the parents and each substituting as parent surrogates for the other, often represent the beginning of viable relationships which can endure for life. The reciprocal reinforcement of self-esteem provides some of the necessary protection during this period of narcissistic sensitivity. (Like the crayfish just after molting, whose skin has not yet toughened into a protective shell, the adolescent, having shed his shell of latency, is also defenseless.) His vulnerability is additionally increased by casting off the protection afforded by the parents. In this way the peer group comes to assume transcendent importance, providing a measure of protection and stability for the adolescent who is, both internally and externally, psychologically adrift.

Though to adult eyes the adolescent appears to be fiercely independent, as in the way he dresses for example, closer examination reveals that his bleached, frayed blue jeans are actually part of a "prescribed" uniform of the day of his peer group. That this compulsive conformity functions as a reassurance of belonging is masked by his focusing on the disparity between the mores of the peer group and the "establishment." How else can one understand 300,000 youths herded together for a rock festival, living in mud and rain for several days, each feeling he is "doing his own thing"? The need for denial of any dependent leaning fosters such blindness as regards the slavish adherence to group expectations. At times this can be a harder task than meeting the requirements set by the parents for their approval. Some of the delinquent acts and antisocial behavior of otherwise law-abiding adolescents have their origin in the group pressure for allegiance.

In turning forcefully away from the parents the adolescent must have somewhere to turn. There is no more lonely position than to be estranged from the parents with no one to fill the void. Clinically, it is a poor prognostic sign to learn that a youngster cannot make or keep friends. For whatever other pathology there might be, this capacity for object relations provides access for the continuation of adolescent individuation mediated by the group. Parents mistakenly construe the friction they encounter with their youngster as a measure of his pathology, not realizing that they are, "so to speak," innocent victims of a development crisis.

## ADOLESCENT DEPRESSION

Mood fluctuations so characteristic of the age are another indicator of the disruption of the previously established ways in which the adolescent judged himself and knew where he was in latency in relation to his peers. There are as yet no well-established standards by which one can judge one's behavior or one's worth. The ebb and flow of moods with evanescent elation dissolving in a moment to painful depression is the price extracted for emotional growth. The sense of urgency combined with self-centeredness characterizes this period. Adolescent creativity often subserves the ego as a weapon against these feelings of depression. Artistic expressions of real merit or creative intellectual achievements can result from this struggle to counteract feelings of worthlessness that characterize adolescent depression. The same relationship between depression and creativity has been noted in the lives of talented artists and scientists.

It is a vexing problem to try on grounds of mood swings alone to differentiate phase-appropriate adolescent depressive episodes from more malignant affective disturbances indicative of serious narcissistic disorders.

Case #10. Robin came to treatment at sixteen after being "busted" by her parents for using "pot." She was an intelligent girl who, however, was hardly interested at all in using her considerable talents, as her marginal record in school attested. It soon became clear that her attraction for marijuana was only one effort she made to relieve chronic feelings of depression. She led an intensely active social life with rapidly changing alliances and flirtations. There was a driven quality to Robin's socializing which represented an attempt to keep herself diverted from inner feelings of emptiness and worthlessness that threatened to erupt if she allowed herself to sit still too long. Naturally, on this score alone, studying was out of the question. Prior to getting caught with pot there was little external sign that Robin was a troubled youngster. The superficiality of her friendships compelled by her fear of letting anyone get too close achieved protective coloration against the ordinary fickleness of her peers. Her need for pleasure and fun caused her to be considered a leader and a pacesetter. Robin could always be depended upon to think up something "great" to do. Boys found her challenging and exciting but they quickly drifted elsewhere, not realizing they were being driven to do this by her own design.

It required a long period of therapy to expose the outlines of Robin's narcissistic problems. Early childhood exposure to the primal scene (parental intercourse) combined with intense conflicts about her own sexual feelings to make her acceptance of femininity fraught with difficulty. Infantile masturbation was complicated by actual urinary tract infections requiring examinations and treatment procedures which were both stimulating and frightening. In adolescence this already shaky foundation for her feminine sexual identity received further assaults in the form of menstrual irregularity with severe cramps and recurrent vaginal infections.

Robin's devil-may-care behavior was her attempt to stave off depressive feelings related to these difficulties in accepting herself as a woman and a worthwhile person, for these two ideas in Robin's mind were contradictory. Psychologically she strove like Peter Pan to be forever an asexual child. And the disparity in her behavior grew more marked the older she became.

It is hard to see how one could have differentiated Robin's depressive feelings from the phase-appropriate mood swings of many of her more fortunate contemporaries (who were going through the "blissful" unhappiness of the age) without extended contact in a period of exploratory psychotherapy. Robin's ability to remain in treatment itself was indicative, for it meant reversing the flight away from the parents as well as the need to keep from letting anyone getting too close. For many adolescents with obvious unhappiness and other evidence of disturbed functioning, treatment remains unavailable to them because of their inability to relate to an adult in a constructive way. It is a challenge therefore to the therapist's acumen to maintain the distance which his patient at any moment requires.

### SOCIAL AWARENESS

There is a more constructive aspect to the teen-ager's exquisite sensitivity to feelings. His acute awareness of his own inner turmoil resonates easily with much of the turmoil of the real world to which the adolescent of today is exposed. This accounts for the extraordinary empathic capacity of this age group for the suffering of others. It underlies the interest which begins to emerge, in the mid-teens particularly, in social and political issues. Youth culture in the United States used to be quite different from either the European or Latin American variety. The aims were frivolous, removed in any realistic sense from the social scene. The direction has shifted, however, in recent years, with increasing social and political activism and seriousness of purpose. Regardless of the form, the tendency to activity is a consistent feature of adolescence. In large measure the need is fed by the pressure to externalize some of the inner strife with which the teen-ager is afflicted. Reflection and introspection are difficult to maintain since they can so easily shade over into brooding despair. This tendency to action combines with the previously mentioned empathic capacity to maximize in adolescence the interest in "causes." Therefore the adolescent, by virtue of his own personal psychological position, can easily identify with the underdog—the weak, the poor, the oppressed, the victims of any superior and presumably selfish force in society. But one cannot conclude, however, that the essential validity of any cause is diminished because it happens to echo the adolescent's own vulnerability and feeling of being oppressed.

Youth protest today is more often than not directed against real injustices and inequities. The point to be stressed is that the adolescent process sharpens perceptions of social injustice and sensitizes the youth to external events which mirror his own individual struggles. Disillusionment with the "establishment," i.e., the people who run things, is thus intensified as the adolescent begins to assess the quality of life around him and sees the disparities between what society professes to be its concerns and values and what in practice occurs. This disillusionment provides outside reinforcement for the separation from the parents. There is thus a synergism between the estrangement from the parents because of their social values and the repulsion from the parents as sexual objects which the libidinal awakening of adolescence has produced. Thus, both from within by fear of his own drives and from without by devaluing his parents as part of the "establishment," separation from the parents is accelerated and the adolescent is impelled to search for his own identity among peers.

From the point of view of the relationship of the group structure to the individual personality, one can delineate positive aspects for growth and maturation which are independent of the particular social function or aim which the group may be designed to serve. In latency boys, in particular, there are cliques and clubs of sorts, but they are transitory and have no real social function to keep them going. Adolescent groups are more viable. The adolescent who joins a club must learn the ropes of the organization and submit to the authority of the leadership. The process of socialization is thus enhanced as the club member is exposed to the petty politics, the stresses and strains, and the necessity to compromise, i.e., to settle for less. Some close observers of recent campus unrest have noted the sobering effect, even among the most activist groups, as they saw the real limitations of disruptive confrontations and pre-emptive demands for instant reform.

Experience forged in these peer group activities, be they pleasure-oriented or grimly political, provides the adolescent with the necessary tools to rebuild and consolidate his fragmented superego. New ego ideals (that which one aspires to be) are formed to replace the discarded infantile images derived from the parents. New value systems emerge which can differ markedly from those of the previous generation. And it is in relation to these new values that self-esteem is regulated. For at the end of adolescence self-regard should be totally emancipated from dependence on parental approval.

It is a challenge to the parents of the adolescent to "grow" along with him and to be able to maintain a relationship not based on the old authority established in childhood. Rather, the relationship should be forged out of mutual respect. The twenty-year-old son or daughter should be able to be viewed as a young friend and not a grown child. The development task of the parent during this period is to remain a viable object for continued representation as an ego ideal, rather than the archetype of what is to be avoided or opposed. This calls for the capacity to respect the adolescent and tolerate the necessary excesses and inconsistencies in his behavior. To the extent that the parent himself is above suspicion in the conduct of his own life and to the extent that he is himself free of hypocrisy, he can hope to maintain credibility in the eyes of his adolescent youngster.

## THE DRUG SCENE

The widespread use of drugs by the current teen-age population is justifiably the subject of attention and concern on the part of health experts, educators, and legislators. While the addictive and deteriorative effects of "hard" drugs (morphine and heroin), barbiturates, and amphetamines have been known and studied extensively, albeit in older populations, there is still divided opinion regarding marijuana derivatives. There is some evidence that the use of "grass" several times a week for only a short period *may* produce severe behavior deterioration (promiscuity and suicide), personality disorganization (psychosis), and evidence of organic brain damage detectable even up to a year after use has stopped (8). But there are also outspoken investigators who claim that they can find no evidence of physical damage and who dispute the causal relationship attributed to marijuana (6).

But there seems to be a unanimity of opinion that the use of drugs does affect the adolescent process in a potentially deleterious fashion. The way in which "grass" or "speed" is used may vary from time to time, but in general the aim is to seek an altered state of well-being that is as deliberate as it is artificial. The ease and passive way by which this generally exciting and pleasurable mood is reached enhances its attractiveness as compared to activities which require some application, some difficulty, and also the risk of failure. Schoolwork and even athletic or constructive hobby pursuits go by the boards.

Case #11. Asked to describe his typical day regarding drugs, Ronnie, a fifteen-year-old, replied as follows. Feeling bored and anticipating some strife because his homework wasn't done, he'd share a "joint" on the way to school. Later in the morning, if he had a test for which he was also unprepared and felt uptight about, he would have another. After the test, to celebrate, he might have some more; either that or in order to develop an appetite for lunch he'd smoke again. This youth attended a suburban high school and came from a middle class intact family of comfortable circumstances. Most of his smoking was casual, unplanned, and shared with friends so that there was great group reinforcement in the activity. At his high school there was a strict division between the users and the nonusers, with the feeling of esprit, brotherhood, and belonging symbolized by smoking which was reminiscent of the ritualized peace pipe of the American Indian. After school and in the evening, more smoking naturally occurred. It was interesting to note that pinning Ronnie down to an actual account of his daily drug use was both surprising and disturbing to him.

This youngster had dropped precipitously in school standing and had given up any athletic competitive endeavors—all as part of his embracing a new "drug-oriented" life-style along with a different set of friends. This new life-style, currently quite in vogue, derives from the "hippie culture." It espouses a romantic idealism as part of an opposition to the crass materialism and the complicated, pressured, urban life-style of an industrialized society. Motifs and values crystallize around peace, pollution, and the return to a simpler way of life closer to nature. Obviously it offers to the individual adolescent in rebellion a ready-made subculture through which he can express, in an organized way, his opposition to the world of his parents and their values as he sees them.

This young man, like many of his friends, though intelligent enough to understand, and exposed to educational programs on drug abuse both in school and out, remained impervious to any real concern. It is also simplistic to believe that much can be accomplished with these youngsters in treatment by attempting to forbid drug use in an authoritarian way. But the therapist as the arbiter of reality has a right and a duty to inform his patient of the risks he is taking and what the effect of continued drug use may be, both physically and emotionally. From there, it has to be dealt with as any behavior or symptomatology with attention to its meaning to the patient, both conscious and unconscious, and the dynamic way in which it operates in his life.

Tony (case #3) at twelve had already experimented with hash and grass, though he did more talking about it than anything else. One day he announced that he had purchased five "uppers" (i.e., stimulants) from a classmate. He did not know what they were, but was led to believe the capsules contained "some hash, some morphine, some speed, and some other stuff." The pills were examined and were able to be identified in the office. Tony was shown how to use the PDR (Physician's Desk Reference), a compendium of products of all major drug companies, which includes color plates of many of the most commonly used drugs. They turned out to be Dilantin. He then "read up" on

Dilantin in the PDR to learn what its uses, effects, and side effects were. Tony was then able to see that he had been cheated, being sold an anticonvulsant, antiepilepsy drug as an "upper."

By his own efforts and motivated by his own curiosity, this youngster was able to begin to appreciate the complexity of pharmacology and the need to be cautious about what he might think of taking. Following this experience, Tony was able to be more open about his interest in drugs. He was surprised that his doctor could understand the allure, the excitement, the mystery, and the temptation to experiment with them. This attraction was identified as part of his wish to be grown up, which in other days would have taken the form of interest in sex, smoking tobacco, or drinking alcohol. The therapeutic task was to detach Tony's wish to be grown up from use of drugs as a symbolic "equivalent." In this way the legitimacy of the wish could be retained for which less harmful means of expression could be found. Simple condemnation would have been interpreted by Tony as a simultaneous condemnation of his desire to be grown up. This unintended condemnation of legitimate desires accounts for the imperviousness to educative efforts which only stress fear and employ such heavy-handed tactics. Another teen-ager reported he had been shown a sex education movie. He said, "They emphasize all the gory details of childbirth and abortion to scare the kids from doing anything." Many well-meaning "drug abuse" programs and films suffer from the same heavy hand. The youthful audience is thus prevented from identifying, which is necessary for any meaningful education to take place.

Within the framework of an ongoing therapy situation, one can see how drug use operates as an attempt to defend against anxiety and anticipated anxiety.

Charles (case #6) tried to relieve his sexual anxiety before going to a prostitute by having several drinks. Another teenage boy related how he had solved his intense anxiety about a blind date. He got "stoned" beforehand with the result that he acted silly on the date. The drug had made him indifferent to the girl as well as oblivious to the way he looked. The evening was a disaster except that he didn't know it. Thus a valuable experience, albeit normally expected to be anxiety provoking, was aborted. This young man had missed an opportunity to master a reality situation which was an age-appropriate task. Emotional growth takes place by just such repeated experiences, and the development of confidence in one's self in heterosexual situations is achieved by such incremental mastery of anxiety. Therefore one of the main "toxic side effects" psychologically of drug use is the way in which it is used to bypass such important experiences and to avoid conflict situations. Tolerance of conflictual tension and using this tension as a source of motivation for adaptive resolution is a most precious ego asset in adolescence. And it is at this vulnerable point that the most frequently used "soft" drugs take their toll.

In addition to regular channels by which illicit drugs are made available, many teen-age girls initially get involved with "speed" (amphetamines) through efforts at diet control. They quickly appreciate the euphoric side effects. The response to "speed" readily meets the adolescent's impatience for results with which psychotherapy cannot compete in lifting a depressed mood. It has to be recognized that intolerance of delay and a proclivity for action rather than introspection are phase-appropriate attitudes only slowly overcome as adolescence proceeds. Once again it is therapeutically sterile to issue a fiat against diet pills or "speeding" as a precondition for treatment. The slow but better road is by the action of the therapeutic process under the aegis of a developing transference.

Case #12. It took Rita many months to acknowledge that her dieting was consistently being sabotaged by forces within herself which she didn't appreciate and therefore could neither understand nor control. During this time she wasted many sessions because she was under the influence of her diet pills. It took quite a while, with repeated demonstration that her "fantastic insights" during these sessions were like "writing on water"; that she could not remember them the next day was obvious, but she still could not give up the diet pills. The complicated meaning of her feelings about her body weight had to be sufficiently unraveled before it could be seen that the diet pill was both a substitute for and a defense against eating; and for Rita, eating was the expression of unconscious oral pregnancy wish. Stopping the diet pill was like stopping birth control pills. She, therefore, had reacted to previous statements by the therapist about the pills as an attempt to make her give in to her sexual wishes. What appeared superficially as a superego admonition ("You ought to stop the pills. They are bad for you.") unconsciously had the meaning of seduction to indulge in a forbidden wish.

In some instances drug use has its main effect as an interference with the therapeutic process itself, aside from many other meanings it may have.

Case #13. Linda readily admitted her interest in drugs, having come for help at seventeen because of difficulties at home and general unhappiness with her life. It was noted that in some sessions she was flighty and given to fits of giggling. One time she reported to her therapist that his face looked like a gopher. She was able to admit, when confronted directly about it, that she had smoked on those days, but denied vehemently that the effects of being "high" were still present. Descriptions of her behavior at school, with indifference to discipline and giggling while being reprimanded by the principal, were also correlated with smoking pot at school. The therapist acquainted Linda with the incompatibility of the mental state of her "high" and the required mental state for therapy to be meaningful. She was shown how she repeated herself from one session to the next, not being able to remember that she had described these events already.

On days when her sessions were in the morning, Linda would often be facile with flight of ideas and euphoric; she also expressed paranoid thoughts. She admitted to "speeding," but explained that she couldn't sleep the night before because she had been out. At other times she admitted using "speed" to combat the fatigue and lethargy of "grass." She began to complain she wasn't being helped by the therapist and she was too busy to come twice a week. One session, six months or so after she had entered treatment, Linda quit without notice.

It had become clear that one of Linda's main problems was a fear of her own passive wishes. She had to fight off any temptation to succumb to them and her therapy foundered on the rocks of an unmanageable transference resistance, for the more she was helped and felt understood, the more frightened she became of getting too close. Her usual methods of provocation, which worked with her parents and her boyfriend, were not successful with the therapist. There were enough data to suspect that the transference was so intense because of the seductive and stimulating relationship between Linda and her father. For example, the parents' sexual difficulties involved father running after mother, who would take refuge in Linda's bed to escape his sexual advances.

Linda turned increasingly to drugs, both to bolster artificially her feeling of being in control of her life (the well-being and expansiveness was provided by speed; the alleviation of anxiety by marijuana) and to alienate herself from the therapy, for she had correctly assessed the antipathy between drugs and treatment, but was using the information perversely.

The final chapter on the drug scene and its utimate impact on the younger generation has yet to be written. While it remains, illegitimately or legitimately (as some would have it), it will constitute a serious obstacle to the propitious unfolding of the adolescent process as it is currently understood. This process as preparation for the assumption of an adult role in society requires hierarchical growth and consolidation of the ego, which in turn depends on resolving basic problems of personal identity and the closing of certain issues with some finality. Bisexual conflicts (sexual identity) as well as vocational or educational goals should be established. Passive strivings related to infantile wishes to be taken care of must yield to an emerging capacity and desire to be the caretaker. Drugs interfere with the adaptive process of conflict resolution and the concomitant growth of necessary ego skills. These psychological effects alone constitute a powerful force against such closures and consolidations, fostering continued passivity and infantile characteristics in the personality.

PROLONGED ADOLESCENCE

Failure to terminate the adolescent process can occur without the influence of drugs. This has been described clinically as the syndrome of prolonged adolescence. It was first described by Bernfeld in males (1923); and the condition has been further examined and discussed by Blos (2).

In essence, the adolescent position, which is of a transitory nature, becomes perseverated into a way of life. "Instead of the progressive push which normally carries the adolescent into adulthood, prolonged adolescence arrests this forward motion with the result that the adolescent crisis is never abandoned but kept open indefinitely" (3b).

By clinging to an unsettled transitory position, basic decisions are postponed and final accountings of achievements are delayed, as are the assumptions of complete responsibility for one's actions. The narcissistic gain of eliminating the risk of failure offsets the continued exposure to shame. Efforts are directed at "the contriving of ingenious ways to combine childhood gratifications with adult prerogatives" (3b).

The preponderance of cases with middle-class social backgrounds and college education indicates that the family's capacity to tolerate and support prolonged dependence operates as a sustaining and contributing factor. The family history further reveals the influence of maternal overestimation leading to expectations of great achievement which have been incorporated into the self-image. Many of these adolescents are rather gifted and intelligent. Bernfeld (1) described them as "having tendencies toward productivity whether artistic, literary or scientific, and by a strong bent toward idealistic aims and spiritual values." Under the continual encouragement from the parent (usually the mother) they come to expect great things from themselves. But they do not regress in the face of failure, which differentiates them from the more severe narcissistic disorders; rather, they continue to try to operate, but without reaching a final decisive end point. In their object relations there is a shallowness and fickleness. Sexual relations tend to emphasize forepleasure; the girl chosen is either strikingly like or opposite to an important incestuous object (sister or mother), and is usually unacceptable to the family. But they cannot emancipate themselves in this way from the family nexus, for it is in this context that they continue to derive narcissistic gratification in being a *wunderkind*; and such admiration is not forthcoming from the external world where deeds, not promises, are rewarded.

Because of the close ties to the adoring mother, these young men show also strong passive feminine identifications, and they lack masculine assertiveness and competitiveness in their character. The normal bisexuality of adolescence is prolonged so that a final sexual identity likewise is avoided. The adolescent crisis is kept open as a necessity in order to avoid regression and a rupture with reality (psychosis) or regression and symptom formation (neurosis). These young men avoid facing conflicts by use of denial. But this avoidance is what perpetuates adolescence itself, since conflictual tension acts as a motive force for personality integration and differentiation as well as for active coping in the mastering of reality problems. This driving force for progression and synthesis is systematically drained off; what arouses strong feelings are narcissistic slights, as when others do not confirm their own high opinions of themselves and the praise which they require is not forthcoming.

Case #14. John was the youngest of three and his mother's favorite. Expression of musical talent was encouraged by his mother who herself was a frustrated singer. John came to think of himself as a budding genius and shared avidly his mother's daydreams of worldwide fame as a concert pianist. The focus shifted in pre-adolescence when he showed an artistic flair for the encouragement of which private lessons were immediately arranged. The accumulation of these extracurricular lessons was used as rationalization for John's lack of friends. He was led to believe by his mother that they were beneath him and that he was destined to greater things. The leveling off of his development in both of these talents was obscured by his sudden accession of interest in chemistry and science in general, which occurred at thirteen on the threshold of puberty.

John did very well in high school, but not as well as one would be led to believe. He had few friends, no girl friends, and socialized superficially at school, usually in relation to academic work. He had a tendency to push beyond his level in any given area, bypassing introductory basic work in favor of more abstruse, advanced, specialized topics. This worked well for him until, at a college level, his basic defects began to show through. In general examinations he did brilliantly but erratically, spending extra time on certain questions and showing himself surprisingly ill informed in other areas. John began to talk of medicine as a career, disparaging the isolation of "pure science." After switching his major in his junior year, he then began to decry the crude competitiveness of the premedical students.

After one year of medical school John presented himself for treatment. He was having great difficulty studying, and deplored the pressurized atmosphere which prevented proper scholarly understanding of his subjects. He had also become interested in the sociology of medicine and was toying with the idea of studying law or taking an advanced degree in social science, with the idea of applying his knowledge to a total revamping of the American health delivery system. He had a girl friend who was a student nurse whose name was the same as his older sister. She came from a different ethnic background and lower social status than the patient, both of which combined to make her unwelcome at his home. He came for help because of severe tension leading to eruption of temper and irritability and difficulty studying. There was also some evidence of somatization with stomach pains and bowel disturbance.

Despite the tendency to expect immediate relief and be given immediate interpretations which would clear up all of his difficulties, John proved amenable to therapy. Treatment was aimed at helping him face conflicts rather than avoid them and he was thus emboldened to complete his adolescence without recourse to the narcissistic defenses he had used to shield himself from discomfort and put off solving basic problems and making basic decisions about his life.

The combined influence of the drug culture, affluence, the tendency to prolong financial dependence justified by the pursuit of graduate studies, all act to make it easier and easier for middle-class youth to remain in the developmental limbo of protracted adolescence. And there is even less hope for the undereducated, unemployed ghetto youth who are on a one-way road to nowhere and who likewise feel no compulsion to resolve basic personal issues appropriate to the adolescent years.

In adolescence, the fires of rebellion are fed by the need to separate from the parents. This need is created by the fears of closeness due to the resurgent oedipal drives, with the parents now as real sexual objects as compared to the fantasies of the oedipal period. In addition, the pre-oedipal passive wishes directed also to the parents must be staved off. Externally there is friction as the parental (adult) mores are flouted in superficial matters such as dress and personal habits. Internally new tensions are set up between the ego and superego, which was fashioned on the parental model. The adolescent ego is thus beset on two fronts: by the need to defend against the ties to the parents as oedipal objects, simultaneous with the related need to defend against the general upsurge of the drives—both aggressive and sexual, both oedipal and pre-oedipal.

Much adolescent pathology concerns conflicts expressed in terms of failure or difficulty in accomplishing these related developmental tasks. The observed upheaval and turbulence is the inevitable by-product of the necessary transformation of the personality by which further growth and development to maturity can be achieved.

# 5

## Juvenile Delinquency

SIDNEY L. COPEL, ED.D.

### Introduction

The history of civilization is the story of man's efforts to tame the ferocity of his instinctual and combative energies and direct them to the needs of social living and group survival. From his earliest beginnings man has always been a social animal. His need for mutual dependence has always been felt, if not explicitly defined, and it can be seen in his efforts to adapt himself to life in increasingly complex social groups. All of the ruined civilizations of antiquity are a historical testimony to his attempts and to his failures.

Society derives the energy for its existence by subtracting a certain amount from the power of each person and this entails some sacrifice for the individual. It is taken for granted that whatever is lost through the renunciation of one's own wishes is more than offset by the greater benefits that society will bestow. This now assumes that an agreeable compromise is possible which is compatible with the desires of the individual and the requirements of his social milieu.

All societies depend for their survival upon a certain measure of social control. There is no society that allows complete individual freedom. The complexities of modern living and the problems of governing large masses of people have necessitated the development of regulatory measures that are economically feasible and can be practically applied. In democratic societies, representative government, together with judicial safeguards, is the means whereby an attempt is made to afford equal treatment to all. However, the problems of present-day society differ in kind and in magnitude from anything ever experienced in the past. Legislative efforts at solution have few precedents to follow and the increasing numbers of laws and authority of government hardly keep pace with social change.

Each new legislative enactment means greater conformity within the group and subtracts something from the freedom of the individual. Societies differ greatly in the amount of control exercised by the central government. Just as there is no society which permits complete freedom of expression, neither is there any society which is totally repressive. The political organization of the society defines for itself just how much individualism it will tolerate and this set of boundaries becomes part of the myth of freedom.

But no set of laws can ever completely regulate social behavior. It is impossible to anticipate every circumstance or to curb the aggression of every individual. The body of law is the heritage of the past and as such is often in direct conflict with the emerging generation and the needs of the present. There will always be those who defy convention and act in opposition to established authority. Defiance of the rules can range from verbal protests to criminality and the state in turn reacts with a punitive vengeance of its own.

The term "juvenile delinquency" is a relatively modern concept describing the condition of the youthful offender in relation to the state. It is a legal rather than a psychological term, and lacks precise definition. Delinquency as a criminal offense covers a broad spectrum of behavior ranging from school truancy to homicide. Just who and what is a delinquent varies from society to society, and even in this country, down to the individual community.

That juvenile delinquency is a major social problem almost goes without saying. From a statistical standpoint the number of juvenile offenders is increasing far more rapidly than the rise in population. From a qualitative standpoint, the increasing savagery of juvenile crime can be read in any daily newspaper. In this country, somewhat paradoxically, delinquency has escalated rapidly in spite of major advances in the living standards of most Americans. In spite of governmental efforts at slum clearance, improved recreational facilities, efforts to provide adequate low-cost housing, and increasing application of psychiatric insights, delinquency remains a perplexing problem (2).

It is difficult to arrive at any sort of accurate estimate as to the incidence of juvenile offenses. Most statistics that are available are vulnerable to major criticism. For one thing, the definition of delinquency varies with the locale. What is legal in one area may be illegal in another. A second factor is the efficiency of local law enforcement. A more effective police force will probably make more arrests and keep more accurate records than an understaffed force. It is the belief of many who work in this field that the quoted statistics on delinquency seriously understate the problem. Estimates have been made that up to three fourths of the juveniles who have had some contact with the police because of a presumed delinquency never even get to juvenile court, and a large number of young lawbreakers escape the attention of the police entirely (23).

Because of the individual suffering created and the general disruption of community life, delinquency has not been a neglected social problem. The search for the causes of juvenile delinquency has, in fact, been a long one. In past centuries, in keeping with traditional doctrines of free will, it was always assumed that the individual was responsible for his own behavior. In many ancient civilizations, when a serious crime was committed, children received the same punishment as adults. Later, when philosophers began to turn their attention to the problems of social living, it was assumed that crime could be simply dispelled by an increase in understanding. Typical of these notions are the words of Hobbes, " . . . the source of every crime is some defect of the understanding, or some error in reasoning . . . erroneous opinion . . . ignorance . . . of the law" (24). The naïve assumption was that some small increase in "understanding" would lead to social betterment since it was assumed that man as a rational animal would always want what was best.

In modern times the search for the causes of delinquency has ranged from the subtle to the truly ridiculous. In keeping with tradition, many efforts have been directed to pinpoint a single cause for this complex problem. If a single cause could be found, then it raises the possibility that an appropriate remedy would be near at hand. As a result, an exceedingly complicated psychosocial problem has become the concern not only of the social scientist, but of the politician and every conceivable type of pressure group. Passionate political sloganizing has, to a disturbing extent, been substituted for methodical scientific inquiry, and the failure of all sorts of governmental programs that have followed has resulted in only more frustration.

The search for the roots of delinquency has led to criticism of many ordinary areas of human involvement. These have included the literature that children read, living conditions in a neighborhood, and lack of "relevance" in present-day education. Appeals have been made to keep "sensational" books out of the hands of children, in spite of the fact that about the same number of delinquents and nondelinquent children read books of this kind. In fact, more than 20 percent of all delinquent children hardly ever read books at all (7). The alleged laxity of our courts has been considered as contributory to delinquency. Yet everything has shown that punishment has little deterring effect on the delinquent. The whole concept of crime and punishment and its deterrent value has meaning mainly for those who are law-abiding in the first place (17). Severe poverty has frequently been cited as a direct cause of delinquency. Poverty is an undeniable contributor to all sorts of psychological problems, but even in the most impoverished neighborhoods, the vast majority of children never become seriously delinquent.

From this brief review, it can be seen that delinquency is not a simple problem linked to a specific etiological unit. The delinquent offense may be a symptomatic expression of just about every kind of psychopathology. The increase in juvenile delinquency can be roughly correlated with a general breakdown in adaptive behavior in the population at large. This all seems part of a general social trend toward the externalization of conflict.

## Environmental Factors

The obvious fact that crime, immorality, and antisocial behavior of all sorts flourish in the slums seems to suggest that a substandard economic setting is the major contributor to juvenile delinquency. This concept provides a general indictment for society as a whole and lifts the burden of responsibility from the individual and the immediate family. It also proposes a simple solution to a very knotty problem. However, the chain of cause and effect is actually more apparent than real.

It can easily be demonstrated that poverty by itself tends to be harmful to the personality. When a child is raised in obviously disadvantaged economic circumstances, certain stimulations will be lacking and full opportunities for healthful expression and relationship may not be found. However, this, by itself, does not necessarily lead to delinquency, per se. For one thing, it does not account for the factor of variability. Raised in the very same neighborhood, why does one boy sell newspapers while another will steal? Even in the most deteriorated urban environments, some 80 to 90 percent of the boys do not become serious delinquents. Therefore, the slum condition itself is a determining factor in only a small number of delinquencies (19). In other words, poverty, by itself, does not explain the so-called "choice of neurosis." It does not explain why delinquency is the characteristic reaction, rather than depression and apathy.

It would seem that it is not so much the slum condition itself, but the psychological factors operative in slum surroundings which are related to delinquent behavior. In the slum situation the child is raised in the confines of a narrow behavioral climate which is in many ways cut off from the mainstream of American life and, to a large extent, at odds with the fabric of our social structure. The slum condition seems to breed standards of its own in which the main emphasis is on individual survival, and this to be accomplished by whatever means happen to be available. Most of the usual mores of contemporary society are ignored. Exposure to incidents of violence and law-breaking of all kinds is commonplace. Occurrences such as illegitimacy, which are often regarded with shame and guilt among the middle class, are either ignored or not regarded as out of the ordinary. The magnitude of the latter problem is to be seen in the fact that for the year 1970 it is estimated some 350,000 illegitimate children were born in this country, most of these in deteriorated urban settings (50).

In the slums the chief identification figures available to the growing child are often people with deep-seated personality disorders, such as gang leaders, who may tyrannize their local neighborhoods and also develop strong, loyal followings (31). Almost from the moment he is born, and throughout most of his formative years, the child is raised under the influence of people whose style of life is in conflict with authority and this inclines him in the direction of antisocial behavior without attendant feelings of guilt (46).

In recent years the rapid advances in mass communication, mainly television, have markedly worsened the situation. In a materialistic society such as ours, the main status symbols are the accumulation of wealth and the possession of objects. The constant outpouring of television commercials has made the ghetto dweller even more aware of the few things that he does have and the misery of his condition. Incessant bombardment with tantalizing advertisements—shining cars with glittering gadgets—gives the impression that there is another world of leisure and wealth that is markedly different from his own. It serves to estrange him further from society at large and makes him even more its enemy. It further whets his appetite to get those things that he feels have been denied him and to acquire them through whatever delinquent means he has learned.

## Familial Factors

Most writers seem to feel that the basis of delinquency is to be found in a history of disorganized family experience. In fact, an unstable familial background seems to be the hallmark of delinquency, whether the child has been exposed to the gross violence of the slums or the subtly destructive conflicts of the upper classes. Common to both is an atmosphere of insecurity in which consistency and demonstrated affection are often lacking. In place of love and understanding, the delinquent has often grown up in a climate of indifference and rejection without clearly articulated values and ideals (47).

Frequently the delinquent child has been raised without the benefit of two parents. Death, desertion, and illegitimacy all play their part in contributing to the single parent family which is so often the background of many delinquent children. Typical studies of delinquent populations have shown that about half of the offenders have come from broken homes (1). Usually this involves the absence of a father from the home. The highest rates of delinquency are found among those boys who were living only with their mother (20).

The absence of a father figure in the home throws the entire burden of child rearing and of establishing controls upon the mother. Characteristically, it has been found that the mothers of delinquent children demonstrate very pathological child-rearing attitudes. Research has shown that they differ significantly from the mothers of healthy youngsters in matters relating to control of behavior and the expression of authoritarian demands (35). In the delinquent family unit, the mother may not only be the child's first model of humanity, but for a long part of his life, the major available object for identification. Therefore any pathology in her attitude toward the child is doubly destructive. If she is cold and rejecting, it may render all future relationships for the child quite tenuous. It may close the door to the possibility of corrective experiences and/or the development of closeness or capacity for real affection (8).

In this type of family the child often does not have the opportunity of seeing modulated expression of feeling. Instead, such expressions of emotion that he does see are likely to be in the form of sudden, intense outbursts and hostilities which are explosive in character and frequently uncontrolled. Relationships among family members are apt to be intensely rivalrous and feelings of belonging to a family as a unit are often completely absent. Competition for the dominant role is often quite marked and this frequently results in a lack of clear-cut role differentiation. There is uncertainty as to who is dominant and who is submissive and who is the father and who is the mother. Each person in the family unit is often in conflict with the other members and roles are alternately abdicated and asserted (44). Communication among the family members is often impaired since the parents themselves may be weak in language and conceptual development. As a result, discipline is not administered with any standard of consistency or explanation of rationale. It is more likely to appear in the form of unexpected eruptions and physical abuse, without adequate verbal justification. At times the parents may even be vindictively punitive toward the child for his delinquent behavior. However, they are typically unable to see any connection between the antisocial behavior and their own actions in regard to the child.

Legal involvements with courts and welfare agencies additionally complicate the problem. They further reduce the power of the family in the eyes of the child and make the lines of parental authority still more obscure. By repeated example the child sees his family members relate to welfare and legal agencies with mixed feelings of awe, fright, and anger. This continually detracts from the strength of his own parents and eventually the child relates to these agencies as the main authority figures and turns his conflicts and rebellion toward them (30).

In sum, the home of the delinquent child is highlighted by an atmosphere of instability in which there is no real clear-cut differentiation of roles and in which opportunities for healthy identification are often absent. The frequent lack of availability of a parent of the same sex and the opportunity to observe and to experience control functions exercised by this parent is critical in the development of delinquent behavior (20a). The lack of a stable family unit also makes it impossible for the child to live through the normal rivalries of the oedipal conflict and to resolve these by identification. The male child raised in the single parent home finds that the only object available as a model is the parent of the opposite sex. For the growing boy, exposed repeatedly to feminine attitudes, it may mean the beginning of a lifelong quest to separate himself from his basically feminine leanings. He may have to drive himself toward a compulsive type of masculinity and attempt to prove this through all sorts of delinquent acting out (51).

## Object Relations

The characteristic disturbance of family relationships, which the delinquent experiences as a small child, seems to permanently affect his capacity to deal later with other human beings. If the beginning relationship with the mother is one marked by a chronic coldness on her part, it will hamper his ability to trust others in the future. For one thing, it may result in the child's inability at a later age to relate with affection to his father (8a). Often the personality of the delinquent's mother is found to be very unstable and her marked changes in mood and mercurial outbursts of temper do not permit the growing child to experience a feeling of object constancy. Instead, they may lead to the incorporation of peculiar contents in the superego and make the establishment of consistent inner controls well nigh impossible. Since the relationship with the mother is often tenuous and inconsistent, the child's energies tend to be deflected back upon himself and he also becomes predisposed to a narcissistic fixation (28). This partly accounts for the self-centeredness, immaturity, and lack of ability to empathize which are featured personality traits among delinquents.

These early relationship difficulties tend to perpetuate themselves and the results can be far-reaching. The capacity to trust, to relate, and to appreciate the sufferings and anguish of others is often, in some sense, lacking. The delinquent's early difficulties with identification make it very difficult for him to put himself in the place of others. It is perhaps partly for this reason that some of them are capable of really sadistic assaults upon others without genuine feelings of remorse except for a fear of getting caught.

It has frequently been observed that delinquents do not tend to differentiate people accurately. Instead, they are inclined to perceive the world in more or less indiscriminate terms. Individuals are not viewed according to their specific roles, but are rather vaguely regarded in terms of stereotyped activities and stereotyped forms of relationship (42). Since the delinquent's ability to trust is developed only in a vestigial sense, the capacity for deep relationship is impaired and he is afraid to trust someone for fear that he may be proven wrong (27). This, of course, would constitute a dangerous blow to his narcissism and therefore has to be warded off at all costs. In place of ordinary communication, the delinquent attempts to resist relationships by all means that are at his disposal, particularly where authority is involved. If subject to questioning, he tends to be passive and uncommunicative, even in response to innocuous questions. His pent-up hostility gives him a feeling of righteous indignation and for him this is sufficient justification for whatever he has done. This seems to take on an extreme form in those cases of solitary delinquency where the offenses are not committed in the company of others. Generally these delinquents are found to be more uncommunicative and psychologically more disturbed than the social delinquents who come from a criminogenic social environment (10).

Because he is so narcissistically involved, the delinquent tends to be the child of the moment and lives largely in terms of the pleasure principle.

The capacity to strive for some sort of long-term goal is generally found to be damaged. Not too much concerned with past experience, he is difficult to motivate toward goals in the long-term future (28a).

## Identification and Diagnosis

The diagnosis and classification of delinquent behavior are more complicated than appear at first glance. Generally, it has been assumed that most delinquents can be roughly divided into two categories. The first would include those where the delinquent behavior is considered to be on a characterological basis. These are children whose problems are largely ego-syntonic and who come from the type of criminogenic background already described. In many respects they seem to be psychopathic.

At the other end of the spectrum are those children where the delinquency is felt to be on the basis of unresolved neurotic conflicts. In theory these children suffer from an unconscious sense of guilt which is quenched through all sorts of delinquent acting out. This is usually considered to be a seeking out of punishment (38).

In actual clinical practice, however, the problems involved in making even the grossest kind of differentiation are often quite substantial. First of all, the external behavior in both the neurotic and the psychopathic delinquent may be quite similar. Therefore a diagnosis made on the basis of the delinquent act itself can be quite misleading (4). The whole gamut of feelings of inadequacy and inferiority, which are the usual hallmark of neurosis, is found generally in delinquent populations at large. Any random group of delinquent children will show clusters of neurotic traits, homosexuality, excessive alcoholism, or any combination of these (1). Probably the only definitive way of establishing a final diagnosis is through a trial period of psychotherapy, such as was proposed by Aichorn many years ago. He felt that if a youngster failed to develop any sort of an affectionate relationship with his therapist, did not respond to treatment, and showed no evidence of guilt or anxiety after a period of treatment, then he could truly be considered a psychopathic character (28b).

As a speculation, the possibility of some type of organicity as a contributing factor to delinquency has been raised by a few writers. For example, characteristic EEG patterns have been cited as one possible corollary to delinquent behavior; but this has not held up under further scrutiny and investigation (34). At least one writer has suggested that when the symptomatic behavior is deeply entrenched and where there has been little response to therapeutic intervention, then consideration should be given to the possibility of a total failure of cerebration as a possible cause of the delinquency (30).

In the usual clinical manner, some efforts have been made to gauge the severity of delinquent behavior by evaluation of case history material. In this approach the investigator looks carefully through the record to try to determine the age of onset of antisocial behavior. Some researchers have reported that age twelve seems to be a critical time for official delinquency and that few cases are brought to court attention before this time (33). Most likely, this is a considerable underestimate of what really goes on. Many children at quite an early age show characteristic patterns of behavior that may herald later delinquency. The child may show problem behavior early in school, although this may not be of a sort that would ordinarily result in court attention. Histories of early school failure, disruption of classroom activity, and inability to adjust to normal social routines are all found frequently. They attest to an early failure of inner controls and the inability of the child to deal adaptively with age-appropriate life tasks and to tolerate early stresses. Since the classroom situation is the child's first confrontation with a major societal institution, failure to adjust satisfactorily at school may, in many instances, be the first indication of a later antisocial trend.

Attempts to arrive at a differential diagnosis of delinquent behavior with psychological tests have generally met with equivocal results. Although some positive findings have been reported, these, for the most part, could have been anticipated purely on the basis of clinical experience alone. For one thing, it is characteristically found that delinquent children tend to exhibit a higher performance IQ than verbal IQ (22). This, in itself, is hardly surprising, since it is in keeping with an action-oriented background and a characteristic inability to deal adequately with verbal material. Delinquent children have also been found to exhibit basic feelings of extreme insecurity. They also develop typical modes of compensation for these feelings, and it is often these compensations which are the distinguishing features of their antisocial behavior (36). Delinquents have been tested for their ability to abstract general principles from proverbs. By and large, they do not seem to show any characteristic deficiencies in this respect (21). Some efforts have been made to pick out delinquents on the basis of their potential for aggressive behavior. One test of this type has successfully demonstrated an ability to differentiate up to 70 percent of assaultive delinquents (48).

## Internal Psychological Processes

The delinquent child typically does not internalize conflict. He experiences his inner tensions as a struggle with outer reality and uses rebellious antisocial solutions as a means of dealing with them (9).

As already noted, a critical feature in the background of many such children is a loss or frequent separation from a parent during the early formative years. It seems to be not so much the loss but rather the ego's reaction to the loss and the time of its occurrence that are the important considerations. An early loss may be misconstrued as a sadistic act against the child and may leave behind a depressive nucleus (29). It seems to leave the child with a lack of satisfaction and can produce a continuing oral need. Therefore the child may incorporate the image of a bad and depriving mother, whether or not this was actually the case. She may have been experienced as such by her failure to gratify the pressing needs of this particular child (15).

A constellation of experiences of this kind creates an imprint of loss and a core of unfulfilled passive wishes that must be continually warded off. The ego of the delinquent seems to react to this along the lines of the repetition compulsion. Only the most archaic type of defenses seem to develop and frequently these consist of denial, acting out, projection, and distortion of objects. The whole focus of defense turns in an extrapunitive direction and the unconscious resentment becomes displaced onto substitute figures in reality (18). The delinquent then seems driven to guard against tensions which might touch on his depressive core. As a result, close human relationships, which always involve the risk of loss, must be avoided. Often the delinquent becomes suspicious of anyone who acts toward him in a friendly and affectionate way. To help seal off the underlying depression and the possibility of being overwhelmed by this, the child must translate passivity into activity. He reverses his unconscious image by acting out a vigorous, aggressive role in order to assure himself that he is not really the passive victim of circumstance.

Another result is to be seen in the distortion of the capacity to love. In the case of the female delinquent, a maternal disappointment is often a decisive cause of illegitimacy on her part. By involving herself sexually, and producing an illegitimate child, she once again re-establishes the mother-child unit. However, the delinquent mother only seems to find satisfaction so long as her infant is very much dependent on her. She usually turns against the baby whenever independent assertions begin to show themselves. Continued infantilization of the child is a frequent result (9a).

## SUPEREGO FUNCTIONING

The lack of object constancy in the delinquent child's early years results in distortions and/or poor identifications in the formation of the superego. This is an additional factor which makes for lessened control and further inclines the child in the direction of motoric discharge of his tensions. The absence of a father in the family unit may make identification with a suitable masculine figure well nigh impossible. Where the family is intact, the father himself may present a delinquent image and therefore the child will incorporate delinquent characteristics in his own superego and ideal. In other words, the critical identifications themselves may be of a pathological nature. Where such is the case, the child will do things against society and have no feeling that this is in any way wrong (16). Rapidly changing parental figures during the formative years may give rise to peculiar contents in the superego in which inconsistency and instability of objects are prominent traits. This, too, will steer the child in the direction of delinquency since it will make it impossible to develop well-modulated controls or to form lasting attachments.

Delinquents from upper- and middle-class families often do not show the gross lack of superego structure found in children from the slums. For example, there does not seem to be the characteristic chaotic lack of progress in almost every area of age-appropriate experience such as school achievement, social relationships, and so on. Rather, these children tend to show special gaps in their superego structure which allow the acting out of rather specific forbidden impulses. Ordinarily, these are children from so-called "good" families. These children are often in some way or other acting out vicariously forbidden wishes of what their own parents would unconsciously like to do (25). Something in the quality of the parent-child relationship and the experience of this has conveyed to the child an unconscious message that certain ordinarily forbidden impulses are really not taboo and would be condoned by the parent. For example, constant distrust and false accusations will get across to the child the idea that an alternative image of him as a delinquent already exists in his parents' mind (26). In line with this, the parent may not show an adequate negative reaction when the child has acted out some forbidden impulse. Instead, he may express disapproval in a halfhearted way, often accompanied by a smile of tacit pleasure, and this conveys the message that the parent is unconsciously pleased with what the child has done. When repeated serious transgressions are dismissed as insignificant, the child does not have a feeling that they are in any way wrong. Since the parental image is the first image of society's values, the child does not get a really clear or consistent picture of adequate restraints. Frequently where this takes place, the parent is finding some type of substitute gratification for his own amoral and antisocial impulses in the acting-out behavior of his child that he is subtly encouraging (32).

Deficiencies in superego standards, values, and ideals make it necessary for the delinquent to find some way to defend his self-image against his consuming rage and depression. He does so by a process of projection and externalization in which his anger is turned toward the outside world and he feels that others hate him or deny him the pleasures that he seeks. Often these children are able to feel bitter hate, and since there is not much ambivalence, there is little possibility for the development of neurotic symptom formation (5). The raw anger is simply accepted for what it is.

### EGO FUNCTIONING

It is not only the superego of the delinquent child that is defective, but the ego as well. The early disappointing experiences in the family make it difficult to establish reliable interpersonal relations. The energies that would ordinarily be used for this purpose remain inwardly directed, and it is probably this which seems to give rise to the increased narcissism and hyperactivity that are so characteristic (28c). Another familiar fact is that the delinquent shows a very concrete conceptual attitude. It is difficult for him to form abstractions of a really high order, and this is another aspect of his primitive ego organization (40).

Very often the delinquent act is some sort of an aggressive expression that is meant to fend off an underlying passivity. However, the basic need for passive relationships and for passive types of gratification nevertheless still comes to the fore. For example, study of delinquents in terms of their free time shows that they often select a rather narrow range of activities. Passive types of entertainment, such as TV and the movies, are frequently sought out, and for girls, the typical pattern is to be involved in some type of desperately unhappy sexual relationship (6).

Frequent confrontation with his own helplessness seems to furnish a constant spur to assert an almost opposite type of omnipotence. Mainly this is due to the fact that the delinquent has never known a secure dependent relationship in the past.

The weakness of the ego is also to be seen in a limited ability to tolerate frustration. The capacity to store anxiety, to delay discharge, or to put up with discomfort is usually in some way defective. When tensions are aroused as a result of some type of impulsive build-up, there seems to be an overriding need for immediate discharge. Thrill-seeking behavior, constant explorations of the unknown, restlessness, and hyperactivity become substitutes for ordinary sublimations and defensive processes. They help the delinquent to counteract the feeling of boredom and depression that would otherwise overwhelm him (14). His constant motoric activity helps to reinforce his image of himself as a powerful person and also to seal off underlying anxieties associated with his real fears of weakness and need for protection. A fantasy of omnipotence also helps to overcome the disappointments that are encountered in daily experience. The frequent use of infantile and hostile methods of dealing with anxiety reveals the extent of the basic insecurity and the gravity of the emotional deficit (41). Aggressive motor discharge becomes an established habit pattern for the relief of tension in the earliest years and becomes more entrenched as adolescence approaches and the new tasks of sexuality and increasing aggression have to be mastered.

## Treatment

There are a number of crucial factors in the character structure and emotional make-up of the delinquent child that make successful therapeutic intervention very difficult. Among the more important are the rather primitive organization of the ego and lack of stability in inner controls. The critical traumatic events of the delinquent's early years, taken together with the frequent absence or inconsistency of parental figures, usually do not allow the development of a typical oedipal crisis. As a result, the possibility for developing transference relationships and for the intense emotional commitment which this entails is usually lacking. The early disappointment in the mother and the vengeful attitude toward authority figures all rule against the establishment of a really trusting relationship with a psychotherapist. In addition, the very nature of the problem, involving as it does constant motoric discharge of tension, is another major obstacle to successful psychotherapy. The shallow development of the inner life also does not lend itself to reflection and introspection. In short, all of the ordinary factors that are usually considered necessary for successful treatment are typically lacking in the delinquent population.

In theory then, it would be expected that treatment of the delinquent would prove to be a disappointing experience. In point of fact, most clinical experience seems to bear this out. Everyday clinical practice, together with formal research programs, have shown the failure rate in the treatment of delinquents to be very high. Even when carefully thought out programs are planned and the best possible personnel are used, the rate of success has been estimated as "poor" to "fair" (11).

Various modifications in treatment technique have been tried in an effort to overcome some of these obstacles. Where the delinquency is found to be deeply rooted, and where the family situation is obviously encouraging the acting out or is grossly pathological, then removal from the home is often found to be an indicated step. However, separation from a noxious environment itself does not solve the problem. It is not the harmful environment that is the direct cause of the delinquency, but rather the effects that have been produced in the child's ego. These will continue to be manifest even when he is placed in a new and more accepting environment. The delinquent child will recreate the past and bring on new situations of rejection, rivalry, and punishment.

The first goal of any treatment is the establishment of a meaningful relationship with the therapist. With the delinquent the suggestion has been made that he must experience his therapist as a clever and omnipotent being if he is to have any respect for him (14a). The idea here would be to recreate the essentials of the early traumatic childhood situation and to allow the delinquent to have a corrective, therapeutic experience with the therapist as parent surrogate. However, in practice, few delinquents allow themselves to become sufficiently involved with their therapist to the point where the relationship ever reaches this intensity.

A high intelligence level has generally been noted to correlate with successful psychotherapy. This apparently does not hold true for the delinquent population, particularly where modified forms of psychotherapy are used which are not verbally oriented or do not aim for direct intellectual insight (43). In his therapy program, the delinquent will probably gain more through the concrete experience rather than through any change that can be brought about through introspection on his own part.

Another suggestion to help overcome the distrustful attitude toward the therapist has been the use of a tape recorder as a substitute for the therapist. Here, the delinquent is encouraged to talk to the tape recorder, and surprisingly it has been found that the delinquent may respond almost as if he were talking to the therapist (45). The problem then would be to find a critical time in which a successful shift could be made from the recorder to an interaction in a helping relationship with a therapist.

The pervasive hostility which the delinquent feels toward authority figures deeply damages any efforts made to establish communication with him. The hostility is frequently expressed through passive withholding of information, minimal response to questions, and indignation at having to submit to something he does not want to do. The persistent defense of omnipotence leaves him with the feeling that in some way or other he will always get away with things and that he can master problems on his own—this in spite of repeated experiences in which he may be caught over and over again. All of this points up his profound impairment of practical judgment and inability to learn from past experience and apply this to future problems.

Group therapy techniques that have been tried with other populations have also been applied to the delinquents with less than enthusiastic results. One such study of youthful offenders showed that, beyond very superficial stages, little real insight was ever elicited, and that at best only moderate changes could be accomplished (49). Another typical report indicates that group therapy should be considered to have accomplished its purpose when a positive relationship between the delinquent group member and the therapist has been established (40a).

Efforts to change the delinquent behavior through vocational activities and/or inclusion of vocational training, together with a psychotherapy program, seem to offer some promise. On the surface, this would appear to make some sense, since the delinquent would be offered a substitute outlet for his energy which would furnish him with opportunity for immediate discharge. Also, vocational training deals with concrete and immediate experience and this is much more meaningful to the delinquent than intellectual abstractions that are beyond his comprehension. In many ways, this type of approach seems to hold the most promise as far as modifying delinquent behavior is concerned. One such study involving vocationally oriented psychotherapy did report major improvements in a number of critical dimensions such as level of guilt, perception of time, and object relations. Here it was found to be of importance for the delinquent boys to be contacted at the time of crisis—in this case, a period when they had just been suspended from school (37). Other reports dealing with training of delinquents in the vocational area have also emphasized the need for a concrete approach and orientation around basic activities. The immediacy of their problems requires outlets in which action and concrete help are essential and perhaps of greater importance than the casework or counseling which the boy may receive (51a). When vocationally treated delinquents are matched with control groups, some important differences are found in relation to perception of time span. Hopefully, it is felt that this would result in some increased prospective thought or fantasy in situations which involve either their self-image or future planning (39).

A number of efforts have been made to predict the success of the treatment of delinquents. Since most treatment efforts fail, this does not turn out to be as difficult a task as it might seem at first glance. When predictions of prognosis are made from psychological reports, more than 80 percent accuracy has been reported (13). Interestingly enough, the presence of guilt and anxiety in some institutional delinquents does not necessarily augur well for a successful outcome. In fact, at least one report has pointed out that the greater the guilt and anxiety displayed, the shorter the length of time on parole until revocation (12). In some instances such as these, the delinquency itself may be the defense against the underlying anxiety, and whenever some guilt is generated, it has to be expiated by further acting out.

# 6

## Drug Addiction

SIDNEY L. WERKMAN, M.D.

---

## Introduction

Drug use among children and adolescents is widespread. The taking of drugs reflects the great variety of changes and transformations that have occurred in the United States and the world during the last decade, roughly the period in which drugs have become a significant part of the youth landscape. This chapter will concentrate on the clinical problems involved in drugs but will comment as well, on the meaning of the drug phenomenon. In order to assess the importance of this phenomenon one must consider a number of parameters including age, socio-economic status, the amount, type, regularity, and social context of the drug used. The term "drug" encompasses a large group of agents, and it is important to define generally what we are talking about.

Young people seek out the exhilarating, mind-easing, euphorogenic qualities of drugs. Most of the drugs we will consider are chemical agents that induce, under fortunate circumstances, changes in perception, a feeling of well-being, a sense of closeness and, in a word, happiness. Most of them are capable of producing hallucinations—hopefully, to the user, pleasant ones. They are pleasure-promoting drugs, ones which young people hope will alter consciousness and help them to reach a different level of functioning. Except for the amphetamines and caffeine-containing drugs, none is used for practical purposes, such as working better, studying, or increasing cognitive effectiveness. Drug users come to the attention of mental health professionals only after "bad trips" and run-ins with authorities, not because of pain and anguish related to drugs.

The following list names drugs that are used to gain mind-altering effects:

### Addicting Drugs
1. Opium derivatives (opium, codeine, Demerol, morphine, heroin).
2. Cocaine.
3. Barbiturates.
### Nonaddicting Drugs
4. Amphetamines.
5. Psychedelics or true hallucinogens (peyote, mescaline, the chemically synthesized drugs such as LSD, IMT, and STP).

6. Alcohol, aspirin, coffee, and the drugs in cigarettes.
7. Anti-anxiety and antidepressant drugs.
8. Organic solvents or "sniffing drugs" (airplane glue, lighter fluid, paint thinner, etc.).
9. Marijuana.

Each of these classes of drugs has important differential qualities which will be discussed. No encompassing term can define these drugs or their actions, for their effects depend significantly upon the subjective state and wish of the user. The "hallucinogenic" drugs do not necessarily result in hallucinations and those not so described often do produce hallucinations. Depending upon circumstances, set, or expectancy, use may result in the experiencing of vivid colors, a transcendental state, euphoria, or depression. But young people take drugs because they want to get "out of my skin," to experience a new level of functioning, out of curiosity and a wish to be one of the crowd, and probably to solve or dissolve pressing emotional problems.

One of the greatest areas of misinformation about drugs concerns the question of addiction. Endless newspaper and magazine articles have headlined this statement: "Marijuana does not cause addiction." However, such accounts merely obscure the medical and therapeutic issues involved in marijuana and other drugs. *Addiction* is a very narrowly defined term in pharmacology. It connotes a state of intoxication and overpowering need to take a drug and tendency to increase the amount of the drug; that is, tolerance to the drugs develops. Most important, if the drug is discontinued, the user suffers withdrawal symptoms such as gooseflesh, sweating, vomiting, fever, or fainting. A drug is not defined as *addicting* unless withdrawal of the drug results in these physiological symptoms. Far more important for young people is the definition of misuse and dependence. As most of the drugs listed above have limited medical usefulness, we must either recognize their societal importance or view them as drugs being misused. A *nonaddicting* drug may result in psychopathological and medical disturbances fully as long-lasting and severe as those from *addicting* drugs.

*Misuse* is the overzealous use of drugs or the exercise of bad judgment in their use. *Abuse* is the use of drugs for other than regular medical purposes and in ways that result in physical or psychological harm to the user. *Dependence* implies the need or desire to take a drug despite untoward consequences and the psychological inability to give up the drug despite one's wish to do so (7).

Though the drugs defined in the table as nonaddicting will not result in physiological symptoms such as vomiting when withdrawn from the user, most of them do create a state of psychological dependence. Most regular users find it difficult to do without them. The drug becomes a crutch in social relations or in certain work situations. The person becomes dependent upon the drug, just as a large percentage of cigarette smokers are dependent upon cigarettes.

## Epidemiology of Drug Use in Children and Adolescents

We must begin with the recognition that accurate incidence and prevalence statistics for drug use and psychopathology resulting from the use of drugs do not as yet exist. A number of studies have attempted to assess the true picture of societal and medical extent of drug concerns, but they still are preliminary (1, 10, 15, 16).

Therefore, we must use the studies that are available and approximate from them and clinical experience where we stand in regard to this problem. In general, the age group we are considering is approximately thirteen to twenty-four years of age, though the age of first use of drugs appears to be progressively decreasing. Other variables of great importance are sections of the country, socio-economic status, and the particular time at which this is written. It is simply impossible to scale drugs in order of their true importance and pathological consequences in a way that would hold true for all of these parameters. Though we know of rare deaths in twelve-year-olds attributed to heroin addiction and, in the last five years, many clinicians have begun to treat upper-middle-class heroin addicts of sixteen or seventeen years of age for the first time, all of these experiences are spotty and, undoubtedly, reflections of individual clinical practices. However, the following trends can be discerned from the professional literature, newspaper and magazine reports, and clinical discussions.

At this time there is little use of morphine and heroin by people until they reach about eighteen years of age. As age increases the use of hard narcotics such as the opium derivatives increases phenomenally and constitutes the primary medical problem in addictions. However, there is growing and legitimate concern that pushers of marijuana sporadically sprinkle the marijuana with heroin, cocaine, and other additives. Thus we are beginning to see the phenomenon of a drug user becoming hooked on a drug he never wanted in the first place. Since access to any drugs is through illegal channels, there is no way for the buyer to assess what he is getting. He cannot trust his pusher because the pusher is usually only a middleman. Even the strength of individual drugs such as marijuana varies greatly. It has been found that drugs bought in the commercial market have widely varying strengths and, therefore, cannot be used for accurate research studies (5, 18).

Amphetamines are often the first drugs used by adolescents. Though sometimes prescribed for medical conditions and, at other times, gotten from a parent's medicine cabinet, approximately one fifth of teenagers will use amphetamines for studying and later for kicks. Pure amphetamine dependence tends to be short-lived, for the user often develops tolerance for the drug and increases the amount ingested or infused into a vein until a pathological result occurs. Nevertheless, the amphetamines are still an enigma to professionals, for many people have used them for long periods of time without untoward effects. In the British Isles there has been great difficulty with an "amphetamine psychosis" syndrome. Young people combine either ingestion or "mainlining" (intravenous infusion) of amphetamines with the ingestion of a great deal of beer over a weekend, resulting in a two- to four-day paranoid reaction of psychotic proportions. However, the reaction is time-limited, if the drug is discontinued, though extremely dangerous (2). We have here an example of a specific syndrome that has not gained great currency in the United States.

Barbiturates are used very little for their pleasurable effects, except in combination with beer, amphetamines, or other drugs. The LSD vogue is primarily in the older adolescent and the young adult. Probably 5 to 10 percent of this population will have tried LSD or its derivatives at least once.

Alcohol and other "adult" drugs have gained little favor with contemporary youth. However, we must note that the decrease in incidence of cigarette smoking in young people that occurred from 1965 to 1969 has now been reversed, and, once again, cigarette smoking is increasing in incidence. Coffee use is declining in young people and has been for a number of years. Similarly, the voluntary use of anti-anxiety and anti-depressant drugs is rather limited in young people. This is an important phenomenon, for adolescents want kicks, excitement, euphoria, while older people seem to want merely to be relieved of emotion or to stay awake. Young people who try the "tranquilizer" type of drug complain about them because such drugs merely quiet them when they want increased sensation, a greater feeling of thrill, or euphoria. The organic solvents or volatile sniffing drugs are most popular with the very young adolescent, probably because youngsters of that age are the ones who are involved in making models with airplane glue and have access to these volatile agents, but cannot get the other drugs described.

Marijuana is *the* drug of use by young people. Research studies suggest that marijuana has been used by a large minority of our youth population (10, 13, 15, 16). About half of the students in most colleges will have smoked marijuana once and 5 to 10 percent are fairly regular smokers. Studies in high school populations suggest that about 30 percent of students have smoked marijuana and figures change radically when a new drug is popularized by the media or underground sources or a drug is reputed to be dangerous (toxic inhalants, such as glue, or the reputed chromosomal damage from LSD). We must assume that drug experimentation and use will encompass about half of the youth population for the foreseeable future. Because almost all drug use is illegal, it is difficult to chart trends accurately. However, the Bureau of Narcotics states that only 6 kilograms of cocaine were seized in 1965, while 33 kilograms were seized in 1969. There has been an increase in the amount seized each year since 1965 (9). Similar patterns are present in regard to marijuana, heroin, and the amphetamines.

Why do young people use drugs? They use them for the kicks that may come from them. Some of the drugs induce a dreamy state of altered consciousness in which ideas seem disconnected, uncontrollable, and freely flowing, and others result in a feeling of great acuity, power, excitement, and confidence. Still others induce vivid color sensations, pleasing, original visual hallucinatory experiences, and sexual stimulation.

Beyond the particular alteration of perception and sensation they induce, the drugs are used by young people for several other overriding reasons. Drugs are used because other people are using them, and young people are notoriously fascinated by any new product. They are moving from a family setting to a larger social setting in which their own judgment must take over. This judgment is immensely influenced by the fads and fashions of the current society. But most importantly, young people are sensation hungry. It is a characteristic of adolescence to want to test one's body, one's possibilities, to the very utmost. As Joseph Conrad put it in *Youth* (3):

I remember my youth and the feeling that will never come back any more—the feeling that I could last forever, outlast the sea, the earth, and all men; the deceitful feeling that lures us on to joys, to perils, to love, to vain efforts—to death; the triumphant conviction of strength, the heat of life in the handful of dust, the glow in the heart that with every year grows dim, grows cold, grows small, and expires, too soon, too soon—before life itself.

Finally, because of a major disenchantment with an adult world that is involved in war, degradation, "making it," and a host of other unpalatable sociological and technological concerns, young people are turning away and groping to find a way into a new experience, a mystical experience that offers escape and a means of increasing sensation and closeness.

Many drugs offer the very things wished for by adolescents—intense emotions, a mystical experience, an opportunity to get closer to other people in a transpersonal or oceanic way. Through drugs young people are able to appreciate perceptions and thoughts on multiple levels and feel the great sense of awe and pleasure of a creative experience. Because drugs magnify experiences, amplify and often pleasurably distort them, the young person feels more free and more creative. There is a de-automatization of experience, a sense of newness and freshness in life. And finally, in his quest for a sense of meaning in life, drugs seem to offer to him a means of insight, of getting close to God, of grappling with questions of death and rebirth. The young person is hungering for belief and seeks it in the combination of drugs, Zen, Yoga, and his often painfully limited and distorted views of other eastern philosophies. So there is a positive searching through the use of drugs. This implies a negative view of the adult world's religions, quests, and values. Part of this is natural and has been present since the beginning of time; part of it may be a desperate reaction to what is seen as a dead end in the adult world. A case illustration will describe both the searching and the pathological consequences of such a search:

A nineteen-year-old male college student was referred to me because of a "bad" drug experience. He enrolled in a college far from his home, hoping to study art and music. His father had died the year before and this patient was pleased to be on his own away from considerable conflict that existed between himself and his mother. However, when he got to college he found that he was not very interested in his courses and had difficulty in studying. He spent a good deal of time sitting around on park benches, visiting museums, and watching the sea. He went on welfare to keep himself going financially and became involved with a number of friends doing the same thing as he. After smoking marijuana heavily, he decided to take some LSD in order to "find myself." "I didn't know where I was going, but knew I had to find a way." After "dropping acid several times," he had a combination of experiences. Though never concerned about homosexuality before, he decided that all of his difficulties were due to a homosexual attraction he had to his father. He was certain that this was the root of his problem and that if he could only reach his father again and have a sexual relationship with him, all life would be "beautiful." He also developed a feeling "deep in my stomach that there is something bad about me."

"I have to get rid of the thing that's in my stomach," he said. "The feeling goes from down there to my head and is all through me and maybe that's why I can't think. Or maybe it goes the other way. When I was most high on the acid everything began to take on a great glare. I walked down to the beach and began to understand how the sea and the sand were related to the sun, and all the water was part of me, because I was made of water and the sun and sand. I began to have a great love of all mankind and just started walking into the ocean to try to grasp it and become part of all of it. I almost drowned, but some friends pulled me out of the water and fixed me up for a while. But if I hadn't gotten these other thoughts, I would have dropped some more acid and gone out there again. That's the ultimate meaning, getting in the sea and being part of it."

On consultation with me he related warmly, immediately, and spoke quickly. However, there was a great deal of blocking, circumstantiality, and inability to organize his thoughts. He needed to stay on subjects on which he had begun but tended to lose the central train of his discussion, and was unable to define accurately the material he was trying to tell me about.

When he returned to his family's house he found that his older sister, age twenty-one, and new brother-in-law were living with his mother. He confided in me that he was quite certain that his sister was really in love with him and that she wanted him to kill her husband so that the two of them could go off and live together. He decided that this would solve all of his problems—the vague dissatisfaction, the painful feeling in his stomach, and the searching upon which he had embarked. He was convinced that having sexual relationships with his sister was what all of his LSD experiences had directed him toward.

This patient is an example of a young man who had functioned reasonably well until drugs seriously impaired his ego capacities, particularly reality testing and the synthetic functions of the ego, turned him back into a world of primitive, primary process thinking, and left him helplessly unable to direct his life except in an alternately impulsive and withdrawn fashion.

The patient described above was in acute need of in-patient psychotherapy and, because of the great anxiety and disorganization of thought processes he was suffering, the use of chloropromazine. Individualized treatment runs the gamut of emergency treatment of toxic symptoms from the use of inhalants, dialysis of drugs in the body, the use of anti-anxiety agents, substitute addiction such as methodone maintenance for heroin addicts, and psychotherapy combining a good deal of reality testing, education, and sympathetic recognition of the adolescent's plight.

The therapist must have thought through his own values and the psychohistorical situation of today before he can hope to engage effectively in psychotherapy with an adolescent on drugs. He must recognize that drugs, regardless of the value placed on them by the society, are means of evading reality.

The most significant point is that young people who use drugs for pleasure tend to give up seeking pleasure in other ways. They become garrulous and feel accepted by others while smoking grass, but do not solve the problems that make them feel socially isolated or anxious when they are not under the influence of the drug. They are like wind-up toys, unable to go through their social paces when deprived of the drug. Drugs are used as a substitute for solving the social and intellectual problems that face them. A person learns how to be a mature social and intellectual being in adolescence and young adulthood. It is a cornerstone of our child-development knowledge that a function in the process of development is most vulnerable to distortion.

The major tasks of the teenager consist of exploring who he is, learning to relate effectively to others, adding to his useful cognitive store, and crystallizing a sense of "career." If these processes are interrupted, it is difficult to reinstitute them. The sixteen-year-old, involved in the process of learning, cannot tolerate interruption of that process. If he cannot study effectively, he will drop out of school and drift away from the necessary task of making decisions about his life.

At a time in life when a teenager needs to imprint on his mind complicated mathematical concepts, drugs scramble his brain. When he is beginning to experience the exhilaration and responsibilities of love and sexuality, drugs tend to make such experiences complicated, artificial, and impermanent. At a time when adolescents must deal with the healthy issues of independence, career decisions, the meaning of life, drugs offer a seductive way of ducking the issues, hiding out and giving up.

Thus the message of the medical and sociological data about most drugs is clear and simple. They are potentially harmful for adolescents still going through formative life experiences. But they are not harmful for all teenagers. Many adolescents can smoke marijuana one or more times and have absolutely no ill effects from this. Similarly the use of other drugs, casually and intermittently, will probably not result in dependence and decrement in function. That is no reason for the mental health professional to turn away from any consideration of the harmful effects of drugs, as the clinical illustration described above and innumerable case histories now document. At this time, when epidemiological data are so inadequate and the chemical effects of drugs have not been researched carefully, we have no way of predicting which particular adolescent will have unfortunate effects from drugs and which one will have none. The concept of the addiction-prone personality, a teenager already schizoid and isolated, simply has not been tested except in the anecdotal experience of individual therapists. But, of greater importance, when a phenomenon has enthralled a large segment of the youth population, we must consider it from another standpoint, that of the defect of the society.

The flourishing of drug use in the last several years reflects many aspects of contemporary America. Law-breaking is more readily engaged in today than it was a number of years ago. The external seeking of thrills is rampant, whether from the shock value of current magazines and literature, the primitive violence on television, or the emphasis on gaudy affluence in our shops and on our highways (20). The demand for immediate relief of tension and the provision of instant thrills and excitement is paramount in all age groups. In this sensation-ridden society, the great direction is one of escape.

All through history, man has searched for drugs that would help him escape from himself, drugs that would help him feel not only healthy, but different, better, less anxious, exhilarated, in a word, happy. This search for drug happiness, for oblivion, has led most often to addicting and habituating drugs.

I am indebted to Dr. Daniel Horn, Director of the National Clearing House for Smoking and Health of the Public Health Service, for many of the following historical ideas (8).

Man found marijuana at least 1700 years ago in China. It may be comforting to note that marijuana didn't overwhelm the world then, as it seems to be enthralling youth today.

A great many forces—social, cultural, and economic—help to mold personal preferences for gratification. Cocaine use was a serious medical problem shortly after the first world war. The college song "Cocaine Bill and Morphine Sue," with its refrain, "Have a little sniff on me," reflects that period. Ether was a frequently used exhilarating drug, particularly among medical students many years ago, and the charming term "Ether Frolic" tended to hide the dangers of the drug. It is merely a historical curiosity in the United States today.

Snuff-taking enjoyed a great vogue in western Europe for hundreds of years. Snuffboxes and snuff spoons were standard accessories of the European lady or gentleman. The handkerchief men wear in their breast pockets—and wonder why they wear it—originated quite practically as a "snuff handkerchief" with which to clean the nose after sniffing snuff. Somehow, snuffing began to be seen as a bad habit and its use declined. A British magazine in 1834 carried the story of a patient asking, "Is it true, doctor, that snuff destroys the olfactory nerves, clogs and otherwise injures the brain?" "It cannot be true," the doctor replies, "since those who have any brains never take the stuff at all."

Chewing tobacco was our parallel to snuff. In 1880 the per capita consumption of chewing tobacco in the United States was three pounds, and by 1894 it had reached a maximum of four pounds per person. By 1910 there had been a sharp decrease in the use of chewing tobacco, and now, for most of us, it is a historical curiosity. Anyone younger than thirty has never seen a spittoon or cuspidor except in an antique shop. An anti-chewing tobacco lobby existed and, in 1883, the *Boston Medical and Surgical Journal* called chewers, "A national disgrace" and said, "As great as this evil still is, however, we believe that it has already lessened, and will continue to grow less as social refinement becomes more widespread."

Our best guess is that chewing didn't decline because social refinement increased, but rather because cheap, machine-made cigarettes became available.

Alcohol has had its ups and downs. Because of a new process for distilling liquor, England was flooded with cheap gin in the eighteenth century. From a production of 43,000 gallons in 1690, a high of three million gallons was reached in 1721. Concomitantly, there was a sharp rise in deaths and all kinds of familial and societal disturbances due to alcoholism. The period was described as a shambles, with thousands of drunks roaming the British countryside. This was the period of Hogarth's vivid etchings and the pathos of *The Rake's Progress*. All England was up in arms and Parliament placed a prohibitive tax on gin. However, the gin producers and consumers had a powerful lobby that kept the Whig government in power by advocating cheap gin. At this point, another powerful group became involved in the fight, the importers and growers of tea. They started a seesaw political battle with the distillers and finally managed to keep the tax on gin. Tea, which had not had a great vogue in England before this time, became the national drink.

Some happiness drugs just seem to die out. Most lose their ascendency because something else has taken their place and not merely because of public condemnation or laws against them. In the long chain of happiness drugs, we have seen gin succeeded by tea, tea by snuff, snuff by chewing tobacco, chewing tobacco by cigarettes, and now, cigarettes by marijuana. Unfortunately, no historical fad in drugs has repeated itself; otherwise, we could attempt to substitute snuff or chewing tobacco for marijuana. However, we can offer some rational advice about the problem.

Facts are important. Yet, until the tragic Greenwich Village murder of Linda Fitzpatrick in October 1967, there was no opportunity to present any of the factual dangers of drugs in the press. If you look back to magazines and newspapers of 1967, you will see many articles glorifying drug use, and statements by prominent Americans sanctioning the use of drugs. Since that time, the press has been more temperate, but misinformation is still the rule rather than the exception.

Gremlins seem to invade the minds of headline writers. A recent research study on marijuana (19) concluded that people using marijuana had difficulty in maintaining a logical line of thought and "tended to go off on irrelevant tangents and forget what they started out to say." Yet the headline in *The New York Times* was "Study Finds Marijuana Effects Mild" and that in the *Washington Post* was "Little Damage Found in the Use of Marijuana."

In addition to facts education, counseling, and treatment are indicated. Also, the society must allow for some experimentation by youth. Now that drugs have become such important factors in our youth society, it is a harmful mistake to throw the book at any drug user or, indeed, to deal with him as a criminal in the same way we deal with burglars and murderers.

Our main job as mental health professionals is to offer facts, information, and counseling. It is a large and not unimportant task; but the real question does go beyond our sphere of interest, and we should recognize that this is so. Drug use will not die out by our efforts alone, but rather by substitution of some other more exhilarating forms of gratification (21).

## Individual Assessment and Treatment

As emphasized in other sections of this chapter, it is hazardous to generalize about drugs and their treatment. Each drug problem must be considered individually. However, I will offer a group of principles that may be used in assessing and treating adolescents with drug problems, recognizing that these principles are inadequate for understanding and dealing with individual cases.

In previous studies of "addiction prone" personalities a great emphasis was placed on early infantile roots, particularly oral ones, of later addiction. Problems of impulse control, difficulty in deferring gratification, and a narcissistic orientation were seen to be present in many drug users. At present, when drug use is such a ubiquitous phenomenon, it is not feasible to look for such characterological determinants of addiction. They may well be present, but if so, are probably pervasive in the environment and more defining of the society than of individual character structure.

More important than the study of individual characterological pathology is the study of the relationship of the drug user and his environment. All assessment must be firmly based on a knowledge of the interaction between the adolescent, his family, school or work situation, and the sociocultural environment. It is impossible to assess a youngster without considering the dynamics of his family. Too often therapists take drug users into treatment in isolation, ignoring the crucial importance of understanding and dealing with the world around him.

Naturally, the drug user himself must be considered the primary focus, but all members of the patient's household must be considered as significant elements in understanding the phenomenon of drug use. When drug use is a casual experience, an experimentation by a youngster along with his peer group, the therapist's role may be one of preventive education for family and child, aimed toward helping the family give support so that the child can turn toward other outlets for his interests and socialization wishes.

If the youngster is a confirmed drug user and suffering symptoms from this problem, a different set of dynamics must be explored. Can the family be counted on to support the assessment and treatment of the patient? Does the family provide an environment that is understimulating? There are times when parents because of their own addiction problem, lack of interest in a child, or excessive punitiveness are such a malignant force that psychotherapeutic work is difficult to initiate even when there is a desperate need for it. Some families are so overprotective that a child remains dependent in every other way and uses drugs as his only mode of showing rebellion and autonomy.

Drug use by an adolescent may be a cry for help, his attempt to assert his independence from his family, an acting out of unconscious parental wishes, a way of defying a parent in an oedipal situation, or a means of regression. All these possibilities must be considered in assessing a drug problem. A vector analysis of drug experience is useful. Does drug use represent a conflict between mother and child or father and child, one of displacement from parental figure to another identification figure in the environment, a conflict of values between parents and children or a reflection of sibling rivalry? Finally, does it represent an internalized conflict within the child that is handled by drug-induced regression? Each conflict suggests entirely different directions for treatment efforts.

Each therapist should make use of the full armamentarium of medical study, clinical interview, family diagnosis, school reports, and psychological testing. Only through the use of these multiple avenues of information can we more accurately assess which adolescents may be helped by individual therapy, group therapy, encounter or sensitivity group work, recreational activity, change of school, or residential and in-patient treatment modalities.

Since many drug problems are seen together with other acting-out symptoms such as running away, stealing, truancy, and fighting, the therapist must make a careful assessment of the potential for working with his patient in out-patient rather than in-patient treatment. Whenever the dynamics of patient and family are primarily of an impulse-ridden, acting-out nature, it is foolish to take such a patient into intensive out-patient psychotherapy. Fortunately, in-patient services are increasingly gearing themselves to the treatment of drug users. In an in-patient service, anti-social problems can be more easily understood and encompassed. The very experience of a short hospitalization can give the adolescent and his family an opportunity to review their situation, impress them with the importance of the drug phenomenon, and give the therapist an opportunity to assess further the seriousness of characterological pathology, while affording an opportunity to plan for future care. In many cases it is necessary to have a dramatic break in continuity of the patient's life in order to help him look at himself in a more psychologically adaptive way and begin to direct himself toward productive goals.

Few adolescents come for psychiatric study on their own initiative and drug users are even less motivated, since the society offers a "secondary gain" by suggesting that drug use is an aspect of the healthy aspirations of young people and the "sickness" of adult society. No matter how much the adolescent may suffer anxiety, depression, or pain, his narcissism is often too great to allow for a voluntary admission of mental difficulty. He certainly does not want treatment. Rather, the adolescent wants help in getting free of the police and other bothersome aspects of his environment so he can continue his drug habit. He often attempts to manipulate the helping people even if they are not identified with his parents. A nineteen-year-old drug user told me:

"I started in junior high school. I first started with alcohol and I quit it because it gave me a hangover. Then I went to marijuana because of the drug scene and then LSD and finally to downers and heroin. When I first started with you, I wanted to get my habit down but not off. I finally realized you can't do that. I always fooled you for a long time. I lied to you so many times. The reason I kept coming was to keep the police off my back."

Individual psychotherapeutic work is based on the patient's motivation for relief of his anxiety and symptoms, his willingness to continue for a considerable period of uncertainty, an interest in understanding himself, and a willingness to consider that his symptoms are problems largely of his own making. The drug user has all the usual adolescent defenses against intense therapeutic involvement and an extra one. He recognizes that the society increasingly condones drug use and looks for psychopathology within the adult world rather than in the phenomenon of drug use itself.

## INDIVIDUAL OUT-PATIENT TREATMENT

Though there are many hazards in this route, psychotherapy is the treatment of choice in some cases. Even so, parental involvement must always be ensured in order that adequate communication and support are available. For individual treatment to be successful, the therapist must accept the limitations inherent in work with adolescents in general (11) and the special difficulties of working with adolescents in today's world.

## SPECIAL PROBLEMS OF THERAPISTS

Drug treatment problems force us to evaluate our own professional value positions and technical therapeutic procedures, for the values of therapists often confront opposing values in their patients and complicate the problem of developing a working alliance. Therapists recognize that they should have a benevolent interest in their patients, but it is difficult to empathize with an adolescent whose life-style, values, and symptoms are antipathetic to those of the therapist. The values of most therapists include those of achievement, the importance of honest work, understanding, freedom, a future orientation, a concern for property, and a belief in education as an important element in life. Therapists in general hold to a number of conventions, if not values, regarding general decorum and dress, language and life-style. In psychotherapeutic work language is critical to the process in which we engage. Symbol transformation is our stock in trade. The adolescent places a much higher evaluation on being "cool" in every way. The very cool society of the drug subculture implies many discontinuities between it and the adult world. The adolescent derides the use of language and cultivates an extremely small vocabulary. He develops a considerable concern for privatism, everyone "doing his own thing," concern about the present only, a lack of belief in or concern with education, career, and the future.

In order to begin to engage effectively with adolescents, therapists must be acutely aware of these differences in orientation between themselves and their patients. They are not necessarily total barriers to treatment. In fact, discussion of them can be of great use. The therapist must recognize, however, that his goal in treatment should not be to steer the adolescent back into the educational process and the "straight" world. The therapist must see his job as one of helping the adolescent to give up drugs and concomitantly find a new way of life that will offer a sense of satisfaction and meaning.

Even the therapist who can confront his own values successfully must also be willing to learn about contemporary adolescent preoccupations. These include a concern with transcendental meditation, rock music, the mystical need for being "on the road," the belief in good "vibes" that make speech unimportant.

Most therapists, at least two generations removed from contemporary youth, had their intellectual world view shaped by the writings of Ernest Hemingway, Fitzgerald, Heller, and J. D. Salinger. For the most part these writers are dead to the youth who, today, read Kurt Vonnegut, John Barth, Hermann Hesse, and myriads of anonymous writers of sadistic sexual books. Young people are excited by protests, the immediate social and warlike problems of the society, and a groping toward the development of a truely communitarian movement.

The therapist must not attempt to invade the world of adolescent drug use entirely, for adolescents need privacy, but he must know something of the habitat in which his patients live in order to communicate with them. It is important that therapists ask themselves if they are truly interested or intrigued by rock music, protests, and meditation. Unless there is a sharing of interests between therapist and drug-using patient, technical knowledge and professional experience will be of no use, for the drug subculture of adolescents in not based primarily on distortions of stages of child development, but on the current social climate. Contemporary adolescents are living a life-style radically different from that of the recent past. We must be careful students of that life-style and of our own values in our work with these teenagers.

A number of special treatment parameters are implied in these concepts. Therapy must be unusually flexible, often intermittent, and tailored to the adolescent's wishes as well as his needs, rather than to the therapist's schedule. We must see such patients immediately when they contact us, and allow them to make their own treatment schedule until they have become involved reliably in the treatment process. Such patients should be permitted to break off treatment without having to fear their own feelings of negative transference or our overt censure. They must know that they can return to treatment when they are ready to make use of it.

If the therapist can tolerate this kind of scheduling and technical preparation, a number of valuable results follow. Transference will be minimized, as will regression. Thus these patients, who already are regressed and wary of adults, will not compound their fantasy difficulties. They can then use therapy to achieve immediate, adaptive goals. If a supportive, developmentally relevant and clarifying relationship can occur, the adolescent will not expect treatment to effect magical, total changes in his life in a short time, but will experience tangible results from this initial phase of work. Following this, the therapist can introduce his patient to the complicated intrapsychic work of analysis of transference and defense structure.

But we engage more effectively with patients if we can enter their own world of interests and concerns. How far we can go in becoming part of this world is defined by our own ability and inventiveness. Just as Anna Freud (6) described the introduction of a child to analytic therapy by showing him that she could tie more complicated knots than the patient, we must use Zen, semantics, ecology—whatever interests coincide between patient and therapist—to show that we, indeed, have some common cause.

In addition, the professional concerned about drug use must understand that drug users demand to be accepted as seekers and learners and not as patients in need of treatment. The concept of "patienthood" is both foreign and demeaning to them to a degree they will not tolerate. However, they usually know when they are troubled and quickly reach out to a telephone contact or storefront center that promises to listen to them and direct them to more definitive help when necessary. We have an opportunity to learn from these voluntary self-help groups, usually staffed by age-mates of the drug users. We can also participate effectively in their activities by offering them some coordination and consultation behind the scenes. Certainly there is no point in attempting to impede them. If there is one sure direction for the future of clinical work with drug users, it is this type of cooperative information and consultation facility.

GROUP METHODS

Since so many drug users see themselves as "seekers" rather than patients, and, indeed, the society agrees with this view, any kind of treatment facility that puts little pressure on the adolescent, gives him an opportunity to talk openly without fear of reprisal, and allows him to explore with his peers and, perhaps, some people a bit older the issues of his life will be useful. Many adolescent medicine clinics, college mental hygiene clinics, and community mental health centers have set up just such open-ended treatment groups, utilizing regular group psychotherapeutic techniques as well as those that are involved in sensitivity and encounter experiences. The important consideration is that the adolescent have an opportunity to communicate, to get across his point of view, and then at the end of his often ideological and polemical tirades be given the opportunity to ask questions like "Where am I going?" It is when this question comes up that the therapist can, again, take a usefully directive role.

NEW TREATMENT AND EDUCATIONAL METHODS

Young drug users shun traditional medical and mental health facilities to seek information and help. Instead they turn to "hot lines," "rap lines," sensitivity groups, encounter groups, and other informal sources for getting their needs met. To them, traditional professionals often represent a concept of rigidity, lack of empathy with their values, and lack of understanding of the wish to use drugs. Indeed, until recently most mental health professionals thought of drug "cases" as they did of alcoholics—

difficult people, unrewarding treatment possibilities, who retained little anxiety or concern for psychotherapy once their immediate drug problem quieted down.

Obviously therapists must study and modify their treatment methods so that greater relevance to the drug user's needs can be achieved. This may suggest a number of alternatives: first, that we concentrate as professionals on pre-adolescents or post-adolescents, rather than adolescents themselves; second, that we may feel a mandate to guide, even coerce, adolescents into codes we believe important; third, that we continue to recognize our therapeutic responsibility for certain teenagers but note that we can only observe and offer advice in many other "forms" of adolescence and youth that are now evolving.

Finally, educational methods and materials have a definite place in prevention and control of drug problems. Despite a torrent of available material about drugs, a great many people, young and old, still have muddled, inapplicable, and dangerously incorrect information. Some excellent summaries of drug information can be gotten easily (4, 12, 14, 17).

A number of these summaries of drug information outline programs of seminars, movies, and lectures that can be useful to young people of various ages interested in learning more about the drug phenomenon. Professionals can be exceedingly useful in organizing and participating in educational progress of this kind.

# 7

# Suicide and Attempted Suicide in Children and Adolescents

JEAN H. YACOUBIAN, M.D., AND
REGINALD S. LOURIE, M.D.

## Introduction

The topic of suicide in the young brings to mind the third act of Wagner's *Tristan and Isolde* and Shakespeare's *Romeo and Juliet*. The uniquely human theme of love and death by suicide—with the infinite subtleties of the powerful feelings involved—finds its best vehicle for expression in the equally unique experience of man's art.

Creativity, so much part of normal adolescent development, has been considered as restitution for man's destructive impulses. Almost all of Gustav Mahler's music deals with the struggle between life and death, which on a personal level reflects his creative invulnerability making restitution for destructive urges. He could be immortal through his music, as he stated in his own text for the finale of his second symphony:

> O Death, all-conquering one, now you are conquered.
> With wings, I have won for myself,
> In fervent love I shall soar
> To the light unseen
> I shall die to live (34).

Throughout the ages the question of suicide has been pondered by philosophers and religious leaders. It has been praised by some as an act of virtue and condemned by others on moral or philosophical grounds. Albert Camus, who met his own death in a speeding car, considered suicide to be the one truly serious philosophical problem. In his essay, "The Myth of Sisyphus," he stated that the judgment whether life is or is not worth living is the fundamental question of philosophy (7).

Views and attitudes about death are central to understanding the problem of suicide. In the young the concept of death develops gradually. According to Piaget, up to the age of six all objects in the world of the child are alive. There is little discrimination between the animate and inanimate.

As the child grows up, this animistic thinking is limited to objects that move and later to things that move spontaneously. He does not have the cognitive ability to appreciate the finality of death until he is ten or eleven years old. Although he may be preoccupied with death prior to this age—expressing his concern through play or verbally—he views it as a temporary and reversible state. Of course, the cognitive lag need not reflect the pain and suffering related to death experienced as separation. In fact, when this cognitive appreciation of death becomes available to the child, it can mitigate the anxiety over separation.

Yet cognitive ability alone does not solve the mystery and significance death has to different individuals. Rare is the person who has reached the level of maturity to understand and accept death as nonexistence. Sigmund Freud wrote:

Our own death is indeed unimaginable, and whenever we make the attempt to imagine it we can conceive that we really survive as spectators. Hence the psychoanalytic school could venture on the assertion that at bottom no one believes in his own death, or to put the thing in another way, in the unconscious every one of us is convinced of his own immortality (19).

In the touching *Songs and Dances of Death* of Moussorgsky, death is the mother giving solace, the lover with promise of bliss, the army chief who conquers all. To some death is the only bridge that can lead to union with lost loved ones. To many it is the eternal enemy to be fought. Saroyan is succinct, "In short, I began to write in order to get even on death" (40).

Death is a prerequisite of passion, the spice of life. Jorge Luis Borges, in his story "The Immortal" wrote:

To be immortal is commonplace; except for man all creatures are immortal, for they are ignorant of death; what is divine, terrible, incomprehensible, is to know that one is immortal. I have noted that, in spite of religions, this conviction is very rare. Israelites, Christians, and Moslems prefer immortality, but the veneration they render the world proves they believe only in it, since they destine all other worlds in infinite numbers to be its rewards or punishments. . . .

Death (or its allusion) makes men precious and pathetic. They are moving because of their phantom condition; every act they execute may be their last; there is not a fact that is not on the verge of dissolving like a face in a dream. Everything among the mortals has the value of the irretrievable and the perilous . . . (5).

Although man has no control over his birth, he can end his life. It is put so well in an early draft of *Herzog* by Saul Bellow:

With one long breath, caught and held
in his chest, he fought his sadness over
his solitary life. Don't cry, you idiot!
Live or die, but don't poison everything . . . (48).

Commenting on the issue of choice, E. H. Erikson wrote: "To be a suicide, although it is a negative identity, is, nevertheless, an identity choice in itself (14)."

The enigma of suicide remains despite various explanations and different approaches. The question "Why?" is still to be fully answered.

## Epidemiology of Suicide

The scope of the problem can be understood if we look at the incidence of deaths by suicide and variations by age groups, sex, and race (46). In this country alone there are over 20,000 suicides a year. It has been estimated that recorded suicide figures are underreported by 25 to 33 percent for the total population; many feel that the suicides of children and adolescents are understated even more because of the stigma attached to suicidal death.

Suicide is a worldwide problem, with the mortality rate increasing in many countries. And the most striking feature of this increase has been the rise in suicide among young persons.

*Age.* There is a direct correlation between suicide rates and advancing age. Suicide is nonexistent under five and virtually nonexistent at five to nine years of age, although about one-tenth of the children under age ten who attempt to kill themselves are successful. Currently there are about 100 suicides per year among children ten to fourteen years of age and the number and rate have been increasing yearly. The rate rises sharply during ages fifteen to nineteen when there is an eight- to tenfold increase; at ages twenty to twenty-four the suicide rate doubles again.

Suicide in the fifteen- to nineteen-year-old age group ranks fifth as the cause of death; there are over 650 such deaths yearly in this age group. Thus suicide takes more adolescents' lives than tuberculosis, appendicitis, rheumatic fever, streptococcal infections, diabetes, and all the contagious exanthems. The accidental death rate, the leading cause of youthful death, is so high that some investigators feel that many of these deaths are probably suicides which are not certified as such. The suicide rate among college students has risen alarmingly until it now ranks second as the most frequent cause of death after accidental fatalities. According to recent estimates, about 15,000 college students attempt suicide each year (33).

*Sex.* In all age groups three times as many males commit suicide as females; the ratio is reversed for attempted suicides.

*Race.* Generally speaking, the rates for nonwhites are below those for whites with two important exceptions: nonwhite females age fifteen to nineteen have very slightly higher rates than white females of the same age; and within the past ten years there has been a striking increase in suicides among young nonwhite males between the ages of fifteen and twenty-four. (Nonwhite males at ages twenty to twenty-four have higher rates than their white male age peers although they are lower than whites at younger ages.)

The larger increase in suicides among nonwhite males may be a reflection of the stresses of migration to urban centers with the accompanying tensions of ghetto living and unemployment; according to another theory, conflicts can also arise from new opportunities and roles.

The concept of "victim precipitated homicide" of Wolfgang (54) could also affect the interpretation of suicide rates among nonwhites. Noting the high homicide rates and lower suicide rates among Negro males, he observed a tendency of certain homicide victims to behave in such a manner as to bring about personal injury to themselves. He related this observation to a prevailing attitude among Negro males that to die by suicide was cowardly and effeminate, whereas death by homicide was masculine, thus more acceptable. Therefore, on the basis of intent, many such homicidal deaths should really be classified as suicide.

## Historical View

There are records of suicides by children in almost every culture. Observers of primitive tribes have told of juvenile self-destruction among the Melanesians, New Zealanders, British Columbian Indians, Sea Dyaks, and others. The writer of the Talmud considered the problem and finally ruled that the children who commit suicide do so unwittingly. There are superstitions in the Bihar Province of India relating to self-destruction by children whose mother, while bearing them, walked over a suicide's grave. Suicide of adolescents appears in English literature from Shakespeare (*Romeo and Juliet*) to Thomas Hardy (*Jude the Obscure*) and Max Beerbohm (*Zuleika Dodson*). In at least a dozen civilized countries, suicide of the young reached sufficient proportions at one time or another to merit lay and professional attention.

The problem has been striking enough to excite comment in medical literature for more than one hundred years. An interesting sidelight in a review of this literature is the periodic shift of emphasis in placing the blame for child suicide. From approximately 1880 to 1900 the chief culprits were said to be the trashy novels and romantic sentimental stories of the time. From about 1900 to 1915 the tendency in the majority of reports was to blame the educational system. From 1915 to about 1935 emphasis was on constitutional factors, stressing the psychotic and the hereditary aspects. It is only in the past thirty years—with the exception of a symposium at the Vienna Psychoanalytic Institute in 1910 (1)—that there have been speculations on deeper underlying motives for children wanting to die.

The earliest figures we were able to find were those of Casper who reported from Prussia on a few child suicides from 1788 to 1797. By the late nineteenth century the rates of youthful suicide had increased markedly (much higher than modern rates). In a survey of nineteenth-century European statistics, MacDonald (1906–1907) reported an increase of young suicides in France and England and an "enormous increase" in Prussia. From 1900 to 1905 there was a worldwide increase in the child suicide rate; Berlin alone had 1,700 cases from 1900 to 1903. It was at this point that the problem was recognized in the United States and began to appear in the literature. This was followed by a general decline in rate, but an upward trend began again about 1930 and is continuing now. The increase has been chiefly in the puberty and early adolescent group, and concomitantly there has been a sharp rise in hospitalization for mental illness of children from ten to fourteen years of age. All authorities have recorded a rise in suicide rate at puberty.

## Child's Concept of Death

Before exploring the dynamics of suicide in children, it is useful to look, from a developmental viewpoint, at the child's concept of death (29). When the thought of suicide comes to a child, this is by no means the first time he has faced the problems of death and dying. He responds even before the end of the first year of life with a reaction to separation. He equates absence with nonexistence of the person who is out of his sight and experiences displeasure and pain. The next step is to be the one in control of his process. When angry, he can turn away and thus remove the person involved in his anger, or he can even hold his hand in front of his eyes and remove that person. When he has faced separation anxiety, particularly with the disappearance of his mother, it is not unusual for the baby to defend himself against the pain he experienced at separation by turning away when the mother returns. When the significant person responds to the child's indifference or turning away by being hurt and rejected, and particularly when this is repeated, the child has learned an important lesson about what can be accomplished by removing himself. Implicit in the older infant's apparent concept is that nonexistence, that is, death, is not permanent: the significant person who doesn't exist when he is out of sight reappears.

When the young child has mastered the question of absence and death as being one which does not leave him helpless but which he himself can initiate and therefore control, he is ready to consider the problem of death in another developmental phase, roughly from two to four years of age; in this phase he has fantasies of multiple magic powers. By his very wish or fantasy he can cause the "death" or temporary removal of anyone who offends him or is in his way—even those he loves. Concomitantly, he thinks he can suffer the same fate; he begins to have thoughts of his own death which then result in fears, particularly as extensions of the normal fear of bodily hurt. Damage to a part of the body or its disappearance can be equated with death in the young child's eyes. Typically, as his bowels can be flushed, mother can be flushed or he can be flushed. At this point death, which he still thinks is reversible, becomes associated in his mind with violence—particularly at ages three and four. Literature for this age group which has been handed down from generation to generation is replete with themes of violence, hurt, and destruction—Jack and Jill fall down the hill, Humpty Dumpty falls off a wall, the cradle falls out of a treetop. In most children of this age we can already see crystallization of the fusion of aggressive and libidinal drives—witness the child's pleasure in these aggressive, hurtful themes. Simultaneously another step should be made: inhibition or dilution of anger and aggression via maturation of love for the mother. Also, aggression is channelized into play and, later, fantasy and sublimated activities. It is this step which is missing in many of the children who attempt suicide, especially when the mother is unavailable and when living situations are chaotic.

Finally, when the family triangle develops and is worked through, usually between the ages of three and six, fantasies of death normally occur again. First they come in the form of death wishes against a loved one who might be in his way. At this point most often there is internalization of these wishes. We then find that the child is relatively more concerned with fear of his own death from the hands of figures that represent humans rather than inanimate objects, animals, or natural forces such as storms and the dark, which he feared earlier. The internalized images— witches, monsters, giants, robots, or men from outer space—are synthesized from TV, fiction, cartoons, fairy tales, the Bible, newspaper stories, and other sources. These developmental patterns of childhood can be carried into adolescence, as will be noted later.

In looking for solutions to these phases of development in which there is this preoccupation with death not only of others, but also of himself, the child learns from these experiences and also from the reaction of adults to his responses: (a) what death means, (b) how it can be used defensively, (c) how it can be used to influence and maneuver others, (d) how it can be a device to relieve helplessness (as in the infant) as a concomitant of struggles with loved ones, and (e) how to use the concept of his own death as a means of achieving importance in the lives of others. Most of all, (f) the fusion of libidinal and aggressive drives as integrated with these concepts of death is accomplished. Seldom do we see a suicide or suicidal attempt at any age in which this fusion is not at least one component, if not the major one.

A developmental area which has been relatively neglected in connection with its relationship to suicidal acts and preoccupations is primary masochism. Whether or not there is such an inborn phenomenon as Freud suggests (20), it is apparent that some infants, born with perceptual distortions, can learn even in the first six months of life that relationship satisfactions are accomplished by hurt to oneself. Because of his strong needs to be dependent on mother, a child born with tactile hypersensitivity will make the first relationship step in spite of the resulting pain and discomfort. One way he can accomplish this is by saying, "If pain in necessary for me to achieve this dependence, then pain must be part of the relationship." In fact, some individuals with this makeup can go further and say, "Pain is my pleasure." One will recognize in this the development of masochism even in the first year of life—shown as a need for and sometimes pleasure in being hurt. Thus constitutional factors can contribute to the specific "patterning life experiences" of Escalona or "coping style" of Lois Murphy. Here again there can be a fusion of drive components which, as development proceeds, can combine in turn with other emerging functions such as the sexual one. We must look in directions such as this to understand the evidence that masturbation is not an infrequent accompaniment of suicide in adolescent boys.

The concept of "chronic suicidal drives" in children frequently appears in the literature. Children will repeat acts which they feel will shorten life. This includes the so-called repetitive accidental self-injuries. Running away has also been found to have many of the same dynamics as suicide in children, and in some cases it has been pointed out that it functions as a suicide substitute with the same symbolic value to the child.

The impulsiveness and apparently little, if any, planning and premeditation in child suicide have been frequently commented upon. All investigators agree that in almost all cases the apparent precipitating cause is trivial, at least to the adult observer. Most of the authors reporting on reasons for suicide attempts of children cite only the immediate precipitating stress (6, 12, 15, 16, 25, 26, 27, 30, 31, 36, 37, 38, 41, 44, 45, 47, 50, 51, 52, 53). However, among those who have looked more closely at psychodynamics (3, 56) the views are not incompatible with the developmental context advanced here. The following cases will illustrate some of these points.

## Case Studies

Of forty children aged three to fourteen who attempted suicide, most of the attempts were based on pressure of the moment in an individual with relatively poor impulse control (29). Closer examination, however, indicated a multiplicity of interacting factors operating in the presence of personality distortions rooted in early life. Following are some representative cases:

*Bob*, ten, was preoccupied with pleasure seeking; he had little supervision, and would be passively defiant and withdrawn when interrupted. Since age four he had been hospitalized at least once a year with head and body injuries, four of which resulted from being hit by cars. When a teacher reprimanded him for taking liberties with a girl, he hung himself with his belt in the cloakroom where the teacher had sent him. "I was sore at the teacher because of my report card the day before," he said.

*Bill,* ten, tried suicide eight times. He called his mother a name. She told his father, who beat Bill so badly that his mother fainted. Bill went to the kitchen and slashed his wrists "to make my mother nervous because she told my father. When she's nervous she makes a fuss over me." He had also taken poison (iodine) when sent to his room for punishment, threatened to jump out the window, and searched the house for sleeping pills. He had run away three times.

*Kermit,* nine, was dull, depressed, and preoccupied with dependency since his mother's death from diabetes a year before. He began to refuse to go to school in his aunt's town where he was overgraded. When the truant officer took him to school, Kermit tried to jump out of the window. At home later that day, he tried to eat a bowl of sugar so that he could die and join his mother in heaven. Sugar, he thought, would burn out his insides.

*Lizzie,* seven, of borderline intelligence, negativistic and resentful, was punished repeatedly by her siblings at their mother's suggestion. When she stole from other children at school or hit them, she punished herself, once by putting her hand in the flame of the stove. Her father talked of suicide every time he was drunk, and finally attempted it by cutting his wrists. The next day, Lizzie cut her wrists and throat.

*Victor,* ten, living in a constantly stimulating environment, was hyperactive, restless, and distractible. He stayed to see a Tarzan movie three times, and lied to his mother about coming home late. When she strapped him, he ran and jumped out of a fifth-story window. His mother reported that a woman on the block had jumped from a window the week before. Victor talked to the ambulance driver about Tarzan's jumping. Victor thought he, too, could swing from clothesline to clothesline. He had tried before to kill himself by drinking glue and wallpaper paste.

DETERMINANTS

In classifying the predominant psychodynamic determinants in these cases, the two most frequent factors related by the children were aggression and escape from an intolerable situation or reality. The aggression most often represented elements of revenge or spite toward one of the parents or the whole family. Some children turned the aggression against themselves as punishment for guilt because of death wishes or masturbatory activities. Inevitably there was a pleasurable result which the child hoped to achieve by turning the aggression against himself. The escape motif was found particularly when the child was made to feel helpless, his dependency was suddenly removed or threatened, or dire punishment was imminent.

Looking at these suicide attempts in a developmental context, we can see that they relate to the child's early ideas of death and represent unresolved elements brought from the earlier stages into the current and sometimes intolerable situation. Thus, in terms of escape, we see a primitive ego defense mechanism emerging. It is particularly in terms of aggression that the child's earlier concepts form nests of psychological experience to which he can return in a later crisis. These are determined by adults' responses which the child can elicit even in the first year of life.

If we add to this the cathexis of oral or anal sadism, or both, the persistence of primary masochism and development of secondary masochism, the libidinization of impulses and relationships, body image concerns, and continuing preoccupation with dependency and/or separation anxiety and their derivatives, we find the ingredients which were present in varying combinations and degrees in the children described here.

### PREVALENCE OF SUICIDAL THOUGHTS

Ordinarily, we would expect that the struggles with the concepts of death of others and of oneself would be repressed at the end of the oedipal period along with other painful fantasies, wishes, and traumatic ideas. However, it is surprising to the adult (who has repressed his memory of painful childhood) to learn how frequently a child is aware of death wishes toward himself during early school age and puberty. This phenomenon appeared during the course of interviews with "normal" school-age children and those with emotional problems. In the literature there have also been indications of the universality of suicidal preoccupations (21).

Since this phenomenon appears in the majority of our children and is not necessarily conditioned by clinically evident emotional disturbance, we might consider that thoughts of suicide, if transitory, are not abnormal. It must also be inferred that these thinking trends are different from actual suicide. Killing oneself is usually rejected as an adaptive device even though there may be pleasure in thinking about the reactions it would produce in others. Such preoccupations appear to be more frequent in children with passive-aggressive character patterns. All this does not apply of course to prepsychotic or overtly psychotic children. Also, these suicidal preoccupations are as common at age six as they are at fourteen.

As we consider the step between preoccupation with suicide and the actual attempt, we have only hints as to how often the step is made. Estimates of the ratio of attempts to successful suicide range from 5 to 1, up to 100 to 1 (24).

## Suicide in Adolescence

Before attempting to understand the "Why?" of suicide in adolescence, it is essential to distinguish between attempted, committed, threatened, "partial," and "probable" suicides. Studies indicate important differences (46). Suicide attempters were younger (modal age range fourteen to twenty-four) than completed suicides, and the sex ratio for attempts was the reverse (females 3:1 over males) of the sex ratio associated with completed suicides. Less than 10 percent of persons who attempt suicide later kill themselves. The problem of suicide attempts is particularly significant in adolescence since it is reported that 12 percent of all suicide attempts in this country were made by members of this age group, and 90 percent of these attempts were made by adolescent girls.

The method used at different ages and by the different sexes could influence the outcome of suicidal behavior. At ages ten to fourteen (for both sexes) firearms and hanging account for 90 percent or more of all suicides. At fifteen to nineteen years the primary pattern is use of firearms by males and poisons by females. The less lethal method of females allows time for rescue and contributes to the preponderance of attempted suicides.

An adolescent may threaten suicide to manipulate the environment. With no self-destructive intent, she might make a halfhearted attempt which could accidently lead to her death. Conversely, another adolescent with serious intent to die might, as commented earlier, invite injury and become the victim of a homicide—thus not be even identified as a suicide.

Dynamically, social isolation appears to be the most effective factor in distinguishing those who will kill themselves from those who will not. While this factor is seen in many types of suicidal behavior, it is more characteristic of cases of completed suicides than attempts or threats.

The diabetic who refuses to comply with the necessary medical regimen illustrates "partial" suicide.

As accidents are the prime cause of death in this age group, it is conceivable that a significant number of victims could be "probable" suicides.

Schneidman's essay "Orientation toward Death: A Vital Aspect of the Study of Lives" takes a much-needed thorough approach in clarifying, defining, and classifying suicidal behavior (43).

In adolescence, as in childhood, it might be helpful to follow the developmental theme as it relates to the problem of suicide.

To become an adult, the adolescent needs to go through the difficult task of relinquishing the dependent and incestuous ties with his parents, and then developing a relationship with an individual of the opposite sex. The process involves not only a shift in objects, but a change in the quality of the relationship. In the ties to the new object genitality comes to its fruition. The earliest imitations and identifications with the mother, whereby the child learns to do for himself what the mother had done for him, pave the way for increasing levels of separation and autonomy leading to the final break from parents and development of a unique identity. The individual who is not flexible enough to make these necessary shifts —because of immature patterns—may be more vulnerable under stress to suicidal behavior.

The ego, primarily concerned with adaptation, is put under great stress not only by the physical changes brought about in puberty but by powerful psychological forces. It needs to mediate between the forces of instinctual drives, demands of the superego and ego ideal, and expectations from the family and environment—to grow up, be independent, achieve in school, assume responsibility, etc. Any factors that additionally influence this balance, like weakening of the ego and of capacity for adaptation through illness or toxic agents (e.g., alcohol and drugs), can increase the adolescent's vulnerability for self-destruction.

Accordingly, in the adolescent in contrast to the child there is an increase in the multiplicity of influencing factors; with the development of personality, the dynamics of suicidal behavior are more complex and similar to that in adults.

## INDIVIDUAL DETERMINANTS

The etiological factors of adolescent suicide can be categorized according to individual, social, and cultural determinants. There are multiple individual factors. Through interaction of constitutional determinants and maturation, environmental forces, and development, suicidal behavior in adolescence is produced.

We will attempt to organize the clinical picture under the following headings: immature adolescents with poor ego development, hereditary tendencies, psychosis, depression, masturbation, identity crisis, drug use, and social and cultural determinants.

*Immature adolescents with poor ego development.* This category demonstrates the dynamic explanations that were presented for suicidal behavior in childhood. Impulsivity, turning in of aggression in stressful situations, identification, imitation and suggestion, spite, avoidance of discomfort, the desire to join a lost object and gain love may lead to attempted or completed suicide.

The strength of resurgent sexual and aggressive drives coupled with a weak ego in the absence of support from the environment is the variable that most contributes to this maladaptive solution.

As mentioned earlier, consideration of Piaget's contributions to cognitive development enriches our understanding of behavior in the formative years. The global "all or nothing" approach and the concrete and realistic oriented-toward-action thinking of the child evolve in adolescence to the capacity for abstract-conceptual, hypothetico-deductive thought.

This transformation allows the adolescent to appreciate relativity and have perspective in his experience. With the acquisition of reversible thought processes, he can introspect and have foresight rather than having to act on impulse. In this vein, intellectualization is a valuable defense to the adolescent in resolving and mastering his conflicts, and later it becomes an essential tool for sublimation (18).

Bollea and Mayer observed poor introspective capacity and hypothetico-deductive reasoning in 90 percent of attempted suicides between the ages of ten and eighteen. Their observations led them to believe the cognitive lag was the consequence of emotional deprivation in early childhood, inability to solve the Oedipus situation, and an absence of valid secondary identifications. "The emotional immaturity clearly determined the impossibility of adopting the principle of reality and consequently implied for those subjects to find an immediate solution to each situation of tension" (4).

*Hereditary tendencies.* Though several studies point to suicides that "run in the family" there is no evidence that self-destructive tendencies can be transmitted genetically. Rather, the issue of identification might explain this pattern.

*Psychosis.* Delusions and hallucinations of a schizophrenic adolescent may lead to self-destructive actions. Balser and Masterson (2), reporting on a study of hospitalized adolescents, and Maria (32) consider schizophrenia a more significant etiological factor than depression in this age group. Lewin points to manic reactions leading to suicide. "The manic does not kill himself for the purpose of dying, but on the contrary to live in fusion with the ego ideal," he writes (28).

*Depression.* Two categories will be considered under depression—first, conflict between dependence and independence, and second, oedipal conflict.

Depression has been considered characteristic in 50 percent of suicidal attempts in this age group (10). Classically, it is associated with the actual or fantasied loss of a loved object. The immature quality of the relation contributes to the primitive anger and resultant guilt. To defend against the feeling of helplessness, the hostility is turned in through the guilt—on the introjected (lost love object) resulting in self-destruction. Though not apparent on the surface, the dynamics point to the wish for union with the lost object (39). The following poem was written by a seventeen-year-old girl who had suicidal thoughts.

### Retreat

Her mother screeched, features making
slight motions.

She cried silently for help
but none came.

a fog thickened around her mind
it was dark and thick—
dappled with white.

she sat wrapped
in a blanket, rocking

to and fro,
in fear.

gradually she left
flying softly away
leaving behind her a rubber body
and a stone face.

The following narrative was written by a sixteen-year-old girl who made a suicidal attempt. The typographic "slip" of "me" before "family" illustrates the turning in of aggression.

### Traffic

The marrow in my bones froze and a hateful, grotesque sensation of suicide swept over my mind. I was no longer content with this life. I held a hatred and loathing feeling for me family. I was no longer stable or at ease living at home, I had had enough. It wasn't fair to be pushed and tormented all the time. I was too strong for them. Their minds were old and weak. I walked the crooked road down to the bridge tressels. The July air was warm but it blew a soothing breeze. I climbed up a little hill with broken bottles and cans, and sat down on the ledge of the tressel. The cars sped under the tressell and the sun reflected on the metalic roofs. I jumped. . . .

The same adolescent displaced her feelings related to parents onto others, re-experiencing the same feelings:

I once had some kittens that I loved very much, but they were taken away from me. The most wonderful woman in the world was my aunt. She was a beautiful, sincere person, but she was taken away from me. My president Kennedy—yes, I loved him, he was a magnificent sacrificing person, but he was taken away from me. The love I once had for a certain boy, and wonderful things we shared, they were taken away from me. And now my ability to love and show genuine care is gone, and my desire to live has now been taken away from me.

Oedipal conflict may be a significant factor in the dynamics of adolescent suicide. In adolescence, when the sexual desire for the parent of the opposite sex and feelings of rivalry and hostility toward the parent of the same sex are revived in full force, the dangers are greater because of the adolescent's capacity for consummation of the act; however, the taboo against incest is equally strong.

The adolescent might try to resolve the difficulty by reversal of affect. Thus it is safer to hate than to love the parent of the opposite sex. When such hostility is not discharged on the object, it can be turned inward, leading to suicide (18). The following excerpt of free prose was written by a sixteen-year-old in treatment who had made a halfhearted suicide attempt and tried running away. Expressing her thoughts about her father, she wrote:

I hate you. Your vile bodies disgust and embitter me. When will you ever learn? Probably never. You don't even know the true meaning of the word love. You are a selfish, cynical person. I can't stand the sight of you, the sound of your overpowering voice, I can't stand to be near you. You are an egotistical society bastard. A member of the so-called Great White Banshees 1965. I hate you. Leave me alone. Oh please God, save me from his bloody sword.

Several authors, including Zilboorg and Schneer and Kay propose that a failure in sexual identity or concern over homosexuality may lead to guilt, helplessness, and suicidal behavior (42, 55). The act of suicide fulfills the need for punishment and gratifies an unacceptable wish.

The ego ideal, too, can be a factor in depression. Where expectations of the ego ideal are not met, i.e., disappointments in love or achievement, depression may result.

*Masturbation.* Fears of loss of control and concomitant guilt resulting from unacceptable sexual fantasies that accompany masturbation also have a significant bearing on adolescent suicide.

Masochism, mentioned earlier—with fusion of sexual and aggressive drives—is observed especially in early adolescent males. There have been reports that pressure on the neck is used to enhance the intensity of pleasurable sensations during masturbation. Several investigators have reported death by hanging during autoerotic or transvestite activity (19, 35, 49).

*Identity crisis.* Negative identity of Erikson (14) may lead to suicide. The adolescent asserts his identity "perversely based on all those identifications and roles which at critical stages of development had been presented to the individual as most undesirable or dangerous, and yet, also as most real."

*Drug use.* LSD is the drug most commonly associated with suicide. Following are some of the ways Cohen says LSD may trigger suicide: delusions and hallucinations resulting from LSD may lead accidentally and without intent to self-destructive action; previously existing suicidal thoughts can be intensified during and after the "trip"; suicide could result from panic accompanying a bad trip (11).

Although experimentation with dosages may lead to fatal consequences, Schneidman considers this type of death accidental (43). He feels these individuals are interested in experimentation, not death; they wish to remain alive but in a drugged or perceptually altered state.

*Social and cultural determinants.* In addition to the individual factors discussed, social determinants are important to note in reviewing the etiology of adolescent suicide. Family relationships are particularly significant in influencing the development and resolution of conflicts in an individual. However, one must be aware that the significance of family factors and qualities is a function of the individual meaning these variables have for the adolescent. Neglect of the individual and intrapsychic approach often leads to simplistic statistical and descriptive explanations and conclusions about the suicidal phenomenon which frequently miss the mark. This is evidenced by the contradictory findings of different investigators regarding the significance of such factors as sibling position, family disorganization, and loss of a parent. Loss of a parent, for example, is significant only in terms of the meaning it has to the individual. This in turn is dependent on the congenital endowment, developmental factors, past experiences, the timing of the loss, availability of substitutes, etc. This does not minimize the significance of loss of a parent especially through suicide, nor does it obviate the necessity to assess the family situation to understand suicidal behavior.

Socio-economic factors such as high suicide rates during a depression and low during war do not seem to affect the rate of suicide in this age group. A number of other social factors, i.e., mass media, religion, racism, have been studied with regard to a possible correlation with suicide. However, the results are not clear. There has been speculation that the reports of high suicidal rates in Eastern Europe could be related to societal pressures and expectations.

The issue of student suicide also underlines the importance of understanding individual dynamics. Students appear to be at greater risk of suicide than their nonstudent peers and are frequently of better than average intelligence and academic performance than nonsuicidal students. However, the key question is whether students are initially more suicidal than nonstudents or whether the school environment makes them more susceptible. The conclusion, drawn from the work of Paffenbarger and Asnes, appears to be that the prior susceptibility of the student is a more critical factor than stresses caused by the school (46).

In looking at the cultural factors related to youthful suicide, we must also incorporate the individual and intrapsychic approach stressed previously. In early development the impact of culture is transmitted primarily through the interpersonal relations with parents. In adolescence the individual has a direct confrontation with his culture and its values, and is both affected by the culture and contributes to its development.

Durkheim used statistics in an organized manner to support his theory that suicide is caused by sociocultural forces. According to him, the suicide potential of a given society varied inversely with the degree of cohesion existing within that society. Accordingly, he described three types of suicides related to the degree of attachment and relationship the individual had within his social context: (a) *anomic*, where a poorly structured, normless society provided few ties and poor regulatory influences for an individual; (b) *egoistic*, where an individual was unwilling to accept the doctrines of his society, leading to lack of integration of the individual into society. The stronger the forces throwing the individual onto his own resources, the greater the suicide rate—hence the high rate of suicide among Protestants (in contrast to Catholics) because of a higher degree of individualism. In relation to the family, the greater the density of the family, the greater the immunity of the individual to suicide; and (c) *altruistic*, where an individual was too strongly identified with the traditions and mores of his social group, leading to suicide because of expected religious sacrifice or political allegiance (13).

Since the publication of his book in 1897, many others have followed Durkheim's sociocultural approach. The high suicide rate among the young Prussians has been related to the rigid, punitive child-rearing practices supported by culture. Hendin (23), too, has related suicide in Scandinavian countries to specific child-rearing practices. Japan, where suicide is the number one cause of death below the age of thirty, has also offered a culturally favorable attitude toward suicide. In the past, the children of the nobility and military classes were indoctrinated at an early age with the belief that suicide was an acceptable, even highly valued, means of resolving demands of honor or duty, e.g., the Kamikaze.

## Clinical Implications

Clinical implications include early recognition, management, and preventive considerations related to the problems of suicide.

There are many prodromal signs that may provide clues to suicidal intentions. This emphasizes the point that no suicidal behavior should be taken lightly. Very often the suicide threat or attempt is a desperate "cry for help."

Social isolation and withdrawal appear to be the most striking feature of completed suicides rather than attempts or threats. As mentioned earlier, it may be seen in many types of suicidal behavior, but it is most characteristic of completed suicides (46). The roots of such poverty in object relations lie in disturbed relations with parents very early in life, but also can be the results of family disruptions such as death, moving, etc.

An adolescent who is delusional and spends much time in fantasy can be a suicidal risk. Depressive neurotic symptoms, anxiety, insomnia, anorexia, and psychosomatic symptoms could also be prodromal signs.

The severity of the suicidal risk can be reflected by the depth of the conflict—degree of guilt, self-castigation, helplessness, primitive quality of aggressive fantasies, and the inner and outer resources available to the adolescent.

Swift and efficient crisis intervention is essential. Caplan says, "During the period of upset of a crisis, a person is more susceptible to being influenced by others than at times of relative psychological equilibrium" (9). Referring again to this susceptibility he writes, "From a preventive psychiatric point of view, this is a matter of supreme importance; because by deploying helping services to deal with individual crisis, a small amount of effort leads to a maximum amount of lasting response" (8). The severity and quality of the problem will dictate the appropriate therapeutic measures to be taken: hospitalization, psychotherapy, psychoanalysis, chemotherapy, and various manipulations of the environment. But in any case, when there is a suicide attempt, the point must be made that the child's life is considered of great importance and will be protected even if it means a short period of hospitalization.

Similar to Freud in 1907, Zilboorg writes, "It is clear that the problem of suicide from the scientific point of view remains unsolved. Neither common sense nor clinical psychopathology has found a causal or even a strict empirical solution" (56). There has been growing interest during the last fifteen years in furthering our understanding of suicide. In 1957, a demonstration suicide prevention center was established in Los Angeles. More recently this pattern has spread, particularly following the creation in 1966 of a center for studies of suicide prevention within the National Institute of Mental Health. Training in suicidology is now part of the N.I.M.H. training programs.

In addition to fostering research, the N.I.M.H. has been making available much needed information to the public, but there is a need for even greater efforts to inform the public of danger signs of suicide and to develop resources in the community. In the framework of the Community Mental Health movement, crisis clinics—especially in the inner cities— mental health clinics in universities, telephone service on a twenty-four-hour basis, etc., have been found to be useful and necessary steps for proper management of suicide both in treating suicidal patients and aiding the survivors of suicide victims. It should be noted that it is not infrequent that a child attempting suicide will reject any communication with a therapist during the crisis. However, this should not be interpreted as a failure; aggression can often be deflected from the original source, i.e., family, and directed outward—not inward. Therefore, resistance should not discourage continuing therapeutic efforts.

Since we must consider the phenomenon of suicide in the social context, programs of prevention can hardly fail to emphasize the maladaptive conditions of our society. Poverty, racism, poor education, unemployment, violence, social isolation of the ghetto, inadequate housing—all produce degenerative conditions of defeat and despair. These are all areas calling for social change. Preventive efforts must be turned to these major social problems as the framework within which other specific programs will operate. Within this optimized social framework, efforts toward improving child-rearing practices should be a major area for preventive services.

# 8

# *The Psychosocial Dynamics of Today's Youth*

RALPH A. LUCE, M.D.

## Historical and Social Context

Few would question that twentieth-century experience is changing human personality. Perhaps psychiatrists first noticed the beginning mutation by the shift in psychopathology from neurotic manifestation to behavioral evidence of character disorder from the era of Freud to the last third of the twentieth century. The breakdown of family, community, and traditional patterns of living and their replacement by a symbiotic attachment to electric age gadgetry in an automated technocracy has turned man away from what goes on inside of himself to a fascination with the multitude of stimuli demanding attention from outside. Before World War II Sorokin (39) spoke of ours as a "Sensate Age," meaning that reality had become only what could be experienced through the sense organs. More recently, McLuhan (29) has described the "nervous system" that man has built outside of himself in the form of the communication media. In a few generations, as indicated by Riesman (36), man has passed from being tradition-directed, through a transitional phase of inner-direction, to the present state of being other-directed. Many of today's youth consider the postponement of present pleasure for a future goal to be chimerical. In our time, overburdened by more responsibilities than he can possibly cope with, inner-directed man, usually a member of the parental generation, has become obsolete. When the stress of isolated individualism becomes too great, other-directedness takes over and man becomes an externalized being, largely alienated from his inner self. The historical process leading to this end was visible to such prophetic thinkers as Kierkegaard (22), Marx (26), and Tönnies (43) as long as a century ago. Perhaps the crucial question for today is whether man can reclaim himself from the historical process, from the alienation, rootlessness, and externalization that threaten his humanity, or whether he will succumb to the monolithic forces of his own creation that take him from himself. It is through an exploration of this question that we shall try to understand the problems of today's youth.

Since 1945, as the culture has become increasingly "sensate," and people more "other-directed," the urgency to live in the Now has accelerated so that neither past nor future seems real to many young people. One causal factor may be that many children must assume, or are given, adult responsibilities prematurely, yet have no real closeness to adults. Halleck (17) has indicated that college students can go for months without speaking to anyone over thirty. Perhaps, as Margaret Mead (30) suggests, "The future is now"; but what about the past? Can the cultural heritage of our civilization be safely jettisoned? Thoreau (41) indicated more than a century ago that he thought the old had little to teach the young. Certainly throwing out the past involves discarding traditional ideas about sex, religion, politics, morality, manners, and other customary patterns of behavior. It involves discarding ancient, medieval, and industrial era concepts simultaneously. If Aristotle and Descartes are dispensable, what about Jesus and Buddha? In times of crisis there tends to be regression to absolute modes of thought, to a state of polarization. Thus wholesale rejection of the past seems just as regressive as mindless clinging to it.

Even if it is true that good and evil can be obscured by Madison Avenue and mystification, probably most would agree that simplistic cause-and-effect reasoning, which is a kind of linear absolutism frequently used in the past to delineate moral behavior, is no longer an acceptable mode in a relative world where each person sees himself within a rapidly changing field or Gestalt. Paradoxically, today's externalized man finds few acceptable values on the outside and so must create them anew or live in an amoral universe. Paralleling the subjective search for values is the rejection of what is objective, intellectual, or cognitive—in short, rejection of so-called scientific data divorced from experience. Experimentation through experience takes primacy over learning from the experience of others, living or dead. Such is youth's reaction to a corrupt present, an inadequate past, and an unpredictable future.

Edgar Friedenberg (12) indicates that the present polarization between the generations is different from that of the past. Previously the young wished merely to replace the old, a threat that no longer exists. Today, according to Friedenberg, the young feel "as if they were locked in the back of a vehicle that had been built to corrupt specifications, was unsafe at any speed, and was being driven by a middle-aged drunk!" The threat to the adult generation is now the legitimate rejection of their world by large numbers of the young. To speak of the rebellion of youth as if it were only a developmental phase and had no validity in itself is a put-down. It is a kind of older generation reductionism which masks its depreciation of youth in intellectual phraseology. It also ignores what is crucial: the horror of the modern world as experienced by young people. A recent cartoon by Cobb (4) masterfully illustrates the point: father and son are sitting atop a nuclear bomb on wheels marked "Western Civilization" which is racing in the direction of a sign marked "Over-population, Over-pollution, Over-kill"; father on top of bomb is watching a TV set and says to son sitting at some distance, "Get a haircut."

The lack of communication between generations is by no means inevitable; nor is it necessarily created by youth to produce distance from the parents so that individuation can occur. It is most pronounced when the young person feels that there is no possibility of the reality of his world being perceived or understood by the parents. Parental attitudes toward school based on selective memories of an entirely different experience twenty-five years earlier frequently block communication with children whose school experience bears little actual resemblance to that remembered by the parents. The initial inability to communicate is further widened because of the young person's feeling that it is hopeless to try to tell the parent what his own experience is like. His own difficulties in articulation are compounded by his conviction that even if the parent listens, he won't hear what is said. The consequence will be a lecture by the parent to the child that is irrelevant to what the child is experiencing. The content of such lectures, usually highly moralistic and overburdened with "shoulds," reveal a parental defensiveness resulting from the threat to parental omnipotence. The child is not doing what is expected, i.e., not following in the parent's image of the child as an extension of himself. Frequently young people find that they can communicate better with other people's parents than with their own. It is not unusual for youth to seek out sympathetic adults who do not let their preconceived ideas and vested interests intervene between them and what the young people are trying to say. Such communication might be called therapeutic.

Another element of obfuscation between the generations is the jargon chosen by the young to communicate important experience. "Getting high," for example, expresses in spatial terms what is most likely a change in temporal sense. "Doing one's thing," far from being a mechanical relationship to objects, represents an intensely personal commitment to something that is meaningful. It is undoubtedly significant that young people choose terms appropriate to older generation experience to express what is not only qualitatively different but what may actually be a polar opposite. Young people accept pleasure without guilt, reject the accumulation of things, euphemistically called "the pride of ownership," in a time of plenty, and place their emphasis on what is scarce in their lives: closeness to others, personal relationships, a sense of community. According to Gioscia (15), what for the older generation is a trip through space is, for those of the young who experiment with LSD and other psychedelics, an exponential experience with time. The new frontier is within, as the young move into what Reich (34) calls Consciousness III where spatial, linear, one-dimensional consciousness is transcended. McLuhan (29) says the young now live mythically, i.e., on many levels at once, and additionally, in one global village where all are world citizens. For the old, as well as the young, it is a world of great complexity, of accelerating simultaneity, of implosion and explosion, a world not unlike that prophetically created earlier in the century in such works of fiction as James Joyce's *Finnegan's Wake* (19). Perhaps "Psychological Man," as described by

Rieff (35), can come of age if he can combine his analytical reasoning powers, which by themselves lead to sterile reductionism, with an integrative attempt to recognize patterns, to live dynamically in a many-leveled mosaic, where dialogue, though often derailed and abortive, is vital to survival. As Tönnies (43) indicated in *Gemeinschaft und Gesellschaft*, first published in 1887, man is moving away from total relationships into an era where most human contacts are impersonal, partial, and frustrating. The American need to deny dependence on others, as discussed by Slater (38), further reinforces the turning away from full human relationship to a dependence on the impersonal support of mechanical gadgetry. People of all ages—but probably more the old and the young—suffer from limited human contacts and from the onslaught of what Toffler (42) calls "future shock," characterized by a triad of incubi: stimulus, information, and decision overload. Some psychiatrists, such as Ronald Laing (23) in London, insist that we are all going insane. Our insanity is due, perhaps in large measure, to our lack of feeling contacts with others, and to being assaulted by technological and bureaucratic garbage, The Big Lie, that numbs us by distorting reality in 1984 fashion, by perverting our values, and by encouraging the helpless receptivity of the perpetual infant.

Even so, the ferment of history as manifested in our common experience is moving the older generation toward the awareness experienced by the young. We must learn from our children, as Margaret Mead (30) says. People of all ages are desperately trying to maintain and reclaim their humanity. One indication is the human potential movement with its interest in sensory awareness, encounter and Gestalt methodology; another is the increasing popularity of Yoga, Zen, and other eastern religious systems and attitudes. The electronic media have done their work well. The reaction against the unfeeling state of isolated individualism, overintellectualism, and overspecialization, manifested by the centuries-old subject-object split inherent in western culture, is spreading. As McLuhan (29) says, the West is becoming orientalized, as the East becomes technologized. The return to what is whole and natural is reflected in changing attitudes, among the young, toward such matters as nudity, sexual behavior, the eating of natural foods, and communal living. The latter obviously does not apply to drug use, which may be viewed as a technique to cope with the problems of growing up in a chaotic culture. It is interesting that many young people renounce drugs completely after being heavily involved for several years.

As a reaction against the predominant culture, often called the Establishment, a counterculture arose during the decade of the 1960s. Emerging from roots in the Beat Generation, the New Movement, as its consolidation is called in the early 1970s, was heralded by the era of rock music, especially the Beatles, the extensive use of drugs, particularly marijuana and LSD, by large numbers of young people, the underground press, and by the development of widespread protest activities directed against such matters as the Vietnam War, the military draft, and an out-of-date college scene that had sold out to the military-industrial complex. According to Slater (38), the polarities involved are almost infinite. Whereas the old culture tends to favor property rights over personal rights, technological requirements over human necessities, competition over cooperation, vio lence over sexuality, accumulation over distribution, secrecy over open ness, striving over gratification, oedipal love over communal love, etc., the counterculture tends to reverse the process. A recent book, edited by Joe Berke (1) and entitled *Counter Culture*, emphasizes the necessity for a total destructuring of America as man's only hope for survival. Many in the counterculture believe that change can be brought about by the cultural revolution taking place in large numbers of individuals who refuse to participate in the Establishment and who live marginally while they "get their heads together" by "doing their own thing." Such a choice may involve dropping out of high school or college, living in a commune, and surviving by making and selling candles, leather belts, or other hand-crafted items.

Another segment of the counterculture, the so-called radical activists, believes that change can occur only by willful intervention in social processes. Such intervention has already manifested itself in a variety of ways such as the burning of the Bank of America, the destruction of draft files, and interference with Dow Chemical recruiting and ROTC activities on college campuses. Many of the less idealistic drop-outs who have severe personality defects may become addicted to hard drugs and survive by selling dope or by commiting acts of burglary and petty larceny. They use the same rationalizations as their more idealistic counterparts to justify their antisocial behavior. It is left to the Establishment authorities to distinguish between authentic cultural change, political action, and delinquency, a task that frequently requires more perspicacity than they possess.

Until recently western science has tended to isolate the object of study from its natural habitat. The artificiality of that approach is slowly being replaced by studying the object in context as part of a living process. The family therapy approach in psychiatry is an example of this phenomenon. The application of similar thinking to historical and social contexts is beginning to evolve by integrative thinking in the social sciences. Although the relationship between alienation, industrialization, and capitalism was well documented by Karl Marx (26) in the last century, it is only recently in the works of such contemporary thinkers as Fromm (14), McLuhan (29), and Slater (38) that the psychological subtleties of the effects of technology on man have been delineated. Man is a highly suggestible and imitative animal. If he is a "naked ape" (31), he is also an upright chameleon. In an era of scarcity when the problems of productivity were foremost, the concept of human productivity assumed high priority, a value that was reinforced by the Protestant ethic. To produce most efficiently, man had to specialize, fragment and limit himself—in short, to become more like a machine. The limitation of function that resulted from the interaction between man and machine helped to foster the split between man and nature, the state of alienation.

Moreover, not only did man subjugate himself to the machine, he also began to idolize it. Idolatry, as discussed by Fromm (14), occurs when man creates an object and then worships it as if it did not come from himself. He renounces his own powers and inner richness by transferring them to what he has created outside of himself, thereby becoming an impoverished "thing." McLuhan (29) speaks of the relationship between man and the objects he has created as producing "narcissus narcosis," a state of numbness that reduces man's capability to feel and to be aware of his immediate environment. Inundated by manmade objects, man becomes a thing, part of the servomechanism. Applying depth psychology to the impact of technology, Slater (38) carries the argument one step further. He believes that the Protestant ethic, as embodied in the authoritarian father, has been transferred to the harsh and punitive, albeit impersonal, qualities of the technocratic society from which we all suffer. Slater (38) cites the unquestioning attitude toward technical progress, regardless of its effects on human living, as a transfer of the punitive patriarch image to technology. Perhaps the greatest significance of the United States Congress voting against support for the development of a supersonic transport in 1971 is that it indicates an attitude of change. It shows that man can say "No" to that punishing father, technology, if he so wishes.

Superimposed on the technocratic society is what Mumford (32) calls the megamachine, a term for the power structure that controls it. The homogenization and absorption of polarized manifestations of dissident culture that rapidly occur through the mass media, via the advertising, news, and propaganda industries, are a particularly powerful part of the control mechanism. They neutralize and destroy by cannibalizing in the totalitarian fashion described by Marcuse (27) as a characteristic of present-day American culture. In the winter of 1971 numerous articles appeared in magazines and newspapers discussing the disappearance of the "hippies." They were purported either to have been reabsorbed into the culture or to have isolated themselves in rural communes. As Slater (38) indicates, because of the prevalent rootlessness, in America everybody is a nobody. One reaction against this anonymity by the more daring of the young was the adoption of unique hair styles and attire that produced maximum visibility. Those who originally accepted this mode also tended to leave home, jobs, and school, thus becoming street people. When large numbers of young Americans grew long hair and began buying bell bottoms at Sears Roebuck, the "hippy" became a nobody again. Those who overextended themselves had a brief flurry as "freaks" or "crazies" but found this stance too exhausting to maintain. To what extent the absorption phenomenon also modifies the culture is difficult to evaluate. What is apparent is that the power structure remains the same, and youth seem more apathetic in the early 1970s than they were during the 1960s.

It is important to understand that the counterculture functions to a significant extent as an antidote against alienation (37). The polarization that it represents is an attempt to reverse the processes of depersonalization and powerlessness fostered by the Establishment. Its rejection by the young as the epitome of "phoniness" is a reflection of the encouragement by advertising of magical and artificial expectations, the distortion of reality, and the pandering to infantile tastes. For example, the tendency of advertisers to sexualize objects such as cars to stimulate consumer appetite is often carried to an absurd, if not delusional, extreme. A recent issue of *Evergreen Review* (9) satirized this tendency by publishing a story of a man who had sexual congress with his automobile. What the young want are not substitute experiences with things but real relationships with people. Pornography and sexuality for its own sake undoubtedly have more meaning for those members of the parental generation who are object oriented than they do for the young who may seem rather casual in their sexual attitudes. For the most part, the young are interested in wholeness, not partial or distorted experience. Unlike their parents, they do not consider the "evils of the flesh" to be evil because they do not separate mind and body. Thus, for many of the young, sex apart from relationship is inconceivable. It is the parents who have not matured emotionally and who project upon the young their own sexual frustrations and tendencies to use people as objects.

If the adults are ambivalently attracted by the behavior of the young, by contrast, the young see very little in the adult world that turns them on. What adolescent children often perceive is an unhappy, guilt-ridden, weak father with coronary heart disease or hypertension who overextends himself during the week as a competitive business executive or professional, and who spends his weekends in a ceaseless round of joyless and compulsive social activity with a wife he barely tolerates. Mother, as counterpart, is often seen as a colorless nag who doesn't understand what went wrong with her life but insists, for highly moral reasons, that her children follow her example. The children who turn to drugs or run away from home are those who cannot identify with parental patterns which seem "crazy" to them. As Friedenberg (13) says, "Today's children aren't fighting their parents. They're abandoning them."

The rejection of family and Establishment values creates a serious dilemma for most young people. They are caught in a psychosocial double-bind which makes it almost impossible for them to solve the essential developmental tasks of adolescence. If there are no heroes with whom one can identify, and no jobs worth doing, how can one find out who one is and what one is capable of? As indicated by Erikson (7), the end of adolescence is signaled when the young person develops a sense of identity accompanied by a degree of competence in some area; when he develops the capacity for heterosexual relationship involving both sex and intimacy; and when he can begin to anticipate at some future date that he or she will become responsible for the succeeding generation. Keniston (20) feels that the inability to be committed, together with the extended period of youth permitted in an affluent society where commitment is not only not essential to survival but may actually be discouraged, are contributing to the development of a new, postadolescent life phase which he calls simply "youth." Margaret Mead (30) agrees that the central problem of today is commitment. What most youth experience is "nothingness" (33) and a fascination with the abyss which, like the reflection of Narcissus, keep them focused on the immediacy of their own personal experience. For them, "to be" and "to enjoy" are much more important than "to do" or "to prepare for," and incidentally, require much less effort and self-sacrifice.

Because the best of youth agree, according to McDonald (28), that full development as a person is possible only within a community, they tend to be contemptuous of whatever in the old culture seems to interfere with the development and experience of community. True community, among other things, involves the sharing of possessions. Things cannot be easily shared if they are considered to be scarce and are thereby overvalued, or if they are being used as projected parts of the self. The young are refusing to impoverish themselves by investing too much value in things; they are trying to stay whole by working only enough to survive, by being nomadic, and by assiduously avoiding the equation: Being equals Having. They see the parental generation as not only consumer-oriented but also using the acquisition of things to fill a void in themselves created by a deficiency in personal relationships and a lack of community. Because the predominant culture puts high value on being young and is also object oriented, parents, as they age, tend to view themselves as obsolescent and replaceable objects, as "things" of decreasing value. The high incidence of divorce in middle life represents to some extent that tendency to project the problem on the marital partner who can then be sloughed off for the novelty of a newer model.

Young people sense the self-depreciation in the older generation and usually take full advantage of its expression as parental guilt. The parents who grew up in the depression years often feel they can never do enough for their children. Relatively guilt-free, the children exploit, often contemptuously, whatever personal and material advantages accrue from this parental attitude. Having been brought up to feel that everything is there for them, many young people not only do not respect "private property" but are incapable of appreciating the amount of effort and degree of self-sacrifice made by the parental generation to produce and acquire the things they enjoy so casually. It is this lack of appreciation together with the envy of the old for the young that help to sour the relationship between the generations. When there is an inadequate intergenerational relationship, the less fortunate young frequently find themselves in an age-segregated peer group whose interest is in momentary gratification and antisocial behavior. The result, according to Bronfenbrenner (3), is "a generation which has not learned what compassion is, and compassion is essential for survival." Indeed, one might add, mutual compassion is necessary for survival; and it is the marked segregation by age group, social status, educational or economic level existing in most parts of America today that has led to increasing intolerance and alienation. Fortunately, the more idealistic of the young are trying to reverse the process by relating to people as people and not because of their appearance, labels, credentials, or possessions.

Whatever the factors are that have led to the other-directedness or externalization characteristic of our time, one effect is to make the world a stage upon which many people act out what in a previous era would have been an internalized conflict. Perhaps as both McLuhan (29) and Slater (38) imply, the collective unconscious has been made manifest in the man-made world. If impersonal technology to some extent represents the disembodiment of the fierce father, perhaps we can extend the metaphor to include the police and the military, those external limit-setters who become the embodiment of the hated and rejected conscience that no longer exists on the inside. With increasing population and decreasing intra-psychic control, a polarization is inevitable between the "crowd" and the "duly constituted officials." As the process evolves, the lack of internal controls by masses of the population is used to justify the increase of control on the part of impersonal government forces. The crowd can then be pacified or repressed, depending on the vicissitudes of the situation and the mood of the administration in power at the time. When the internalized, evaluative powers of the public are weak, the government can lie with impunity and not expect to be challenged in a way that threatens the power structure. Lack of awareness, a passive-receptive attitude, and a dissipation of moral energy resulting from externalization seem in combination to create the appalling apathy of the American public. The question is not why so many young people protest but rather why the majority of those over thirty seem so indifferent.

In 1973 it is estimated that the average American works for the government until May 20. Why is it then of so little concern how the government spends tax money? Why was there so little outrage against a government that waged an illegal and criminal war against the peoples of Southeast Asia? Why does the American public tolerate a nuclear arms buildup that represents not only a tragic waste of limited world resources, but which, if ever used, would destroy forever human life on earth? The inescapable conclusion is that the self-destructive urges of the older generation are centered in a government bureaucracy for which no one takes responsibility and which keeps, therefore, the destructiveness of the individual from being recognized. Perhaps the ultimate question is whether the young can help the old to become aware of and to take responsibility for their own suicidal and homicidal urges before the conditions for survival have been unalterably destroyed.

## Processes of Change

The manifestation of dialectical process in social phenomena is the tendency for the opposite to emerge. As more people have become externalized and automatized, a minority of self-actualizing young people, eager to develop their humanity to the fullest, have emerged to experiment with new life-styles which attempt to deal realistically with the problematical issues of community, involvement, and dependency—crucial issues, according to Slater (38), that have been too long ignored by the established culture. These young people form the core of the counterculture which has sprung into being as an alternative to the dehumanized Establishment mode. A survey made by *The New York Times* at the end of 1970 indicates that there are now at least 2,000 communal living situations in the United States alone (18).

An important consideration is to differentiate between what is response to and what is reaction against manifestations of social change. Sometimes the evolution and the revolution intermingle, and all opposites appear the same. The breakup of forms that began early in the century has undoubtedly been accelerated by technology but was not "caused" by it in any Aristotelian sense. What began in art and literature before the invention of electronic gadgetry is now a well-established psychic trend. For example, among young people there is a shift in emphasis away from cognitive to perceptual thinking, away from intellectual to perceptual experience. The change is both individual and cultural: individual, in that the young show to a lesser degree than their parents the processes of denying and repressing; cultural, in that the emphasis is on maximizing sensory input in the Now and reacting to it, rather than on actualizing the self from inner resources. There is a reaction against what seems too intellectual, scientific, objective, and a response to what is sensual, stimulating, and immediate. Habitual sensory stimulation, a kind of substitute feeding, creates a state of hunger and dependency which is addictive. The young person walking down the street with his transistor radio blaring is a familiar picture. Unquestionably a dependency on outer stimulation encourages the passive-receptive attitude and consumer orientation so well described by Fromm (14). There is also a close correspondence between the increasing emphasis on perceptual experience and the process of externalization, the so-called expansion of consciousness, and the increased awareness seen in the earlier maturation of children, in part attributable to television. The perceptual-cognitive shift suggests a primitivation of personality, a regression back to a state of greater dependency on the immediate environment, albeit manmade and artificial.

As McLuhan (29) indicates, man has built a nervous system outside of himself in the form of the communications media, but leased it to commercial interests; the medium is the message in the sense that the increased stimulation leads to earlier maturation, but the nature of the message tends to provoke a reaction against the culture. The young often reject the trivialities and false myths that bombard them from the media by an attitude of cynicism, coolness, and deliberate negativism that is all-encompassing. The combination of negativism and dependency on sensory input encourages a passivity which tends to inhibit action. Often the cultural rejection by the young ends in stasis; they feel helpless in taking action against what they oppose. The centrum from which effective action can be initiated has been obscured and weakened by the dependency on input. The result is reaction to input rather than action initiated from within, and an overwhelming sense of meaninglessness. The latter is proportional to the inaction. Many young people, unable to overcome their passivity and take effective action, find it difficult, if not impossible, to understand how meaning, like happiness, is a by-product of active involvement.

## Labeling the Mutant

De Chardin (6), Darlington (5), and others have indicated that man now has a primary role in his own evolution. How he will change to some extent depends upon how he wants to change and what he is willing to do or not do about it. Future planning requires a concern for environment, genetic integrity, population control, and other fundamental matters, but it also requires comprehensive consideration as to what kind of human being is most desirable. The titling of this section was done with tongue in cheek because, if anything characterizes his difference, the emerging man is a person who has done away with labels, categories, and hierarchies. Along with the perceptual-cognitive shift, there has been a mind-body integration that is experiential. Just as the new man does not split his knowledge into compartments, he does not categorize the body: he is ONE, not static, but part of an ever-changing cosmic process. Living with continuous change and increasing complexity reduces the new man to a state of elemental flexibility. Supremely adaptable, other-directed, externalized to the point of being inside out, unwilling to be subliminally, symbolically, and superficially manipulated by a multitude of stimuli that impinge indiscriminately, the new man is both sponge and stone, both malleable and immovable. He is indeed a paradox who cannot be categorized. Though his expediency might be condemned as psychopathic, his externalization described as infantile fixation or manifestation of identity diffusion, his behavior described as the acting out of what should be contained or internalized, it must finally be admitted that no contemporary conglomerate of sophisticated psychological labels can adequately encompass him. What he is remains to be experienced. His meaning can be interpreted only in the context of his world. Perhaps retribalized and living in one global village or, at least, megalopolis without family or marriage or church or school as we know it, he may, indeed, not be recognizable were we able, anachronisms that we are, to observe him a few years hence from the comfort and security of our time machine.

Unquestionably, there are many factors that go into the making of today's nonauthoritarian, protean (25), or externalized man. The hierarchies built by centuries of Aristotelian tradition are in shambles. We are witness to what Novak (33) calls "a civilization of massive dissolution." The past is gone; the present is a chaos of inappropriate remnants; the need for community is desperate. As Mumford (32) indicates, "In their unconscious, the young are living in a post-catastrophic world; and their conduct would be rational in terms of that world. Only by massing together and touching each other's bodies do they have any sense of security and continuity." To the young the cherished myths of their elders seem as cruel deception: rugged individualism, a competitiveness which exploits the other's disadvantage, production for profit. The young have reacted by forming their own culture, one based on immediacy, intimacy, and communal sharing. If acting out against what is is their mode, how can the older generation expect to appraise the behavior of the young with any accuracy by thinking in obsolete categories? Even the polar concepts of psychological man such as sickness and health have little meaning in the contemporary context. We must try to be all-inclusive, attempting to see the whole picture rather than limiting ourselves to the vocabulary of one specialty or one point of view.

As students of human development, we know that the past should not be forgotten. The cliché about those who forget the past being condemned to repeat it is as true to the individual life as it is to historical process. The repressed does return in disguised form and demand expression in a compulsively repetitive way until it is recognized for what it is. To deny the past is to be condemned to live a half-life, a life dominated by unrecognized demons. In their desperation to extricate themselves from what seems to be an unspeakable horror, the young often seem to be giving up the logos essential to enlightenment. It can only be hoped that by rejecting the old gods some of the new men will be more god-like themselves.

## Consequences of Historical Process

Although the breakdown of hierarchies appears to occur as a direct consequence of the breakup of traditional cultural values in a technological society, the American character has been predisposed from the beginning to level differences. What began in the seventeenth century as a rejection of

European values and culture has been reinforced in our time by social and geographical mobility, urban anonymity, mass-produced conformity, and a democratic ethos emphasizing equality, the effect of which is often to deny significant differences or, by recognizing them, to condemn them as abnormal or subversive. If American egalitarianism is highly intolerant, it has nevertheless abolished the master-slave relationship. Hopefully, the culture is moving away from anal fixation with its predominance of sadomasochistic relationships into an era of genitality and cooperative mutuality. Youthful contempt for competitive, exploitative, and authoritarian relationships has speeded the dissolution of master-slave relationships in the institutional world of church, school, and business, as well as in marriage and the family. Under the new rules, authority becomes synonymous with earned respect, and no president, priest, teacher, husband, or father is respected simply because of his role. He must earn the authority of his role by treating others, and especially the young, with equal respect, by being open and listening, and by being willing to acknowledge and share both weakness and strength.

The manifestations of hierarchical breakdown are widespread. One example is the recent popularity of a book, *The Student as Nigger*, by Jerry Farber (10), an essay that heralds the end of the traditional student-teacher relationship. No longer is it possible for higher authority to legislate change. Moreover, the days of children being lectured at, whether at home or in school, are over. The dialogue, the mutual exchange between equals, has replaced it. Student participation in school administration and curriculum development is another manifestation of the transition to equality, motivated to a significant extent by the oppressive atmosphere of most public secondary schools and large colleges. Dilution of family influence and a reaction against the overdetermined qualities of the small nuclear family by all the family members are two of the factors that have contributed to the decline of the traditional mother and father roles in the home. Many children in today's world bring themselves up, and such children are not about to subjugate themselves to teachers, priests, or politicians who may know less about the world than they do.

## The Family Context

Just as cultural imprinting occurs within the family, so does rejection of the culture begin within the family. The reduction of the modern family to a nucleus of mother, father, and children, where the spectrum of emotional demands of each on the other is intensified, has, under the influence of accelerated social change, brought the family to the breaking point. It is as if all of the reaction against parents, school, and past heritage is now focused in the family. The young reject totally what previous generations rejected selectively. For many, the rejection is only temporary; for others, the substitution of drugs, alcohol, or alternate life-styles leads in directions from which there is no return. The adolescent who runs away from home to avoid a suicidal depression may be reborn a new person, but one who can never again fit into the value system incorporated in parental expectations. He has become his own man, and if the parents are wise, they will welcome the opportunity to establish an entirely new and quite different relationship with him that will encourage a dialogue between the generations. Parents and children who respect each other can agree to disagree. Where there is no communication, there can only be disappointment, feelings of injury, and hostility.

It is important to make certain distinctions in evaluating the differences between generations. These distinctions can often be elucidated by asking the following questions.

To what extent do the children demonstrate by thought and behavior the consciously acknowledged values of their parents? Such values, though identical, may be expressed in such a unique way as to appear opposed or at least quite different from those of the parents. However, close examination may reveal their similarity. For example, radical political behavior by children often is a concrete manifestation of beliefs verbally espoused by the parents. Such parents may never have acted on their beliefs. Their children are, in a sense, acting for them. An extension of this situation is manifested by the increasing alienation from institutions exhibited by succeeding generations. If the parental generation is disenchanted or lukewarm about participation in a religious organization, for example, it is not unusual to find the next generation totally indifferent to it. Beginning rejection of a traditional form may appear in one generation; total rejection of it may be obvious in the succeeding generation.

To what extent do the children demonstrate by thought and action the unrecognized or unacknowledged values or behavior of their parents? Parents who follow the cocktail hour with aspirin, tranquilizers, and sleeping pills find themselves confronted with children who "do drugs." The children justify the smoking of marijuana as being less harmful than the alcohol which the parents use to reduce their tensions. In the sexual arena, the promiscuous daughter may be acting out the repressed sexual frustration of the mother. Consciously horrified at her daughter's libertine tendencies, the mother may refuse to see any resemblance between her own attitudes and her daughter's behavior.

To what extent is there a genuine polarization between generations? Where there is true rejection of parental values and a sincere attempt to establish an authentic life-style in contrast to the corrupt or unsatisfactory patterns followed by parents, it is possible to see the emergence of a new personality type and distinctive cultural values. If the new or counterculture can magnetize society by providing valid alternatives to the defective value systems and degenerate life patterns of previous generations, perhaps the phoenix can rise from the ashes. A more modest expectation might be that the third generation in succession will represent a balance between the extreme manifestations of the present parental and children's generations. If parents of the depression have overworked and overemphasized security and acquisition of goods to the detriment of their development as whole people, capable of loving and sharing, their children have often "thrown out the baby with the bath water" by refusing to come to terms with the cultural heritage of the past and by refusing to establish and work toward any long-term goals. Perhaps the third generation will be able to live in the present while coming to terms with both past and future. Selective acceptance of contributions from the past are essential to the establishment of competence and identity in the present, both prerequisites for anticipating and preparing without undue fear for a viable future.

Historical trends and cultural variants certainly affect the patterns seen in today's youth, but there is also the more personal intrafamily dynamics which exert a crucial influence. Certain generalizations seem justified from clinical observation. For example, the parental generation, referring to those born and raised prior to World War II, can, at least among the middle-class white population, be characterized as instinctually repressed. Aside from stilted "birds and bees" explanations mouthed to young children, most parents from such families hardly ever openly discuss sexual matters. They do not accept sexual feelings and behavior as something to be integrated into everyday life. As a consequence, such parents are frequently uncomfortable in displaying either verbal or physical affection between each other or with their children, at least after the children have passed the age of early childhood. There is an isolation of feeling manifested by psychic aloofness and stiffness of body posture. In such families, the use of Anglo-Saxon terms to express anger or to describe bodily functions is taboo, with the result that an atmosphere is established which inhibits the direct expression of feelings, especially angry or sexual ones. As a consequence, conflicts between family members are often not worked through to resolution even when they are recognized and acknowledged intellectually. More commonly in the repressed family, there is an ongoing process of denying conflict, the properly tranquil exterior concealing the demonic cauldron within.

If it is accurate to characterize such parents as repressed and alienated from feelings, the most characteristic reactive pattern in their children seems to be depressive. The children feel deeply the lack of affectual response in those who have reared them, often mirroring the repressed feelings of their parents. A common clinical entity is the suicidal adolescent girl with an unresolved dependency tie to a menopausal mother. Such a mother, cold and without affect, might appropriately be depressed; yet it is her daughter who feels for her. In family interviews mother and daughter can often be observed sitting closely together with daughter crying while other siblings and father sit in a more detached manner elsewhere in the room. Often repressed parents have forgotten the turbulence of their own adolescence and the circumstances of their own adolescent marriage, the problems of which may never have been acknowledged, let alone resolved. Such parents are unable to cope with the upsurge of feelings, the need for free expression, experimentation, and rebellion manifested by their adolescent children. Frequently, a critical point in their marriage was reached shortly after the birth of the children or when more than one sibling was in infancy. At such times in the history of many families the parents were on the verge of splitting up, with one parent, most commonly the father, having an affair. In retrospect it appears that the mother in such families may have been depressed at a critical time in the development of some of her children. The recurrence of this kind of history seems important in evaluating how a depressive syndrome develops in many adolescents today. There is not only the reaction to repressed parents, the pressures of a highly competitive school program, and what seems to them an oppressive cultural situation in a chaotic historical time, but also the scarring which has resulted from a relative degree of maternal deprivation early in life. Such adolescents often feel empty and pursue a frantic pattern of drug taking, diverse sexual experiences, frequent runaway episodes, etc. Although some of this behavior may be an attempt to deal with ontological anxiety by the active search for meaningful experience, significant relationships, etc., frequently such behavior seems to function as an attempt to overcome depressive feelings in an active way, by getting out and finding substitute satisfactions in the world at large. It is a kind of replacement therapy.

It is frequently seen in clinical practice, as previously mentioned, among adolescent girls who make suicidal attempts, that they are bound to mother in a state of unresolved ambivalence. It is this dependency which prevents them from actively rebelling and, if need be, leaving home to become actively involved with peers and others in ways necessary for their continued growth and development. Such girls are caught in a double-bind, an ambivalent pregenital relationship with mother. For various reasons, they have been unable to move from mother love to father love, to accept and work through an active oedipal situation where the love of father sustains them while they reject mother, becoming, thereby, able to emancipate themselves, one parent at a time, from the family. After such girls have been treated for the medical emergency following a suicide attempt and after the shifts in family dynamics that follow a suicidal attempt have had their effect, it is often possible to work in therapy with them toward emancipation from mother. They may then move into a more active problem-solving position in which they can begin relating to father and/or peers more satisfactorily, feeling less inundated by the intense, internalized, perfectionistic demands as well as the pressures for academic performance imposed externally by the school system, etc.

A generalization that can be made from clinical observations of this kind is that adolescents who are bound in an apparently insoluble dependency conflict with parents tend to become depressed and suicidal. Those who are able to resolve problems more actively may take flight from the family as an avoidance of depressive feelings. If such adolescents remain within the family, the anger is internalized and they become depressed. Upon fleeing from the family they can find substitutes for parental dependency through drugs, supportive peer relationships, sexual experiences, etc. Usually the active process of seeking out satisfactions relieves the overt depressive syndrome by enabling greater energy discharge in a situation where projection and acting out of conflicts provide relief of symptoms by externalization.

Another variation is observed in those family situations where the adolescent boy or girl continues within the family but refuses to fit into the repressive and overly restrictive patterns prescribed by the parents. Such adolescents are often accused of living in constant defiance of parental rules and regulations. They often do not appear to be doing anything that is particularly destructive to themselves but because they keep irregular hours, often consort with companions not acceptable to the parents, and from time to time resort to drug taking, they are subject to intense and constant hostile criticism from parents. Such adolescents who might have originally taken flight because of depressive feelings find themselves with a problem of negative self-image and low self-esteem, the latter being reinforced by constant criticism from the parents. These are the adolescents who are never able under any circumstances to satisfy parental demands. The reason is of course that the demands are unreasonable and unrealistic and the force behind them is motivated by unrecognized feelings of the parents, such as injured narcissism because the child is not enough like them or simply an unwillingness to let go, to let the adolescent grow up and find himself in his own way. Such parents are often envious of the adolescent, his seeming freedom and sexual powers. The parental reaction is to force such a person into an infantile role and to reinforce a pattern of deprivation where very little happens except homework, school routine that is strictly planned, and parentally approved social relationships that offer little gratification or self-determination. It would be redundant to say that such parents have been unable to recognize that their children have a right to determine their own lives. Such parents often experience their children as extensions of themselves or objects for projection. Consequently they consider all of the child's activities as a reflection of themselves. Because of their own repressions, indicated by shame, guilt, and embarrassment, they often express more concern for "what the neighbors think," a superego projection resulting from too much internalization, than for what is reasonable and realistic behavior on the part of adolescent children in the process of growing up.

The increased turbulence and rebellion of adolescent children is reflected in their cry for more freedom at a time when parents feel they are being extremely lenient. Although part of the struggle is related to the individuation process, another element is focused on different attitudes toward time and mobility. Parents complain that the children will not check in or call to let them know where they are. Young people feel their whereabouts are unpredictable and subject to change depending on what friends they meet, what they decide to do on the impulse of the moment, etc. Rules about the time to return home and what is an appropriate bedtime are even more controversial. Granted that the parent's concern about the young person's whereabouts is proportional to his ambivalence toward the child and to the degree that undesirable parental fantasies are projected on the child, the argument about time has other determinants. Whereas parents have been conditioned to view the day as a time to work and play and night as a time to sleep, the children of the electric age do not make this distinction. Because they do not rigidly associate certain functions with time of day, they often have difficulty in regulating their lives. Parents see the new patterns as disruptive, and often there is no compromise except for the young person to go elsewhere to live. It can be suspected that the pressures on young people, especially stimulus overload, may be partly responsible for their nocturnal alertness. Many young people of high school age speak of the night as the only time they can be quiet and alone. Taking a solitary walk at three A.M. may not indicate either delinquent tendencies or emotional pathology in an adolescent; on the contrary, it may be his way of finding himself apart from others.

The rejection by young people of the depersonalized, object-oriented world accepted by the parents has been previously emphasized. Because object-oriented parents frequently treat people as objects, including their own children, the children usually react with an intensity occasioned by the extent to which their humanity has been violated by the parents, teachers, and other adult figures in their environment. The refusal of the contemporary adolescent to dress respectably according to parental standards, which usually means in expensive clothing, is one example of the contempt for surface values and affluence. With monotonous unanimity, today's high school student would rather dress in blue jeans and what in a previous generation might be considered working clothes than display the status symbols provided by the parents. Although the old guard may feel that the abolition of dress codes has permitted the high school population to regress, it has at the same time enabled adolescents to express their feelings about themselves and the society in which they live through the clothes they wear. The low self-esteem, student-as-nigger status which most of them feel is expressed by the clothing they choose (10). Clinical observation confirms that when an adolescent begins to develop a stable self-image and overcome the self-derogation which has been reinforced by overly critical parents, then he frequently begins to dress in a more colorful and attractive manner. To a significant extent the choice of clothing reflects self-esteem and when seen in perspective provides additional evidence that repressed parents produce depressed children.

## Treatment Possibilities

Meaning is a function of internalized experience. When there is fixation to a state of externalization, there is neither concern about meaning nor a reflective evaluation of experience. The person who is concerned with meaning is autonomous and internalized. Relatively speaking, the externalized man does not learn from experience since he lacks the evaluative equipment that develops as a result of internalizing images, concepts, and values. According to Frankenstein (11), two important causative factors in externalization are a lack of closeness to parents and the impersonal qualities of the educational climate. Both factors have implications for therapy.

If externalized man is heteronomous, the success of individual therapy will depend to a large extent on the personal relationship with a strong person who does not rely on technique alone and who can assume responsibility as necessary over the person's life outside of the therapy hours. Such a person would seem to be the most effective therapist for the externalized man. A nondirective and anonymous therapist who has no actual control over the person's life outside of therapy would be viewed as weak and ineffective. The psychosocial dynamics of the new man requires a reassessment of old therapeutic approaches which tend to see the "patient" as an isolated entity. The emergent personality is inextricably involved with what is outside of him, and does not respond well to limited approaches which depend for their success on the working through of intrapsychic conflicts. If it exists, the "cure" for externalization and the resultant heteronomy does not lie in a limited, permissive relationship, one which repeats the parental patterns; nor can it occur within the context of a distant relationship to absolute authority which is a historically more archaic mode. However, it does involve a concern for total environment of which the therapist is a part. Therapy conducted in a rap center, part of a newly developing therapeutic milieu for young people, may illustrate the direction in which psychotherapy must evolve to remain viable in today's world (40). Laing's (16) experience with Kingsley Hall, a residential treatment center in which the therapists themselves lived on an equal basis with the patients, has served as a model for some of the developing therapeutic approaches now being used in the United States. The experience of Synanon (44) in the treatment of drug addiction by providing total environmental control in which there is no escape from the consequences of one's actions or inactions may be the most practical model for the therapy of the externalized or environmentally dependent man that is now available. Those who do not consider themselves emotionally disturbed increasingly are seeking out "growth centers" like Esalen (8), a special kind of total environmental approach, for self-exploration and integrative experience. Perhaps both Synanon and Esalen represent highly sophisticated, contemporary versions of the religious retreat, a place apart from the world where personal growth and self-renewal are possible.

In spite of all other considerations young people today need ongoing relationships with adults whom they respect and with whom they can communicate. When a relationship is therapeutic, there is both mutual respect and mutual expectation. Lederer (24) makes the distinction between analytic therapy, which is essentially accepting and uncritical, and anabolic therapy, which is essentially demanding and paternal. Analytic therapy, a maternal approach, may be able to deal with problems that have their root in early childhood, but anabolic therapy is more appropriate for conditions arising during adolescence, when the need for paternal guidance is greatest. As Lederer (24) indicates, the anabolic therapist to some extent becomes a teacher, helping the young person to find an aim in life. If the young person can identify with the therapist, the process of internalizing images, concepts, and values can progress until some degree of autonomy is possible. Such an approach might be labeled "replacement therapy" or even "corrective emotional experience," since, to some degree, an attempt would be made to make up for what had been absent in the person's earlier life, namely a close relationship to a benevolent father whom the child feels can comfortably control his world. As with imprinting, experiences missed at critical periods but provided later are somewhat artificial at best and only partially effective. However, as Blos (2) has discovered, the adolescent usually has a second chance to individuate, a phenomenon that provides tremendous opportunities for resolution and growth.

It is apparent that young people today can live with much less structure than their elders. However, the breakdown of hierarchical structure and authority relationships occasioned by rapid social change does pose a threat to many who are in positions of power. Their reaction to institutional breakdown is often to resort to measures of increased control. In one sense, society in its institutional aspects provides on the outside what is lacking on the inside of individuals. Anarchy might work very well in a society of internalized people; however, when the population is largely externalized, anarchy is chaos. When increased control, the opposite of anarchy, develops as a reaction to social breakdown in a capitalistic democracy, it usually evolves into the phenomenon called fascism, often taking the form of military dictatorship. As a social mechanism for righting a society which has turned itself inside out, fascism is defective because it attempts to rigidly fixate what is already essentially static, thus opposing all change. When a problem develops from either too much or too little, any therapeutic endeavor must attempt to withdraw the excess and provide the missing ingredients. When the condition combines excess with deficiency, the paradoxical problems of instigating change are even more subtle.

## Concluding Remarks

I used the term psychosocial dynamics in the title of this chapter in an attempt to encompass three concepts that seem important in understanding many of the phenomena observed in today's youth. However, the danger in formulating any categorical sequence is that it may lead not only to fragmentary thinking but also to an overemphasis on the pathological aspects of processes that may be temporary, developmental, or perhaps moving toward some kind of progressive resolution. Alienation, anomie, and externalization are terms which describe either states of being or processes; they do not exist as separate entities. Neither existence nor essence, they are higher-order generalizations which have a relative and descriptive intent that is neither all-inclusive nor exclusive. Hopefully, they help to describe important aspects of that field or complex context in which many young people today have their being. Their existence apart from the totality of life processes is purely fictional.

By its simplest definition, alienation can be considered as estrangement from prevalent values and social processes, a state of being out of tune with the times, to mouth a cliché. According to Pappenheim (26), it can be understood only when it is considered as a part of the social situation as a whole. Such estrangement does involve a splitting between self and other and a restriction of positive affective response, which, by engendering frustration, may intensify negative reaction, i.e., oppositional or rebellious behavior. It can be differentiated from its counterpart, the schizoid process, by its point of origin and by the fact that the capacity for total response still exists when external circumstances are favorable. Unlike the splitting in the schizoid process which is intrapsychic and between various aspects of the self, the restrictions leading to alienation are in the environmental field. Under altered circumstances, the alienated person can respond with greater spontaneity and in a more wholistic way; the schizoid cannot. Anomie, like alienation, is a state of being. The anomic state is that of rootlessness and is characterized by a restless, chronic dissatisfaction. Kerouac's novel *On the Road* (21) is perhaps the most popular fictional account of this phenomenon among today's youth. The young person who runs away from home to avoid his own depression and to escape the oppressiveness of repressive parents may pass into the anomic state and become a chronic wanderer, constantly searching for his ideal place but never finding it. The older generation too, through frequent relocations that leave them bereft of old friends and relatives, may feel chronic dissatisfaction in every location, despite all outward manifestations of comfort and success. If the parental generation moves from split-level trap to split-level trap, the alienated young person, by contrast, may be on the road to finding roots. A recent historical trend is for young people who escape from the cities and suburbs to find their place in a rural commune, farm or a forestry station. The movement away from the crowded, polluted, and stifling urban environment usually also leads away from alienation and back to the natural world where elemental values can be concretized in the routines of primitive, day-to-day country living. If the anomic Odyssey of youth achieves its purpose, it may not only resolve the alienated state but also replace the externalizing tendencies of modern life with a balance and synthesis between the inner and the outer man. The shared intimacy of the commune, if relatively free from conflict and if accompanied by the time and space for inner development, may be a way of restoration, a way of leaving behind the alienation, anomie, and excessive externalization characteristic of complex city living.

A comprehensive phenomenology of youth today requires a synthesis, a bringing together of pertinent thinking from all of the social sciences, philosophy, and literature. Additionally, as Margaret Mead (30) says, "The future is now," and we must be willing to learn from our children. It is apparent that they are attempting to resist the diseases of alienation embodied in what Lewis Mumford (32) calls the megamachine or the "Pentagon of Power." Because the parental generation is hung up in a state of isolated individualism characterized by the obsolescent nation-state, the children who are living in what McLuhan (29) calls "one global village" will burn flags, draft cards, and the Bank of America to inform us of the dangerous irrelevancy of established values. They will take off their clothes to reveal our stuffiness, they will live in poverty to shame our wealth, and they will eat simple food as an antidote to the plastic, additive-filled diet we have fed them in our mass-produced, assembly-line, and now computerized society. Our greatest hope, as always, is in the best of our youth. We must not only listen to them, but also try to learn from them.

# 9

## Cultural Disadvantage:
## A Psychosocial Phenomenon

THOMAS J. EDWARDS, PH.D.

There has recently developed a flurry of concern about the adjustment problems of the so-called culturally disadvantaged segment of our society. Why? Is this a new horde of barbarians that has suddenly loomed over the horizons of our apathy and now threatens to annihilate us? Is this possibly a problem that has been in existence for a long time but one that we simply haven't bothered to attend to? Are we suddenly activated by the psychology of crisis? Or has our society finally matured to the point of being able genuinely to feel both compassion and objective concern about those among its citizens whose psychic structure is often irreparably marred by their rejection status?

Exclusion of significant numbers within our society has an unquestionably deleterious effect upon both those who are excluded and those who exclude. This phenomenon of exclusion has created various types and degrees of psychic scar tissue, the eradication of which has now become a social imperative.

### Cultural Isolation and Ego Formation

Certain groups within our society have a disproportionately high representation within the disadvantaged population. These groups tend to be identifiable either because of ethnic visibility or because of distinctive last names. This identifiability has made it fairly easy for the in-group majority to isolate the culturally or ethnically different in keeping with what has been referred to as "attitudinal apartheid" that is still prevalent in this country (3).

Children develop self-concepts within a social context that involves not only the primary family group and a bit later the peer group, but also the greater society, from which they learn how to feel about themselves. Awareness of ethnic differences in status begins to develop even at the preschool level (7) and is reinforced by a myriad of subsequent experiences. This author recalls, for example, being required to learn the following rhyme as a first grader:

> Dirty hands are such a fright,
> See, I wash mine clean and *white*.

> Mother says that it's quite right
> To wash them morning, noon, and night.

But non-Caucasian children cannot wash their hands "clean and white." We were also told in elementary school social studies classes that "our Pilgrim forefathers landed on the Plymouth Rock." Whose forefathers? How do black children or American Indian children or children from Spanish-speaking backgrounds react to the apparent fact that our curricula are almost exclusively Caucasian Anglo-Saxon in their orientation? For many generations our communications media have supplemented our curricula in distorting the self-concepts or the total psychic development of the non-Caucasian children who move into adulthood with severe marks of oppression (7). Tonto, the Indian, and Stepenfetchit, the black comic, are illustrations of sterotypic reinforcements of the negative self-images that are the legacy of children who grow up isolated in ethnocultural cocoons. And the effects are often both devastating and irreversible (1, 3, 5, 6, 8, 9, 12, 13, 14).

Probably black Americans are studied most exhaustively and held up as "Exhibit A" in terms of damaged self-concepts because they are socially visible and therefore find it much more difficult than most other groups to escape the psychic blows of racism. Hence, throughout Black America we might find in somewhat exaggerated form helpful indices of psychological trauma, the counterparts of which exist possibly to a lesser degree within all segments of the American population that are excluded and isolated because of ethnic or cultural difference.

Awareness of significant social difference develops at an early age and tends to persist. For example, Goodman made a study of racial awareness in young children of preschool age and found "unmistakable" signs of bigotry on the part of white children and an awareness on the part of black children that they were "marked" (5). Relative to this observation, Grier and Cobbs assert that "for black and white alike, the air of this nation is perfused with the idea of white supremacy and everyone grows to manhood under this influence" (6).

In his *Education in Depressed Areas*, Passow has compiled the writings of seventeen nationally known educators who detail the devastating effects of cultural deprivation and isolation upon the learning process (10). These writings make it eminently clear that these cultural isolates achieve markedly below their innate learning capacities, that ego impairment figures prominently among the several causes of this underachievement, and that a true assessment of their intellectual capacities is practically impossible because lack of stimulation tends to impair intellectual functioning.

In the recent past there has been a tendency on the part of rejected minority groups to turn their backs on both their physical and cultural heritage and make desperate efforts to identify with the majority group.

First-generation Americans of non-Anglo-Saxon origin have in many cases refused to learn the language of their parents. Millions have been spent by black Americans in their attempts to bleach their skins and straighten their hair. As a case in point, an art teacher who was a member of a workshop conducted by this writer reported that she had had a class of black children draw themselves first as they felt they appeared and then later as they wished they appeared. There was a tragically persistent tendency for them to portray themselves as being much more Caucasoid in their later wish-fulfillment drawings. They wanted to escape the stigma of their Negroid features with their attendant psychic pain and damage to their self-concept.

Kardiner and Ovesey (7) and Grier and Cobbs (6) cite numerous case histories that reflect the psychic devastation wrought by rejection, isolation, and cultural deprivation. This devastation is often characterized intrapsychically by self-hatred, marked feelings of inferiority, rage reactions, and minority paranoia. Currently on the American scene there is widespread evidence on the part of black citizens of "spontaneous psychological revolution," a phenomenon that is quite obviously a reaction against the psychic burdens that have been borne by blacks since the beginnings of United States history. Self-hatred is being replaced by the "black-is-beautiful" assertion; feelings of inferiority are being replaced by the chants of "black power!"; and minority paranoia is being acted out in various types of self-assertion in the form of both violent and nonviolent protest, rather than being held seething inside.

There are those who contend that the psychological revolution of rejected minorities is out of proportion to the realities of present-day America's attitudinal climate. This is a matter for further speculation and debate. The fact remains that this revolution represents reactions against psychic trauma and damaged self-concepts resulting from exclusion, deprivation, and outright rejection. If these reactions are exaggerated, they may have to be tolerated until the time that America's attitudinal climate changes and both majority and minority psychological equilibrium become a reality.

A significant question remains unanswered: Can the acting out against frustrated psychosocial expression ameliorate the psychic condition of oppressed minorities? Or is there to remain psychic scar tissue that can only disappear with the coming of new generations who from birth are essentially free from such frustration? At this point, this remains a moot question.

Cultural disadvantage is not only the result of physical isolation but, and probably far more significantly, a product of psychological isolation of a sort that underscores implied genetic and status inferiority. The deleterious effects of psychic damage wrought upon the psychosocial isolate manifest themselves in depressed levels of aspiration, intelligence that is virtually inaccessible to present-day measuring instruments, impaired cognitive functioning, severely limited motivation, and a low achievement expectancy level both in school and in the job arena. The effects of this psychosocial isolation upon society are wasted manpower and social disruption.

## Cultural Shock of the Disadvantaged and Social Disruption

It is a truism that economically and culturally depressed environments contain within themselves numerous conditions that militate against an optimal physical, emotional, and cognitive development. However, to these internal conditions must be added the cultural shock experienced when one dares to venture outside of his safe sociocultural cocoon.

A culturally isolated environment tends in many ways to be a protective one. Contrasts among its inhabitants are likely not to be very marked and customs are relatively uniform, understood, and accepted. Food preferences, social amenities, and language, for example, are essentially the same from family to family. However, this comfortable familiarity gives way to often rather severe and traumatizing cultural shock when one moves out to seek greener pastures. If there is a mass migration of numbers of people from one environment to a sharply contrasting one, ethnocultural conflict and even psychosocial disruption are likely to ensue (13).

Millions of black Americans migrated north in search of greener pastures. They were disappointed that economic opportunities were not as they had anticipated. They were discouraged when they were herded into black ghettos with woefully inadequate housing, even when they were economically able to afford something better. They were embittered by their being barred from many kinds of jobs or denied admission into trade unions.

Black Americans also realized that their dialect of American English was regarded as substandard, comical, and a badge of intellectual inferiority. They realized, too, that general customs, food preferences, and patterns of family life were different. In short, there was severely debilitating ethnocultural conflict. The various forms of discrimination that were leveled against them generated real feelings of persecution. The white man became the oppression stimulus and inevitable stimulus generalization gave rise to the kind of minority paranoia mentioned previously, a syndrome that was destined to distort the black man's perceptions of his own psychological life space (1, 2, 5, 6, 7).

White America reacted to this alien ethnocultural body of blacks in its midst by imposing numerous complicated controls and restrictions. The blacks were culturally different and socially visible. Black America reacted initially with disappointment and seething resignation. However, a series of events occurred against the background of justified indignation and of minority paranoia that suddenly and dramatically changed the black man's self-concept as a powerless social nonentity and unleased black rage (6, 8).

Hence, we see that transplanted cultural isolates experience a kind of cultural shock that can lead to extensive and explosive psychosocial disruption. This can be seen most dramatically in the case of the black American, since he is a large minority and is socially visible. His case is also especially dramatic because the history of his existence in America and the white man's special feelings toward the slave and toward the ex-slave created a special kind of psychic devastation (6). It would unquestionably be revealing to compare the American Indian with the American black in terms of cultural isolation, cultural shock, ethnic conflict, and a possible eventual psychosocial disruption leading to a Red Power movement. The traumata suffered by the Indian parallel in many ways those experienced by the black American and one might therefore predict similarities both in psychic disorder and in ways of coping with ethnocultural conflict.

## *Motivation, Achievement Expectancy, and Level of Aspiration*

One characteristic that is very frequently noted regarding the culturally different disadvantaged student is his underachievement. It is generally held that native intellectual capacity is distributed equally among all ethnic groups. If this be a tenable assumption, why then do we find this disproportionately high degree of underachievement among students from certain atypical cultural backgrounds?

This writer is in complete agreement with Forshay's position that "simplistic answers to the question of the encouragement of bright students are, in the main, inadequate" (12). It is posited here, however, that motivation, achievement expectancy, and level of aspiration are interacting variables in the lives of disadvantaged children that affect profoundly their achievement in school and beyond. To be sure, there are other such variables, some of which will be discussed subsequently.

As was mentioned previously, one very crucial problem seems to be this: growing up with the feeling of being a social outcast has a damaging effect upon ego formation. The self-concept that results may seriously affect motivation, depress one's level of aspiration significantly, and create underachievement.

Motivation to achieve a goal derives much of its power both from the attractiveness and accessibility of that goal and from the organism's perception of his own ability to achieve the goal. Students from culturally disadvantaged backgrounds frequently have a history of failure so intensive that they early become psychological drop-outs, both from school and society. If one fails frequently enough, he eventually comes to expect failure. This depressed achievement-expectancy level is one aspect of damaged motivation: "If I'm convinced that I cannot achieve, then I'll not even bother trying" is the feeling of the culturally disadvantaged learner. This negative concept of self as a nonachiever also has obvious effects upon goal-setting behavior related to level of aspiration: "Why should I even bother to set immediate or long-range goals if I know that I won't be able to achieve these goals? I'll just settle for mediocrity. The hell with trying!"

Repeated emphasis is placed by educators and social psychologists upon the immediate home environment and the family structure as causative conditions affecting the motivation, aspiration, and achievement of disadvantaged children. These are undeniably influential. However, it cannot be held that without ideal stimulation from the home a child is destined to be an underachiever. An interesting phenomenon is the fact that despite numerous negative factors in the experiential backgrounds of certain persons, they achieve far beyond what might have been predicted and "make it." Elsewhere this writer has suggested that this phenomenon of the "cultural breakout" should be studied carefully in order to identify a cluster of factors that typify this kind of personality. This might be instructive in revealing types of persons or types of fortuitous events in the lives of these "breakouts" that alter their motivation, their achievement-expectancy level, their level of aspiration, and possibly their total self-concept, and lead ultimately to what appears to be spontaneous acculturation.

An example of extrafamilial influence in altering the self-concept and raising the sights of disadvantaged youth is Big Brothers of America. This nationwide organization identifies a fatherless boy within a given community and pairs him with a responsible adult male who functions as a "big brother" or a father surrogate. In this kind of a relationship, the boy learns a greater sense of personal worth, identifies closely with his big brother as model and friend, and begins to modify his self-concept. In addition, his experiences—both direct and vicarious—begin to expand, his verbal facility develops, his fund of general information increases, his coping skills diversify, his motivation to achieve grows, and his level of aspiration rises. All of this results in a greater sense of personal worth because somebody of significance really cares. It is a wonder that the federal government has not given massive support to an organization like Big Brothers of America that goes so effectively to the psychological core of a problem of disadvantage stemming from familial disruption.

The newly created organization IN (Interested Negroes) is another example of a direct, frontal attack on the problems of motivation, achievement expectancy, and level of aspiration. Successful Negroes in a variety of service and professional occupations have day-long sessions with black high school youths during which they chat informally about themselves and their work; they explain what they had to go through in order to achieve; and these high school youths get firsthand, on-the-job glimpses of what people like themselves are achieving. This kind of direct contact with a concerned person provides many insights into the vocational world for these students and gives them realistic bases from which to raise their level of aspiration.

Still another type of extrafamilial influence on disadvantaged youths is the direct, one-to-one contact with a concerned adult that is nonorganizational. In countless instances a fortuitous relationship develops between a disadvantaged youth and an older person and there results a significant, positively modified self-concept that produces accelerated achievement and raised sights. As a teen-ager this writer experienced this type of concern from an employer for whom he worked as a houseboy and gardener, and this involvement has persisted even to the present.

Despite the fact that disadvantaged youths need to know that people from ethnic and cultural backgrounds similar to their own have succeeded, it is not a *sine qua non* that this ethnocultural identity be present in all cases. More and more it seems that the concern, encouragement, and specific guidance of an interested adult is the crucial factor, rather than his ethnic or cultural origins. It is apparently the presence of effective mediation (4) that reverses the negative psychological effects of psychosocial disadvantage and this can be done quite often by a variety of types of nonfamilial "adjuvant mediators."

In assessing the achievement potential of youths from disadvantaged backgrounds, it is essential to look carefully at experiential factors within the family, in the school situation, and within the general society that come to bear in the formulation of a child's self-concept and ego strength. These are the factors that deserve prime consideration in any kind of psychological assessment as well as in any program of clinical or environmental therapy.

Despite the low level of motivation that has depressed levels of aspiration of disadvantaged groups in the past, there is currently a trend in the other direction. Recent events have resulted in these groups making reassessment of their status within society, of their own personal worth, and of their potential for self-determination. This reassessment of self appears to be contagious and is spreading throughout various ethnic and cultural minorities. The increased ego strength that has resulted in much greater self-assertion has, in turn, prodded America toward the development of a variety of educational and vocational thrusts. The possibility of academic achievement and occupational security appears to the disadvantaged to be more and more a reality. Hence it might be tenable to predict that America's current *Zeitgeist* will ameliorate much which in the recent past has created within these minorities thwarted ego development and a sense of futility.

## Cognitive Functioning among Cultural Isolates

There is currently considerable speculation among psychologists and educators regarding the cognitive functioning of culturally different and disadvantaged youths. The point is often made that experiential and language deprivation conspire against and severely limit the cognitive development of such youths. This may well be true. However, an alternative point of view might be this: children who grow up in cultures that diverge significantly from so-called standard American culture have experiences and a communication system that determine the direction of their cognitive development, rather than the degree. Within their own cultural cocoons they develop effective coping skills and adjust adequately. However, when they are measured against criteria that are inappropriate and irrelevant to their own special environments, they seem to demonstrate inadequate cognitive functioning.

There is a certain communality of experiences typical of the normally advantaged child. With adequate mediation, a child develops from these experiences a reasonably adequate repertoire of concepts (1). These concepts provide the prerequisite conceptual elements or building blocks necessary for the acquisition of the new concepts that comprise our typical school curriculum. The learning of Standard American English is the linguistic dimension of a child's total development as he readies himself for a barrage of psychological and educational testing and for participation in the educative process.

The culturally different child may appear to be cognitively different because of essential differences in experience, degree, and kind of mediation, repertoire of concepts, and the phonology and patterning of his language. It might follow logically that the kinds of testing instruments and our criteria for adequate development are totally irrelevant to the developmental demands of the culturally different child. His cultural difference may only put him at a disadvantage when he is required to make an intercultural leap for which nothing has prepared him.

The crucial factor is this: Our meager instruments are inadequate in our attempts to assess the intellectual capacity or the cognitive functioning of culturally different children. We must assume a normal distribution of mental ability within this group and then set about to supplement what they have already learned with experiences, concepts, and language learnings that will facilitate their cultural transition and allow them to become cultural straddlers (2). Beyond this, we must help this transition to take place in a setting that will enhance rather than devastate their self-concept and motivation.

Over a three-year period, this writer studied in depth the cognitive functioning, the case history data, and specific learning deficiencies of a twelve-year-old, illiterate, Mississippi-born Negro boy. In addition, an attempt was made to reverse the effects of very severe cultural deprivation and isolation. His was the classic case of the disadvantaged youth within our society.

As was mentioned here previously, intelligence tests tend not to "get at" the true learning potential of cultural isolates. This was the case with this boy, whose "measured IQ" was in the sixties. After a short period of time spent working with this boy and observing his cognitive functioning carefully, it became apparent that his intelligence had been seriously underestimated and that his assignment to a special class for the mentally retarded was an error.

During this three-year period of working with him, constant diagnosis en route was practiced. Both attitudinal and academic problem areas were identified and attempts were made immediately to effect more positive adjustment. Experiences, concepts, language facility, and expanded cognitive power were all goals within his program and undergirding these goals was a relationship that reflected constant concern.

The result of this intensive attempt to reverse the effects of his cultural deprivation was that he could no longer be retained in the special class. He moved successfully through junior and senior high school with a new sense of self, a new and higher achievement-expectancy level, and with goal-setting behavior that attested to a considerably higher level of aspiration. His case underscores the reversibility of sociocultural disadvantage.

Although it can be demonstrated that significant and positive changes can be effected in the academic and vocational lives of persons who have been severely disadvantaged for a number of years, it is the firm belief of this writer that there remains inevitable residual scar tissue on the personality and on the functioning of the sensorium of a person who has remained disadvantaged past the early formative years. It would follow logically, then, that concerted efforts should be directed toward the preschool and early elementary years in order to effect maximal enhancement of cognitive functioning and of self-concept.

## Cultural Difference and Differential Superego Development

A child's superego development takes place within and in terms of the special cultural milieu that spawns him. There is nothing absolute about the values, the customs, or the ethics that figure in the formation of his superego. Within his family and peer group there is a fairly well codified system of ethics; attitudes toward noise and order and social amenities tend to be relatively consistent within a given culture; sex practices and attitudes regarding marriage, family, and home are fairly well agreed upon; and goals worth pursuing are shared communally. A child adjusts to these aspects of his culture, learns them, assimilates them, and develops an ego capable of behaving within the cultural framework that provides the substance of his superego.

Cultural difference and conflict become problems partially because different cultures create different systems in accordance with which superegos develop. A child who grows up within a special cultural cocoon may indeed have no neurotic conflicts as long as he remains in his cocoon where his ego only has to function in terms of the superego that developed appropriately within that culturally distinctive milieu. However, a shift into a different culture raises problems. Confusion results when he encounters a different body of values, customs, and ethics. His self-concept is likely to become damaged if his cultural difference in values is reacted to with derision, rejection, or penalization. Neurotic stresses are likely to result if he does anything that runs counter to the values of his earlier superego system or to the values of the new culture when he begins to incorporate this culture into his total superego functioning.

The problem of cultural difference and differential superego development is not one that has received the lion's share of the attention of either psychologists or educators, although certain psychiatrists and other behavioral scientists are beginning to explore this dimension of cultural differences (1, 5, 6, 9, 11, 13). Yet intrapsychic conflict must be considered and dealt with if it develops as a result of efforts toward cultural transition.

If youngsters are born into a culture whose values run sharply counter to the "mainstream culture," it would follow logically that orientation to this latter culture should begin at a very early age. This, however, should be done very carefully. During the preschool period a child learns a great deal about the values of his own culture and they are bound together inextricably with his feelings toward those who populate his primary group, including himself. If he is forced to turn his back on the comfortable, home-base environment that spawned him, he is likely to experience intrapsychic conflict. Also, if he ultimately rejects his native culture for a new one, serious feelings of guilt may result.

The answer to this dilemma of intercultural conflict is not an easy one. In working with teachers of culturally different children, this writer constantly makes the plea that children be helped gently and skillfully to become cultural straddlers, a concept that was alluded to previously. In essence, this involves their developing a kind of cultural versatility that allows them to move freely and selectively back and forth between their native culture and that of the mainstream within the society. This is not an idle plea, since there are countless examples of individuals who are very effective and comfortable as cultural straddlers.

## Psychopathology and the "Caucasianization Phenomenon"

Although our primary concern here is the behavior pathology of childhood and adolescence, such pathology should be viewed within a context that explains both its etiology and its consequences. Therefore the apparently neurotic conflicts manifested in adulthood need to be traced back to childhood and adolescence to be understood in terms of causation.

The phenomenon that might be referred to as "Caucasianization" begins early, especially if it is to be successful. The parents of blacks and other non-Caucasians see that the way "upward" or "ahead" is by way of a path toward the emulation of successful, dominant Caucasians. "Don't be like us," they admonish their children. "We want you to have it better than we had it." Thus the "Parent-Child Caucasianization League" is formed.

It is crucial that we view these dicta imposed by well-meaning parents upon minority children, examine the internal conflicts that result from cultural ambiguity, and also consider how these parentally imposed dicta are reinforced by the realities that these children face in their everyday life experiences. One such child might easily engage in a monologue that would go like this: "I've got to make it. My folks want me to and I want to. I can't talk the way my parents do. I must look around carefully and see what people do who do make it. I must watch my manners and my dress. I have to get good grades in school and go to college to be 'acceptable.'" The monologue would then continue—an unconscious recitation of the middle-class values of the dominant culture, and one that is rarely if ever articulated overtly.

The "Thou Shalt's" and the "Thou Shalt Not's" infiltrate surreptitiously into the child's superego structure, dictate his every move, and determine his levels and areas of aspiration. He is on his way. He has disaffiliated himself from the culture that has spawned him in his quest for "upward mobility." All of this may well be the genesis of pathological conflict in the early childhood of a non-Caucasian.

If a child is cradled, loved, spoken to, and fed in one cultural milieu but learns early that he must reject this milieu if he is to thrive or even survive, how does he reconcile conflicting *modi operandi*? Having ingested and assimilated both, is his psychic situation not fertile soil for a neurotic conflict?

Again, the black American serves well as "Exhibit A" from which we might generalize to various non-Caucasian minorities who have had to go through similar psychic gymnastics. There are those, of course, who have not been subjected to the stress of conflicting cultural adaptations. Having remained essentially within their comfortable cocoons, they experience no major intrapsychic conflict. Resentment? Yes. But not the stress of the "Ultra-Caucasoid Non-Caucasian."

A special type of pathology has emerged among certain black intellectuals. Having grown up during the first century after the signing of the Emancipation Proclamation, theirs was an "acculturation quest." That is, they accepted and strove to achieve those aspects of General American Culture that had previously been alien to their enslaved forebears. This involved, of course, moving through traditional educational processes, becoming comfortable and articulate in Standard American English, and becoming integrated into the mainstream of Americana. These were their levels of aspiration.

Increasingly the black intelligentsia became a special psychosocial entity within the United States, and a substantial schism developed between its members and their black brothers who had moved less rapidly from the mores, the values, and the language of their common forebears. The thrust toward Caucasianization has been obvious and increasing numbers of blacks are achieving this goal. But as this process gets under way during early childhood, there develops a separation away from the primary ethnic group without a compensatory acceptance by the dominant group. Two potentially pathological dangers may result from this thrust toward Caucasianization. First, severe guilt may develop as an individual realizes that he has abandoned, forsaken, deserted his ethnocultural brothers. Second, as he attempts to become a "cultural straddler," anxiety may result as he experiences ethnocultural ambivalence, ambiguity, and the loneliness of finding one's self in a no man's land. The potential rewards of Caucasianization propel him onward, reinforce his efforts. But these efforts become severely tempered by feelings of guilt and anxiety and the fear of ultimate rejection by the dominant group that may indeed control his destiny.

Again it must be underscored that this is not a uniquely black experience. This same phenomenon of conflict in the quest for Caucasianization can be observed among Americans with Spanish surnames, among American Indians, among Eskimos, among Americans of Southern European extraction, or among Americans of totally non-European ancestry. They are seen by themselves and by their ethnocultural brothers as deserters and this results in the Caucasianization syndrome.

It should be indicated here that the breaking out of one's cultural cocoon is rarely conscious. The many motivations for this phenomenon operate insidiously. Much of what is communicated by parents is never spoken aloud, only implied. By the same token, the greater society rarely ever spells out its reservations regarding the acceptability of non-Caucasians who attempt to disturb or usurp its special prerogatives of territoriality and its special ethnic birthright of privilege. Hence, motivation toward Caucasianization and its attendant conflicts and anxieties are absorbed and assimilated primarily by inference but are nevertheless very real.

The ultimate problem for the individual engaged in Caucasianization emerges when he thinks he has "made it." What rewards are there for all of this effort and conflict? To what extent has he become freer now to live where he wants to, to operate and compete freely within the job arena, or to declare without reservation, "Now I am a first-class citizen of a free society!"? Is his apparent acceptance real or, he asks himself, "Am I simply window dressing, a pawn in an insidious game of tokenism?"

## The Black Revolution and the Return Home

Factors in our recent history that have led up to the Black Revolution have been carefully analyzed and reported by other writers (8). It might be interesting and instructive, then, to examine certain of the psychodynamics that have accompanied this revolution. Again, such an examination might provide insights into the psychodynamics inherent in the activities of the Mexican-American "Chicanos," in some of the territorial takeovers of American Indians in their quest for "Red Power," or in the emerging assertions of "Eskimo Power" within our forty-ninth state.

Apparently within the collective psyche of non-Caucasian America a decision was reached. If this decision were articulated, it might go something like this:

Our attempts at a steady, quiet assimilation into the mainstream of Americana have been essentially futile. It has been a quest for Caucasianization during which we have turned our backs on our original cultures. We have rejected our heritages because we made the erroneous assumption that they were inferior. Only Northern European, Anglo-Saxon, Caucasian culture had any place in the American sun. Hence, we have been in the process of betraying ourselves and our cultures. We even made a mockery of ourselves which further intensified the feelings of inferiority imposed either through rejection or stereotypic ridiculing of us by the dominant population. Even when we have been entirely successful in many instances in achieving total Caucasianization we have been either merely tolerated or viewed as a rejectable oddity—like a baboon playing a fiddle.

The non-Caucasian pronouncement continues: "We have had enough! If all men are created equal, as it is alleged in 'our' Declaration of Independence, then we want to participate equally in our common destiny as a nation, in the evolution of our common cultural growth. We no longer intend to grovel worshipfully at the Sacrosanct Shrine of Caucasian Culture. Rather, ours must become a Coalition of Cultures. We shall quickly revive those aspects of our various cultures that we were on the verge of losing. In this there will be sharing and cultural reciprocity. Also, together, with mutual respect, we must go on with the business of advancing the social and technological and cultural goals of humanity. We all have much to give and to share: 'One nation indivisible . . .'"

Although not verbalized as such, this is the apparent essence of the pronouncement of non-Caucasian Americans.

And what of the children and adolescents? Within the black community of the United States, concerted attempts have been made at every chronological age level to develop, absorb, and assimilate attitudes, convictions, styles of life, symbols, and slogans all aimed at the evolution of a new sense of self that will supplant self-rejection of the sort that in the past has been psychologically destructive. Whereas black adults carry within themselves psychic scar tissue that at this point may be ineradicable, it is their hope and the intention of an emerging generation that no psychic lesions will be inflicted in the future that will result again in such scar tissue.

So, black youth within the United States make the signs and chants of "Black Power" and wear Afro hairdos and garb and become immersed in Black Studies courses in an attempt to learn those aspects of their ethnic past that have traditionally been left out of their curriculum and which they feel must be woven into the fabric of a common but diversified cultural heritage.

Again, this "reidentification phenomenon" being experienced currently by blacks has its counterparts within a number of non-Caucasian minorities that have been at a disadvantage because of their cultural differences. It is apparent that the major thrust is not against all that is Caucasian. This would be both futile and impossible. Rather, the goal seems to be toward true recognition, exchange, and respect within the mosaic of a diversified American culture. The baton is being passed on to the children and adolescents within the various minorities who prefer diversification to Caucasianization.

## Reaction-Formation in Reidentification

If the ultimate fulfillment of our destiny as a democratic nation is full and equitable representation and participation in the continuous process of growth, we have fallen considerably short of the mark. To minority groups who have been at a disadvantage because of their cultural divergence from the Northern European Anglo-Saxon norm, this has been particularly apparent. It has seemed that Caucasians have been saying to non-Caucasians, "Be like us. We are the prototype of America. We have fashioned America in our own image. Love it or leave it!"

So, in the past, seemingly powerless minorities have attempted to conform to this dictum, have striven for "integration," even as they have questioned its meaning. However, having sensed the futility of the concept of integration on the terms dictated by Caucasians, non-Caucasians began to question and then to rebel: "We demand full participation!"

There developed an abrupt about-face on the part of minority groups. There was a frenzied rejection of the tactics that had previously been employed in attempting integration. It was something like a reaction-formation. Behavioral tendencies were in many instances in direct opposition to what they had been previously.

The credo of the very militant seemed to be something like this: "Anyone not totally militant or hostile against the Caucasian is an Uncle Tom." (The Indian counterpart was "Uncle Tomahawk!") And further: "No Caucasian is to be trusted. No Caucasian can help our cause because they mean us no good. We must remain separate and do our own thing." There was some pathos in the drama of the militant, especially the militant who had been a member of the elite, the intelligentsia, because he suddenly struck out against all that had represented his aspirations during childhood and adolescence and early adulthood. Apparently the conflicts that had seethed within were relieved. It was now possible to be one's self, not have to reach for the apparently "unreachable dream," to go home again and "set loose."

Among somewhat less militant black Americans there was still another strategy: the Black Caucus. Whites were baffled as blacks within their midst, intellectual black friends, asserted that there was a need within many organizations, such as integrated churches, for the Black Caucus. The essence of this psychological tactic was this: "We need time to think and time for dialogue among ourselves. We must examine our own feelings, unimpeded by the restraints that we have felt consistently when we were with whites. We must establish our own identity firmly, not have it established or dictated for us by whites as has been the case in the past. Temporary separation is imperative so that we can work through the differences and confusions that have been characteristic of us during these three and a half centuries of subjugation. White Man, leave us alone for a bit. Let us do our own thing. We'll be back. But when we return we will have achieved internal integration and will thus be able to get on with the business of a harmonious coalition of diverse cultural and ethnic groups. So we caucus now for the sake of our own integrity."

There are not only black caucuses but also brown caucuses and red caucuses. All seem to be aimed at the alleviation of the stresses that have plagued non-Caucasians and at the creation of mental health through the development of a clearer sense of self through the realization of true identity.

What might seem in Freudian terms to be an unhealthy reaction-formation is probably a necessary interim moving-back (not retreat) for the purpose of an ultimately firmer and psychologically and sociologically healthier full participation in the self-determination of a nation.

Very young members of these various minority groups are watching attentively and are absorbing much of the new philosophy that these minorities are evolving. Their forebears have experienced much by way of intrapsychic conflict, culturally disadvantaged because the culture that nurtured them was non-Caucasian. The youth will observe and then ultimately participate in the new psychosocial destiny of their nation.

# 10

## Psychosomatic Disorders of Childhood

A. SCOTT DOWLING, M.D.

### Introduction

In contrast with the enthusiasm of its early proponents, the psychosomatic or psychophysiologic concept has turned out to be an embarrassingly complex and recalcitrant area of investigation and therapy. The promise of therapeutic effectiveness and of a conceptual bridge between psychological and physical medicine has yet to be realized. At best, our theories are intelligent efforts to penetrate the outer layers of an enigma; at worst we have simplistic explanations which convey little of the richness of either the psychology or the physiology of man. Although the *Diagnostic and Statistical Manual* of the American Psychiatric Association defines psychophysiological reactions as "[A] group of disorders characterized by physical symptoms that are caused by emotional factors and involve a single organ system, usually under autonomic nervous system innervation" (6), few would say that emotions "cause" ulcerative colitis or asthma or even the abdominal pains and vomiting of childhood. There is no reason to ascribe a direct, simple, causative relationship between emotions (or their physiological components) and physical illness. End organ susceptibility, intermediary mechanisms, multiple etiological factors, and the intricacies of human psychology must be considered in all instances and have proven especially stubborn to elucidate.

A final embarrassment is the profusion of opinions of what is and what is not psychosomatic. The concept has been closely but variously defined by such authors as Alexander (4), Fenichel (35) and Schur (90), but has also been so broadly defined by other authors that every aspect of human illness appears to be included (61, 75).

The purpose of this chapter is to selectively review, assess, and comment upon the present state of psychosomatic investigation and theory as it applies to children. Although there is general agreement that differentiation of those phenomena which we call psyche and those we call soma occurs principally in the earliest years of life, much less consideration has been given to the disruptions and distortions of this differentiation in infancy and childhood than to the better known disorders of older children and adults. The youthfulness of our patients allows a developmental viewpoint which is less available to those who study adults.

Viewed broadly, all of man's activities, awake or asleep, healthy or ill, involve both mental and physical processes; they are, in this sense, "psychosomatic." Looking more closely, we can delineate eight forms of mind-body relationships; only the last three will be considered psychosomatic disorders in the discussion which follows.

First, a smooth coordination of mind and body in thought, affect, and action characterizes a balanced psychophysiologic state. Both exteroceptive and introceptive impulses may achieve conscious or unconscious mental representation, thereby influencing the executive functions of the mind. These executive functions, in turn, direct, modulate, inhibit, or facilitate bodily processes through their modifying influence on efferent impulses, both corticospinal and autonomic, to achieve a balanced "mind-body" state.

Second, in physical illness or injury, mental processes may be affected: (a) by direct injury to the organs of sensory input or of motor discharge, or by direct injury to the physical substratum of the mind, the central nervous system; (b) by flooding the ego with sensory input which may reach unmanageable proportions; (c) by the symbolic meaning of the illness or injury, or by the symbolic meaning of diagnostic procedures and treatment.

In each of these instances personality functioning may be compromised; special measures, such as ego or drive regression, may then be utilized to safeguard personality cohesion. Some of these effects in young children are described by Anna Freud (37) and the pertinent literature is reviewed by Prugh (75).

Third, physical damage to the body may occur as an accidental accompaniment of a psychological state. The deformed skull of an inactive, depressed infant who rarely moves his head from a single position and the development of finger deformity with nail-biting are examples. These accidental complications of a psychological state are not considered "psychosomatic."

Fourth, consciously or unconsciously directed self-injury is a frequent symptom of severely disturbed adolescents.

A fourteen-year-old impulse-ridden boy frantically sought to limit aggressive actions toward his caretakers by openly carving his own and his girl friend's initials on the skin of his legs and abdomen.

A fifteen-year-old boy whose two older sisters had died in a fire and whose older brother had died by drowning, accidentally burned himself and repeatedly suffered broken bones and lacerations.

The extreme instance of mental infringement on somatic integrity is suicide.

Fifth, the body may be used by the mind for symbolic expression of unconscious conflict. Although the difficult problem of differentiation from nonsymbolic accompaniments of drive discharge or affective states will be considered, these pure neurotic conversion disorders are not considered "psychosomatic."

Sixth, when the psychological milieu is disturbed, optimal psychological and physical development may not occur. These are disorders of development usually seen only in early life. Certain instances of failure to thrive and institutional death, in spite of adequate physical care, are extreme examples; colic, restlessness, and vomiting in the early months are more common examples. Somatic vulnerability, on either a genetic or experiential basis, may be a precondition for some of these diseases, e.g., eczema. These are the earliest psychosomatic diseases.

Seventh, the physiological accompaniments of drive discharge or affective states may occur without conscious recognition of the drive impulse or affective state.

These affect equivalents (35a) are simple psychosomatic disorders.

A fourteen-year-old girl whose deceased grandmother had been, until age five, a loving and attentive "mother" to her and whose mother was a cold, ungiving, obsessional woman, experienced incomprehensible symptoms on entering a "food store." On looking at "all the food on the shelves" she began to weep with no awareness of sadness; in contrast, at the meat counter she experienced palpitations and a sense of dread. In analysis in her early twenties, these symptoms, which had continued into adult life, were found to be related to intense but unconscious feelings of deprivation with a desire "to be fed" by grandmother or mother and to an overwhelming experience of anxiety and excitement at age three or four when she was genitally seduced by her grandfather.

Eighth, in some individuals, reversible physiological changes may occur which are unusual autonomic accompaniments of emotion or are the reactions of the body to a fantasy. Bronchiolar constriction with asthmatic wheezing may occur at times of unexpressed anger, urticaria may occur with fantasies of being whipped (86).

A seventeen-year-old boy, while recounting a vivid recollection of being beaten and choked by his father, threw his head back and clutched his hands over his throat. As he talked in an agonized way of these experiences, erythema and extensive linear wheals appeared over his neck.

Chronic tissue changes may eventuate from these functional responses, as in the "psychosomatic diseases" of ulcerative colitis, asthma, and rheumatoid arthritis. In contrast with affect equivalents, somatic predisposition or vulnerability is postulated. These disorders, both transitory and chronic, are considered psychosomatic and will be described in greater detail below.

Our discussion in this chapter will be limited to the sixth, seventh, and eighth points mentioned above: developmental problems of early childhood in which somatic disturbance is linked to psychological states of mother and infant; the physiological accompaniments of drive state without conscious recognition of the impulse or affect (affect equivalents); and the transitory or more permanent disturbances, both functional and with tissue damage, which are unusual accompaniments of affect or bodily reactions to fantasy.

## The Relation of Psyche and Soma in Infancy

At birth there is little or no differentiation of psyche from soma. Functions which later become part of the older child's or adult's mental functioning are totally in the hands of his mother. Recognition of danger and need, provision of bodily care and nourishment, and investment of the infant's person with a sense of value are maternal functions. In the early days and weeks of life, stimuli and responses to stimuli have only rudimentary and largely subcortical representation. The infant's congenital equipment, both perceptual and expressive, is modified through maturation and development to allow more mature responses which do achieve central cortical representation and control. The infant's participation in feeding is a particularly clear and instructive example of this progression. Nonspecific, inborn, reflex patterns of rooting and sucking become modified to the particular mode of feeding (bottle or breast) and even to the characteristics of the individual nipple or breast. Conditioning of feeding responses to external stimuli associated with feeding, e.g., the smell of the mother or the sound of the bottle being prepared, regularly occurs, promoting greater specificity of both perception and response, as well as establishing an alertness to external events. With progressive development of ego functions such as memory, perception, control of motility, reality testing, etc., feeding moves from a conditioned response to an ego-directed activity. It becomes a meeting of inner needs and outer requirements under the direction of the mind.

Both noxious and gratifying events elicit reflexive, automatic, often global somatic responses in the neonate; these change toward increasingly differentiated, specific, limited responses which are partially or totally mental in character. This process of "desomatization," a substitution of mental for somatic events, can be considered to follow a developmental line toward controlled action rather than automatic action, toward consciously felt affect rather than somatic response alone, toward signal anxiety rather than traumatic anxiety, toward secondary process rather than primary process thought, and toward the use of a more neutralized energy as contrasted with a more libidinized or aggressive response. These and other aspects of the process of desomatization and resomatization have been most fully conceptualized by Schur (90, 91) and will be discussed below. The progression along this path from the newborn's somatized responses to the largely desomatized response of the adult cannot yet be traced in detail. However, several critical points can be identified. In general, these steps will parallel the development of secondary process thought, of the capacity to neutralize psychic energy, and of the transformation of anxiety from felt danger to an ego alerting signal. It is apparent that the importance of the availability, consistency, and quality of maternal care in initiating the early steps in this process is enormous—for example, in shaping a rhythmicity of somatic need and satisfaction, and in meeting a need before discomfort becomes exhausting. Another later step is the acquisition of an ability to use words to identify, differentiate, and communicate feelings, an important component of verbalization (53).

With these considerations in mind, psychosomatic disease in infancy and young children may be viewed as a developmental disorder, that is, as a partial failure of a developmental process toward desomatization, due wholly or in part to a lack of those aspects of maternal care which assist the infant in acquiring less fully somatized forms of response.

## Psychosomatic Developmental Disorders of Infancy

It has been recognized for some time that somatic integrity is not assured by providing the known physical requirements for food, water, warmth, etc.; the multiple stimulations and gratifications of regular, repeated, responsive maternal care are necessary for physical as well as psychological growth (73, 100).

Spitz studied ninety-one infants who were separated from their mothers at three to four months of age and subsequently were cared for by a nurse in groups of eight to twelve. They received adequate bodily care but were "emotionally starved." Bowlby summarized related studies in a classic W.H.O. report (15).

The children became completely passive, lying in their cots in a supine position. They did not even reach the stage where they could turn around sufficiently to perform a withdrawal by lying prone. The face became vacuous, eye coordination defective, the expression often imbecile. When motility returned after a while, spasmus nutans in some, and bizarre finger movements in all were manifested, reminiscent of decerebrate or catatonic movements. The developmental level regresses by the end of the first year to 45 per cent of the normal; sitting, standing, walking, talking are not achieved even by the age of four.

The progressive deterioration and the increased infection-liability lead in a distressingly high percentage of these children to marasmus and death. Of the 91 children followed by us for two years in Foundling Home, 37 per cent died. In contrast, in another institution, Nursery, where the children were cared for by their mothers, not a single death occurred among 220 children observed during a four year period. It appears that emotional starvation leads to progressive deterioration, which is in direct proportion to the duration of the deprivation which the child has undergone (101).

Less extreme deviation from fully adequate mothering results in a variety of less severe and often transitory somatic disorders. The mildest of these "problems" occur frequently and simply reflect the temporary imbalances of an ongoing developmental process. Spock, in his discussion of such transitory physical symptoms as irritability, crying, fretfulness, and hypertonia, states:

But we don't know the meaning of these patterns of behavior. We only know that they commonly occur and that they gradually peter out—usually by three months of age. Maybe they are different variations of one condition. In a vague way we can sense that the age period between birth and about three months is one of adjustment of the baby's immature nervous system and immature digestive system to life in the outside world and that a smooth adjustment is harder for some babies to achieve (102).

Although they receive scant attention in the pediatric literature, infants with similar but more severe disorders are regularly admitted to pediatric hospitals with poor weight gain, "spitting up," vomiting, or inordinate crying; these infants have no apparent physical cause for their symptom. If physical development is noticeably affected, these babies are termed "failure-to-thrive." Many of these infants are, in a sense, "treated" by the hospital admission; they gain weight, keep food down, and become more contented. Designation of the mothers of these babies as "nervous" or "overanxious" fails to define the maternal attitudes and forms of care which prevent smooth physiological functioning. Unfortunately, the hospital cure does little or nothing to ameliorate these attitudes. A helpful approach, both diagnostically and therapeutically, is to consider these symptoms an expression of problems which are not the mother's or the infant's alone, but rather spring from their relationship. These problems are expressed, on the one hand, by maternal attitudes and forms of behavior, and on the other, by the psychophysiological symptomatology of the infant. Viewed in this light, a proper study of the illness would include three areas of inquiry, the mother, the child, and their relationship. One way a diagnosis can be made is by joint admission of mother and child to a homelike hospital setting where observations can be made and therapeutic measures effected. This viewpoint sees the mother as the infant's "auxiliary ego," affecting both his somatic and psychological development. As we shall see, somatic disturbances in the older child rest, in part, on attributes of his "internal ego" which are quite comparable to the inadequacies of the external "auxiliary ego" which adversely affect the infant's development.

### COLIC

An examination of two relatively common infant disorders, colic and eczema, will illustrate these points and extend our inquiry to other problems and considerations. Colic, a regular and protracted fussiness, usually occurs in the evening, beginning during the second or third week of life and fading away at about eight weeks. Colic occurs most commonly in first-born children and in those who are breast fed. It is practically unknown in institutional environments; an involved mother is a requirement for its occurrence. Wessel, Cobb, Jackson, and coworkers (106) report on their experience with forty-eight colicky infants whom they contrast with fifty unaffected control infants. Birth weight, weight gain, sex, educational level of mother and father, and a family history of allergy did not distinguish the fussy from the contented babies. Family tension was judged as an important causative factor in twenty-two of these babies, allergy was similarly judged to be important in six. Both family tension and allergy appeared to be important in nine. In eleven cases no cause could be determined. They concluded that colic is " . . . possibly one of the earliest somatic responses to the presence of tension in the environment" (106a).

They suggest an interesting explanation for the spontaneous termination of colic at eight weeks of age: "As the infant grows older, the evening fussy period yields to a play period, or a period when the child seems restless and demands extra attention, but does not actually cry as if in pain. The cessation of the 'paroxysmal fussing' may be related to the achievement of a certain level of motor and social development" (106a).

Treatment methods have run the gamut from monotonous stimuli to medications such as antihistamines, phenobarbital, and alcohol, to use of a pacifier and relief of the mother's tension. Colic often ceases when the infant is hospitalized or cared for by a different person (106b).

Rene Spitz classifies colic, together with eczema, as a "psychotoxic disease," a disorder resulting from the wrong kind of maternal care, in this instance anxious overpermissiveness, as contrasted with the "deficiency diseases" of anaclitic depression and marasmus due to absence of any maternal care (101). Calling upon studies from the pediatric and psychiatric literature as well as his own observations, Spitz suggests that the colicky infant is unusually hypertonic from birth, requiring extensive opportunities for discharge of tension through oral activity. Spitz believes that if the mother of such an infant is unable to distinguish hunger need from the need for tension discharge, she may well provide the wrong kind of maternal care, attempting to feed when food is no longer needed. The excessive tension is then relieved through screaming and motor restlessness. A more appropriate form of relief, Spitz believes, would be obtained through use of a pacifier.

## ECZEMA

A discussion of eczema will bring us to many of the complex and troublesome issues which arise in assessing published reports of psychosomatic diseases. Pediatricians, allergists, psychiatrists, and dermatologists of various theoretical persuasions and with varying degrees of experience, knowledge, and understanding of other medical specialities have written voluminously and sometimes dogmatically on this, as on other "psychosomatic" topics. The discussion will formulate some of these problems.

Infantile eczema or atopic dermatitis is a disease entity usually beginning in the first two years of life. Its onset is typically during the first six months; in 30 percent it is evident by three months of age (48). To paraphrase Wise and Wolfe (108), "Eczema is a reaction form—an allergic response on the part of a susceptible individual to something to which he is sensitive. Eczematous eruptions are characterized by polymorphous lesions consisting of erythema, scaling, papules, vesicles, and at times lichenification, accompanied by more or less itching." Eczema affects the face and flexural surfaces of the extremities, especially the antecubital and popliteal fossae. It is characterized by remissions and exacerbations but generally is limited to the preschool years, at least in the more severe forms (92).

Foods have been implicated as specific allergens, and standard methods of treatment include elimination diets and efforts to prevent entry of allergens through the affected skin. Its association with a family history of allergy and a positive correlation with the later occurrence of hay fever and asthma are widely quoted in support of its allergic origin. Some allergists give no evident consideration to possible psychological factors in the causation or exacerbation of these diseases. For example, Glaser, in his text (48), speaks of body type, eye color, and eruption of teeth in relation to onset or exacerbation of eczema, but makes no mention whatsoever of developmental psychological factors.

Much of the time-honored evidence for the allergic concept of eczema is being challenged. Leider (57) states that the elimination of allergens does not halt the disease, nor does the free-feeding of allergens, as determined by skin test, lead regularly to an exacerbation of the disease. Among egg-sensitive patients, ingested eggs lead to urticaria, not eczema (64). Ratner and Silberman (80) have questioned the hereditary concept in allergy; in very few families can one find convincing evidence of its hereditary occurrence. Most cases of "allergic" disease are single cases, or one of only a few cases in large families.

Lipton, Steinschneider, and Richmond (58) discuss and extend a suggestion of Jacquet that "it is not the eruption that is itchy but the itchiness that is eruptive." Is itching the result of pre-existing lesions or does the itching and scratching come first, initiated by central mechanisms, and followed by lesions in individuals with susceptible skin? Several studies have emphasized the special vulnerability of the skin of eczematous persons (55, 85).

Although recent studies have confirmed the increased incidence of asthma and hay fever in individuals who have had eczema (71), this finding is open to various interpretations. The classic position of the allergist is that each illness—eczema, hay fever, asthma—is adequately explained as a manifestation of an underlying hypersensitivity. An alternative or supplementary viewpoint is that the usual processes of maturation away from the discharge of psychic energy in somatic symptoms are incomplete; in regressed states these pathways of discharge are facilitated with susceptible peripheral organs serving as points of discharge (43, 50). Of special interest is Pasternack's finding (71) that there is a higher incidence of asthma in infants who develop eczema before six months of age as compared with those who develop it later—a possible result of early fixation of energy discharge via somatic channels.

Spitz's discussion of eczema (101) takes a very different position than that of the allergist. He studied twenty-eight infants with the disease, utilizing 165 other infants in the same institution as controls. These babies, raised by their mothers in a penal institution, were examined at birth and at regular intervals thereafter. Developmental studies were done at three monthly intervals. Spitz notes two findings that, taken together, were specific for the infants with eczema. Compared with controls, the eczematous babies had shown an increased responsiveness when cutaneous reflexes were tested prior to the onset of symptoms. In addition, their mothers, although manifestly anxious and concerned, betrayed strong hostility toward the children refusing to permit cutaneous contact with them. The infant's need for cutaneous contact was frustrated by the mother's hostile inability to provide this form of care.

Maternal characteristics were investigated in descriptive studies by Mohr (70) and Rosenthal (84). Mohr found that mothers infantilized their eczematous children as a defense against hostile, destructive impulses toward the child. Furthermore, the mothers tended to disengage themselves emotionally from the child, encouraging others to take over the maternal role. Rosenthal reports similar findings of maternal inaccessibility in his study of twenty-five infants with eczema. Independent of Spitz, he concluded that these infants receive insufficient skin contact from their angry mothers.

Evaluating retrospective reports, such as those of Mohr and Rosenthal, is complicated because, unlike Spitz, these authors had no contact with mother or child prior to the onset of disease. It is difficult to distinguish the attitudes which existed prior to the onset of symptoms from those which have resulted from living with the illness, in this instance a disease with visible, weeping, and sometimes bloody lesions over much of the body. Does the mother hesitate to pick up the baby because of an early "rejection of motherhood" or is she frightened, hurt, and saddened by the plight of her child?

Anna Freud raises an additional and important question in her introduction to a book by Spitz (39).

. . . Dr. Spitz goes further than most in ascribing specific psychotoxic disorders of the infant to specific emotional disorders of the mother—an intriguing suggestion which might prove less controversial in the case of the complex personalities of the mothers if assessment of their behavior was based not on observational methods but on analysis.

Furman, a child analyst, describes his experience with two preschool children: a boy, Chuck, with eczema beginning at fifteen months, and a girl, Gretchen, with an allergic rash beginning at age two. They and their mothers were participants in a unique investigative and therapeutic program of supervised nursery school and analytically oriented "treatment via the mother," a form of therapy for preschool children conducted by the mother under the direction of a child analyst. A recent book describes both this program and its findings (43).

Chuck's eczema had been of such severity during the two and a half years prior to therapy that cortisone had been used for a year to achieve some relief. Hospital treatment had been of help in clearing the lesions prior to admission to the therapeutic school. Furman describes Chuck's behavior, visible skin reactions, and the course of the skin lesions thus:

> The emphasis at the start of the work was on the separation problem the mother and child shared. Chuck dealt with the situation in a controlling way, either refusing to leave his mother or leaving when he was ready, after delaying to count the buttons on her coat a number of times, for example. He also used passive-into-active in abruptly leaving her on other days. When the teachers or his mother tried to help him with his feelings around separation he either withdrew physically or else emotionally with no evidence of any recognition or acknowledgement of what was said to him. His every fiber seemed to say, "If it's unpleasant, I'll say it isn't there." At times when anger was anticipated his skin would flush and he would soon be scratching. Later, as some of his denial lessened and he could acknowledge what was said to him, he would just start scratching without there being a preceding skin blushing. The scratching stopped when he could verbalize his feelings and his skin became essentially clear for good after about six months at school. During this period his self-imposed dietary restrictions offered an avenue to discuss his previous dietary restrictions; his insistence on the miracle of clear skin offered entry to the earlier miracle of his body changes with the cortisone; and his focus on the then-current name of the nursery school—The University Hospitals Nursery School—gave a chance to review his hospitalization (43a).

Furman stresses the limited range of defenses open to Chuck—a very controlling type of passive-into-active defense and denial; these gradually gave way as sublimations and verbalization became available outlets for him. His greater mastery of aggression and his new-found capacity to verbalize feelings and experiences were thought to have kept his eczema inactive. At the five-year follow-up Chuck had no suggestion of eczema or other psychosomatic disease.

Gretchen's rash began during an intense training struggle toward the end of her mother's pregnancy. Later, particularly severe exacerbations occurred in her fourth year as a response to separation from her parents.

The therapeutic program had relieved her allergic rash by the age of five. Greater freedom in recognizing and verbalizing aggression and a shift in defensive structure from widespread inappropriate reaction-formation, denial, and reversal to more age-adequate defenses were important psychological changes that preceded the clearing of the skin lesions as well as the relief of other symptoms. It appeared that Gretchen's skin had offered a site for discharge of feelings which she found impossible to master by other means.

## Infant Disorders: Discussion and Problems

Even this limited review highlights problems of evaluating results associated with different theoretical and methodological positions, problems which arise repeatedly in the literature of psychosomatic disease. Investigators from sciences of human functioning as disparate as skin physiology and psychoanalysis, utilizing investigative methods as diverse as enzyme biochemistry and "treatment via the mother," have studied and reached conclusions about the etiology of eczema and other psychosomatic diseases. Properly integrated, this multiplicity of approaches to the same problem is, of course, highly productive. Still, without some judgment as to the relative value and significance of different types of studies, the net result on the reader can be one of confusion.

Questions often arise in assessing reports which seek to link a physical symptom or syndrome with a specific psychological process. The intermediate links from psychological process to symptom are usually unclear, and an adequate understanding of the psychological process is often lacking. In contrast, a basic science text such as Rothman's study of skin physiology (85) defines its area of competence and Glaser's clinical text (48) emphasizing descriptive and physical therapeutic aspects of eczema is quite straightforward, if myopic.

The author of this chapter is a practicing psychoanalyst of adults and children with a background in general medicine and pediatrics. His bias is that of the psychoanalyst who has worked daily for years with a number of patients who have psychosomatic disease. The analyst who becomes deeply familiar with the psychological life of relatively few patients, the psychiatrist who evaluates and provides psychotherapy for a larger number of patients, and the pediatrician or internist who sees many patients and has a shrewd eye for human relationships, make complementary but quite different contributions to an understanding of psychosomatic ills. If the different type of experience is not kept in mind, there is danger of confusing descriptive or epidemiological studies with studies of individual psychological mechanisms such as that by Furman.

The literature abounds with psychologically naïve reports of x number of cases of a given disease. Impressions gained from a few interviews or a series of psychological tests become the raw data for conclusions about a mother's unconscious attitudes toward her child, the present and past meaning of a symptom, and the vicissitudes of the affective life of the patient and his famly. There is value in these studies, but that value is in drawing attention to a link of undetermined significance between an illness and easily visible aspects of personality functioning. They are not valid statements of psychological events. Similarly, in-depth study of a few patients cannot establish epidemiological characteristics of the natural course of a disease.

At present, two psychological approaches appear to promise further understanding of these disorders: learning theory and psychoanalysis, especially as modified by ego psychology during the past thirty years. The data required for conclusions within either theoretical framework are extensive and require specialized training and experience on the part of the investigator.

Two further problems of these and of other reports should be mentioned. Some of the psychologically oriented reports suffer from a lack of documentation of the illness being investigated or treated. Spitz's reports on "infantile eczema" are clouded by a lack of diagnostic precision. Melitta Sperling has written astonishing and extremely valuable reports based on analytic treatment of sizable numbers of children with ulcerative colitis (95, 97, 98). The validity of the psychological mechanisms and therapeutic results which she describes are marred, however, by a lack of medical documentation of diagnosis or therapeutic results.

Finally, there is a paucity of prospective studies and a failure to describe, in detail, the circumstances surrounding the onset of illness prior to the inevitable psychological complications engendered by medical investigation and treatment, by the child's experience of chronic illness, and by the disruptions of family functioning which occur with protracted illness. Prospective studies by child psychiatrists and analysts and careful psychological diagnosis at the time of onset would be of inestimable value.

## Psyche and Soma in Latency and Adolescence

Latency and adolescent children have achieved a structured personality, that is, a consistent differentiation of id, ego, and superego functions. The child's drives and his parents' efforts to guide and restrain those drives toward socially acceptable forms are no longer the personae of conflict. Instead, the conflict is predominantly internal, a conflict between personality components. Anxiety is experienced when internalized standards and expectations of danger are in conflict with drive derivatives pressing for discharge. At this new level of development we find a variety of psychosomatic phenomena which, as in the younger child, ranges from transient symptomatology of varying and uncertain significance to severe, protracted disturbances of life-threatening proportions. In an infant the disordered physiology is a result of an inability of the mothering person to respond to the infant's need, often in association with a congenital or acquired somatic vulnerability. In the older child symptoms occur when ego mechanisms are inadequate to mediate between need (drive impulse) and superego or reality requirements. Again, a congenital or acquired somatic vulnerability may be present.

## Psychosomatic Developmental Disturbances of Latency and Adolescence

A wide variety of physical symptoms such as dermatitis, increased incidence of infection, and muscular aches and pains may appear during the period of establishment of superego functions in early latency (11). Similarly, adjustment to the drastic psychological and physiological changes of early adolescence is frequently accompanied by vague somatic complaints (44).

Disturbances of growth have been described in circumstances of emotional upheaval in both latency and adolescent children (42, 83) as well as when an older child is making delayed efforts at structuralization of his previously undeveloped personality (12, 83).

## Affect Equivalents in Latency and Adolescence

Affect equivalents, usually of minimal significance, occur with great frequency during these years. In some instances the disturbance is of special importance.

After a severe but unacknowledged loss, a fourteen-year-old boy suddenly developed "watery eyes" due, he said, to "getting something in them." In therapy, his sadness was revealed and its connection with the watery eyes established.

Under extraordinary circumstances a persistent affect equivalent, unmodified because of its unconscious meaning, may lead to disaster.

Seventeen-year-old Marlene, afflicted with cystic fibrosis and moderately severe pulmonary disease, was admitted to a pediatric hospital for routine examination and a course of intensive pulmonary care. Physical examination, chest films, and pulmonary function studies indicated that her pulmonary pathology was not significantly more severe than at the time of her last admission for routine studies, nine months previously. Although underweight and chronically ill, she attended school regularly, worked as a counselor at the local cystic fibrosis camp, and was involved in a variety of social and academic interests. In the hospital she complained of "nervousness" about her condition but was active and frequently left the hospital to visit and eat with her family. One week after her admission, a young man, her close friend and fellow counselor at the summer camp, died in the hospital of advanced pulmonary disease. Unknown to hospital personnel, Marlene witnessed his death from the corridor. Soon after she complained of a sore throat and lack of appetite; there was no evidence of physical disease of her throat but she remained severely anorexic in spite of attempts to help her to eat. Six days later she was hyperventilating, complained of weakness, and refused to leave her bed. Her psychogenic anorexia had resulted in metabolic acidosis compensated by the hyperventilation. Laboratory studies gave no indication of progression of her pulmonary disease. Neither anorexia nor weakness could be explained in terms of physical disease.

I saw her at that point. She appeared severely depressed and ill, breathing rapidly and barely able to lift her arms from the bed. She told me of her friend's death but said she felt no sadness about it. It didn't bother her. Her throat, she said, was all tightened up like a lump. She just didn't want to eat or get up. In my discussion with her then and on a subsequent visit, I attempted, with little or no success, to help her find a conscious awareness of the sadness and fear that were evident in her symptoms.

Still she refused to eat. Her breathing became more variable and was no longer a direct response to the metabolic condition. She hyperventilated when slower breathing would have been metabolically appropriate and vice versa. Medical regulation of the fluctuations from acidosis to alkalosis became extremely difficult. In this unstable metabolic state she suddenly expired.

Autopsy revealed only the moderate pulmonary disease. It was concluded that the affect equivalents of anorexia and lassitude, complicated by respiratory fluctuations, also on a psychogenic basis, were responsible for the metabolic disturbance which preceded her death.

## Unusual Autonomic Accompaniments of Affect or Fantasy without Tissue Damage

In an outstanding series of publications, the English pediatricians John Apley and Ronald MacKeith (7, 9) have delineated a group of psychosomatic disorders of childhood whose frequency and importance were previously unappreciated. These are the recurrent pain syndromes of childhood including recurrent abdominal pain, recurrent limb pain, and recurrent headache. Taken together with recurrent vomiting, they constitute what Apley and MacKeith call "the periodic syndrome" (9a). These studies are a model of careful collection of descriptive and epidemiological data and illustrate the value of this type of information in assessing "psychological" illness. It is equally true that these studies are not themselves "psychological"; they provide very limited help in understanding the psychological processes involved.

A small proportion of children with these syndromes enter the hospital for further study. Presumably these are the youngsters with more severe or protracted disability. In 200 cases of severe abdominal pain studied by Apley (7) only 7 percent were found to have a causative organic disorder. In these the diagnosis was made by simple diagnostic studies such as careful history and physical exam, urinalysis, and hemogram. In commenting on the use of more elaborate studies, Apley states, "The physician may himself become a pathogenic agent in perpetuating the illness by his well-meaning but never-ending efforts to find a physical cause" (9b). The continuation of medical myths such as "grumbling appendicitis," chronic nonspecific mesenteric adenitis, and pinworms or giardiasis as causes of abdominal pain, and the misapplication of concepts such as intestinal allergy and abdominal epilepsy to conditions in which abdominal pain is the only symptom, have done much to obscure the diagnosis and treatment of significant psychological disease. Apley provides compelling reasons to oppose mythological misdiagnosis and mistreatment. Thirty adolescents and young adults were interviewed eight to twenty years after being studied in a hospital for recurrent abdominal pain and were compared with a control group of children who were in the hospital at the same time for a specific physical illness. At follow-up, one third of the "pain" group had lost all symptoms, one third had lost their abdominal pain but other bodily symptoms had developed, and one third retained the recurrent abdominal pain together with additional symptoms such as severe headaches. Phobias, incapacitating anxiety, and other psychological symptoms were "several times [more frequent] than in the control group" (7).

Studies of other recurrent pains have yielded similar results. Recurrent limb pain was found in 4 percent of unselected schoolchildren (10); hospital study of 213 of these children revealed only seven instances of even questionable organic causation. Recurrent headache occurred in 14 percent of unselected schoolchildren; of eighty children with severe recurrent headache studied in the hospital, a convincing physical cause was found in only four (8). Mythological explanations and misapplied diagnoses abound for these pain syndromes; limb pains are ascribed to growing pains, rheumatic fever, and subacute rheumatism; headaches to eye strain, sinus disease, and migraine.

Apley and MacKeith find a consistent association of these symptoms with "emotional stress." They note the frequency of family history of similar symptoms, either on an organic or psychological basis, and they present findings of the efficacy of relatively brief psychotherapy in relieving the symptoms.

What can we say of the psychological events in children afflicted with these disorders? The literature is of little help. General descriptive terms abound: "emotional stress," "overprotective mother," "tense child," etc.; but these are gross external manifestations of undetermined inner events. Without claiming generality for the findings, the following case history of a ten-year-old girl seen in psychotherapy, not analysis, provides evidence of neurotic mechanisms which have been consistent among the small group of children with severe recurrent abdominal pain whom I have treated.

Beryl was ten years old when referred by her surgeon for evaluation of severe recurrent abdominal pain which prevented her from attending school. Her symptom began one year previously after she stayed with an aunt and uncle while her parents were out of town at the maternal grandparents. Pain was described as sporadic, intense, and generalized or left-sided. Her pediatrician examined her, diagnosed abdominal epilepsy, and treated her with Dilantin without improvement. She was then hospitalized where a GI series, barium enema, and intravenous and retrograde pyelograms were done. During her hospital stay she was very upset, especially following the anesthesia for retrogrades. There were no positive findings and she was discharged with no improvement in the daily recurrences of pain. Admitted to another hospital, she again had a GI series and barium enema and, in addition, electroencephalogram, sigmoidoscopy, and skull films, again without conclusive diagnostic findings.

Abdominal epilepsy was diagnosed and she was given larger doses of Dilantin. Although her pains diminished, she became more withdrawn, with poor school performance and renewed periods of anxiety. Pain began again, Dilantin was increased, and Compazine was added without change. Parents sought another surgical opinion and the referral was made.

Beryl was then the third of six children, aged seven to thirteen. In the evaluation interviews her father was affable, articulate, and concerned. He proved to have a quick temper and was given to sudden outbursts of rage and spanking with his children. Beryl's mother was a nurse at a local hospital for alcoholics; she stopped work during times when her daughter had the pain. They described Beryl as "very good," never complaining, always obedient. They couldn't remember an angry outburst from her.

Prominent characteristics of both parents were their own inability to talk or think in terms of feelings and a sense of disbelief and discomfort when, in the course of treatment, suggestions were made that they talk to Beryl in these terms. Prohibitions of anger were justified and reinforced on religious grounds. No education about sexual facts or feelings had been given.

Beryl was a chubby, pretty child who could, with help, express her distress in seeing me, yet another doctor. The evaluation and the later course of psychotherapy disclosed a number of relevant aspects of the problem. Uppermost in her mind were the ideas and feelings about her illness and its treatment during the past year; they focused on the sigmoidoscopy and "when they painted me pink," her term for the perineal preparation for pyelograms and the unexpected pain with urination which followed the procedure. Confusion and a sense of damage to genitals and mind (epilepsy) were the initial reactions; much later in therapy we learned of anger and a sense of punishment when left by her parents for these procedures. As we continued talking of the medical treatment, she described events prior to the pain but associated with it. She recalled that her parents' trip, just prior to the symptom, had been to her maternal grandfather who had recently become ill with cancer of the "peanuts" (penis). Her memory of him was of an old man who once put her to bed for not eating everything. When he died, she was told his death was "just as well since he couldn't think and do things right." She also remembered that her mother had openly wondered, before the trip to visit her dying father, if she would die young of cancer. Cancer, Beryl said, is "something inside that makes you fat and is hard to get out."

During her parents' trip Beryl stayed with an aunt, uncle, and cousins whom she did not know well although they lived in the same community. Now I learned that her aunt had been in the final stages of pregnancy and her uncle was a physician with books about having babies which she explored with her cousins. In this home pregnancy was openly discussed. Sexual questions arose but left only confusion as they were not answered at home. With parental permission we discussed babies, their origin, and the process of birth. Fantasies of oral impregnation and abdominal birth came more openly and were modified by these discussions.

Although Beryl had now returned to school, her pains continued in a less intense form. Expression of aggressive fantasies toward siblings and parents and their modification through discussion with parents and therapist resulted in cessation of pains. Beryl imagined that little men were fighting in her stomach and made her hurt. Much of the anger centered on her mother, for being so busy with work and other children, for leaving her for trips and later in the hospital, and for treating her "unfairly." Beryl retained a painful literal belief that these angry thoughts could make mother get sick or die; in particular she believed, and used religious teaching to substantiate her claim, that being angry could make her mother die of cancer. Repression of angry fantasies and reaction-formation in being good had temporarily resolved both these angry feelings and her sexual concerns—and both reappeared in the symptom.

In this instance, we can distinguish psychological processes familiar in neurotic symptomatology: dissolution of previously effective defenses (repression and reaction-formation), return of the repressed, elements of satisfaction of impulse, defense against recognition of the forbidden thoughts, and self-punishment for the impulse. The symptom was overdetermined; pregnancy fantasies, aggressive thoughts and fantasies, punishing ideas of being sick and damaged, and identification with the pregnant aunt, her mother, and the sick grandfather, all contributed to the onset of the symptom. The misguided medical procedures intensified and confirmed many of these meanings, prolonging and worsening her problem.

It seems likely that, in many instances, the common pain symptoms of adult life—low back pain, headache, and wry neck—are also minor psychosomatic disorders, unusual autonomic accompaniments of affect or fantasy.

It is apparent that in this instance, as appears to be true with other somatic symptoms of organs with autonomic innervation, one can distinguish psychological mechanisms familiar to us from the study of conversion disorders. The rigid, descriptive separation of conversion disorder from organ neurosis or psychosomatic disorder is giving way to recognition of widespread overlapping of these categories. See especially the writings of Engel (26, 31) and Sperling (95, 96). Perhaps the basic requirement for a bodily function to participate in a conversion disorder is that it be capable of cortical representation and that the function in question be subject to modification by cortical mechanisms. Many autonomic functions have been thought to be excluded from cortical representation and control. The revolutionary work of K. M. Bykov in Russia (17) and of Miller and coworkers (66, 67, 68) in this country has challenged this assumption.

Further, these authors have established that functions under autonomic control can be modified by learning procedures. Earlier studies of patients under hypnosis (18, 93) make the same point. A dramatic example of a conversion-like autonomic disorder is erythrocytic autosensitization (2, 3), a capillary bleeding disorder which can occur during adolescence.

## Other Autonomic Accompaniments of Emotion or Fantasy without Tissue Damage

Bodily functions which influence temperature regulation, cardiac rhythm, and susceptibility to organic disease appear to be influenced by psychological states. Secondary utilization of the symptom to represent elements of psychological conflict or affect may occur as learned responses.

### TEMPERATURE REGULATION

In a careful study of 2,529 patients admitted to the University of North Carolina Hospital, White and Long (107) determined that ninety-one patients or 3.6 percent of the total had temperature elevations without discernible reason. Temperatures were corrected for diurnal variation and route of determination. Rigid criteria were used to exclude other causes of fever; clinical or laboratory evidence of physical illness, whether diagnosed or not, excluded the patient from the "psychogenic" group. In all cases the temperature returned to normal without use of medication. The mean temperature elevation was 1.15°C. These patients were found on all services in the hospital but, proportionately, the greatest number were admitted to the psychiatry service. Slightly more than 2 percent of pediatric patients had "psychogenic" fever by the authors' criteria. No effort was made to determine the psychological characteristics of the affected group.

Van der Bogert and Moravec (105) studied body temperature variations in apparently healthy children and found temperature elevations of up to 2°F. with "excitement."

Renbourne (82), in an extensive review of many aspects of temperature taking, describes temperature elevations averaging 1.4°F. at times of anticipatory anxiety or excitement in young men.

Apley and MacKeith (9c) address themselves to this problem, conveying with anecdotal evidence their conviction that elevation of temperature may occur not only as an accompaniment of excitement or anxiety, but as a recurrent accompaniment of emotional stress. They describe the case of an eight-year-old girl with recurrent pyrexia believed to be due to chronic pyelitis.

On reviewing the case it was apparent that urinalysis had never shown more than a few white cells, and organisms had not been grown. When the home was visited it was found that the father had suffered from tuberculosis of a kidney and was terrified that Sylvia might have the same disease. Reassurance and explanation, based on a comprehensive approach, produced a lasting cure of her episodes of pyrexia and frequency of micturition (9d).

They conclude their discussion with the following comment:

Overindulgence in laboratory tests is harmful—to the doctor as well as to the patient. The mother's habit of using the thermometer, or the thermometer itself, should be broken. The emotional background may need further exploration. Explanation, reassurance and counseling may be successful in abolishing the fever, thus confirming the presumptive diagnosis; at the least it should help the patient and family to live amicably with the fever (9e).

## CARDIAC ARRHYTHMIAS

Falstein and Rosenblum (34) in their review of psychological aspects of supreventricular tachycardias in children conclude:

Sinus tachycardia, extrasystoles, auricular tachycardia, paroxysmal auricular fibrillation and paroxysmal supreventricular tachycardia are included among those symptoms which can be significantly related to emotional stress, and for which no structural cardiac pathology can be ascertained by any of the tests available to us at the present time.

They distinguish three types of paroxysmal auricular tachycardia: an accompaniment of the Wolff-Parkinson-White Syndrome associated with congenital or acquired anomalies of conduction; an infantile variety occurring early in the neonatal period associated with significant mortality; and, lastly, a variety which occurs in older children with recurrent attacks of variable duration. This last type occurs without known organic disease and is resistant to therapy. Predisposing factors are said to include infection, fatigue, and emotional disorder. The authors present two cases, both boys, who from the evidence presented would appear to have been strongly counterphobic with extreme castration anxiety. An appealing hypothesis is presented:

It would appear that the element of fearlessness and the need to deny the underlying terror is associated with enhanced vagus activity resulting in vagus inhibition of the primary sinus node (34a).

They suggest that an initially specific response to a specific stimulus becomes a learned response with symbolic meaning:

At first the stimulus is relatively specific. Later, symbolic or related situations, visual stimulation, and even fantasy can serve to set off attacks once the pattern has been well established . . . and a ready irritability of the subsidiary pacemaker is produced (34b).

Although other authors are in agreement that psychological events may precipitate cardiac arrhythmias (20, 62, 99), present studies are insufficient to establish this hypothesis.

## SUSCEPTIBILITY TO INFECTIOUS DISEASE

There is growing evidence that psychological states are contributing or immediate causes of certain infectious diseases. Freud, in 1905, stated:

The major affects evidently have a large bearing on the capacity to resist infectious illness; a good example of this is to be seen in the medical observation that there is a far greater liability to contract such diseases as typhus and dysentery in defeated armies than in victorious ones (40).

The more recent evidence has been of a statistical or epidemiological nature.

In their study of streptococcal infections in families, Meyer and Haggerty (65) point out that "for many common infections, commensalism or peaceful coexistence between [the] organism and its human host is the rule, while disease is the exception." Although almost 30 percent of well schoolchildren are colonized by the beta hemolytic streptococcus, the risk of developing illness is as low as 20 percent. Meyer and Haggerty studied 100 persons in sixteen families for a period of one year. Throat cultures were taken at three-weekly intervals and at times of illness. Serial interviews were conducted with the families about past and current medical and social factors that might influence the incidence of illness, and a diary was kept of illness, therapy, and life events. A variety of host, agent, and environmental factors were studied as dependent variables for the independent variables of streptococcal acquisition, illness, and antistreptolysin O titre rise. School-age children had the highest rate of colonization and illness. Host characteristics of sex, allergic history, and tonsillectomy bore no relation to illness. Acute family or personal crises bore a strong relationship to the onset of streptococcal illness: 35 percent of illnesses occurred within two weeks of such stressful events as loss of a family member, serious illness in family, minor illness with serious implications, or a nonmedical family crisis. A temporal relationship of such grossly disturbing events and susceptibility to streptococcal illness was established. The mechanism through which this susceptibility is effected is not known, although the authors speculate that increased amounts of adrenal corticoids in association with stress may have been of importance.

Kaplan, Gottschalk, and Fleming (52), in a pilot study of changes in oropharyngeal bacteria with psychodynamic state, describe an increase in oropharyngeal streptococci at times of intense dependency wishes with associated shame and rage in their study subject, a 32-year-old hospitalized woman. Saul (87), in a study of adult patients in psychoanalysis, similarly links colds, coryza, and sore throats with "the thwarting of strong receptive demands."

The comings and goings of the lowly wart, a virus-induced epithelioma, have long been known to be influenced by suggestion. Ullman, and Ullman and Dudek (103, 104) have reviewed the literature and presented further evidence that a crude authoritative form of suggestion can terminate many cases of warts. It would appear that in this instance a variation in local tissue response to a previously present virus is induced by suggestion.

Herpes simplex is another viral illness in which changes in host susceptibility play a most important role in determining the presence or absence of clinical disease. Recurrent herpes is a painful, disabling illness, affecting skin and mucus membranes, especially of mouth, nose, and vaginal region. Crops of painful vesicles may occur almost continuously or at intervals of a few days or weeks.

Although I can find no report of this condition in the literature of children's illnesses, I have treated a young woman who developed the recurrent vaginal lesions at age fifteen. Blank and Brody (13) report dermatological and psychiatric findings in six men and four women with recurrent herpes. All were said to be immature, passive, highly suggestible, and overreactive to small stimuli. With the development of positive feelings for the therapist, there was rapid and continued improvement of the herpetic lesions; when feelings of shame and guilt were more evident, the lesions tended to recur. Although the therapeutic results reported by the authors are most impressive, therapy was not of a type to allow detailed examination of the psychological processes involved. As with the studies of changes in oropharyngeal bacteria and the incidence of streptococcal disease, the nature and mechanism of relationship between psychological state and tissue change remain obscure.

## The "Major" Psychosomatic Diseases

Most discussions of psychosomatic disease in adults begin with observations of the most severe disorders, and develop theory and therapeutic formulations from this grim and complex perspective. Discussion of the "major" psychosomatic diseases of childhood—asthma, ulcerative colitis, regional ileitis, hyperthyroidism, duodenal ulcer, and rheumatoid arthritis—has been delayed to this point to emphasize a developmental perspective and the wide variation in severity of psychosomatic phenomena at all ages. We have emphasized the continuity, the imperceptible shading of normal to pathologic psychophysiologic events in infancy, childhood, and adult life. This is most clearly seen in infancy when inevitable and developmentally necessary fluctuations in psychological functioning are reflected in crying, restlessness, and variations in gastrointestinal activity. With increasing disproportion between infant need and subtle or not so subtle aspects of maternal care, we find a series of physiological "symptoms" of increasing severity: colic, continual spitting up, and restlessness occur at one end of the spectrum; vomiting or poor weight gain and intractable crying occupy a middle ground; and failure to thrive and institutional death occur at the upper end of the spectrum. Smooth physiological functioning is dependent on more than calories or prevention of physical harm. A repeated readiness and adequacy of maternal response to infant need are also necessary. With maturation of mental functioning, these maternal functions of satisfaction, modification, and assistance in delaying gratification of needs are increasingly taken over by mental mechanisms. On this more autonomous level, disproportions between need and adequacy of response also arise. As in the infant, symptomatic evidence of this disproportion may be of varying degrees of severity. One need not hypothesize a massive regression to infantile forms of physiological or psychological functioning to understand these symptoms; susceptibility of specific functions through constitutional factors or conditioning, the retained accessibility of the body to the mind, and selective regression of specific ego functions will suffice.

Unlike the affect equivalents, disorders in this category require the presence of one or more additional factors that will render the organ or function vulnerable to influence by the psychological process. More than sixty years ago Freud wrote,

The affects . . . are often sufficient in themselves to bring about both diseases of the nervous system accompanied by manifest anatomical changes and also diseases of other organs. In such cases it must be assumed that the patient already had a predisposition, though hitherto an inoperative one, to the disease in question (40).

The literature devoted to this question is extensive. Innate autonomic variation and other genetically determined factors such as allergic hypersensitivity in asthma are of unquestioned importance. Intrauterine and infantile experiences may contribute to organ vulnerability either as psychologically fixating events or at a time when somatic injury renders the organ more susceptible to future damage.

Recent studies by Miller (66, 67, 68) and by Shapiro *et al.* (94) have attacked the traditional "inferiority" of the autonomic nervous system as inaccessible to cortical influence and have demonstrated the possibility of "learning" pathological autonomic responses. Unusual autonomic responses such as wheezing or elevated blood pressure could become available for expression of conflict or affect by this means, possibly with unconscious primary symbolic meaning.

ULCERATIVE COLITIS

Studies of ulcerative colitis by child psychiatrists and child analysts have uniformly been drawn to the mother-child relationship as a central issue in the development of the disease. There is considerable agreement about the descriptive nature of both this abnormal relationship and the child's personality. There is much less agreement about the optimal mode of therapy and the outcome of therapy. Findings of several investigators will be considered together with the methods of investigation employed.

Prugh (74) reports sixteen cases, age four to nineteen, eight investigated in once-weekly psychotherapy, the others less frequently. Of those seen in psychotherapy, he says, " . . . a much deeper insight into the dynamic psychological mechanisms involved [was obtained] than was possible with the other six cases merely seen in consultation."

The children were, without exception, "emotionally immature" and had great difficulty in establishing comfortable social adjustments. More specifically, he states:

The least common denominator of these personalities appears to be their relative inability to express effectively or in a balanced way strong feelings of anger or resentment, particularly in relation to parents or other figures in authority . . . (74a).

Prugh found parents to be overindulgent and often inconsistent. The outcome of these attitudes was an "overwhelming domination" of the child, usually by the mother.

The observed relationship of an emotional component to the child's symptoms is summarized as follows:

. . . an emotional component was operative in all of the twelve cases seen in this series. The evidence for such a component was based on the observed or historically inferred correlation between the appearance of spontaneous or experimentally induced angry or aggressive emotions and an immediate activation of a hypermotile colonic response leading to trismus and diarrhea (74b).

With resolution of angry feelings in a more normal way, the gastrointestinal symptomatology subsided.

Mohr, Josselyn, Spurlock, and Barron (69) described their findings with six children, aged seven to eleven years, who were in individual psychotherapy and were observed on an in-patient ward for children. Following the suggestions of Margaret Gerard (46), the authors placed special emphasis on the mother-child relationship, extending their study to the mother's relationship with her mother as described in interviews. Results were presented mainly in descriptive generalizations. For example, the authors believe that the patients' mothers "consistently felt unable to win the love and approval of their mothers," and "see the world as a dangerous place in which one survives only as a result of one's own efforts." These unhappy mothers were superficially domineering and controlling toward their sick children:

> . . . this effort at control is motivated by deep fear that failure will have disastrous consequences. The potential disaster stems in part from their own destructive wishes toward the child. . . . The effort at control proves to be unsuccessful and the mother suffers the narcissistic pain, anxiety and discouragement of a sense of failure in her actual inability to meet the child's needs as her mother had failed to meet her needs (69a).

Children react to this domineering ineffectiveness with efforts to meet their own needs, efforts which account for the overstriving of the children as they attempt to control the danger of abandonment. Symptoms and feelings of helplessness increase when these efforts to assume parental responsibility do not succeed.

George Engel, in his discussion of this paper (23), points to the similarity of these findings to his own study of adult ulcerative colitis patients and their parents. He raises an interesting question. Greene and Miller (49) have noted that in cases of childhood leukemia there is a disturbance of the mother-child relationship which is similar to that in ulcerative colitis. In both instances the child assumes a "surrogate ego role" for the mother. In both ulcerative colitis and leukemia this abnormal dependency "intensifies the symbiotic part of the mother-child relationship and places both mother and child in great danger of loss" (23). In this setting of danger an actual or fantasy loss may precipitate overt disease. Is there a common psychological background to be found with many organic illnesses—are many diseases "psychosomatic" in this sense? Engel and the Rochester group discuss this complex question in later papers (27, 31, 33, 88).

Finch and Hess (36) report their findings in seventeen children, aged four to fourteen years, investigated by detailed case history and family evaluation by a caseworker, by psychological testing, and by psychiatric evaluation. Eleven of these children were followed in psychotherapy for periods of four months to three years. In all cases the mother was aggressive and dominating while the father was passive and ineffectual. None of the parents could express overt hostility in an appropriate manner. Outwardly the mothers were concerned; they nevertheless required complete submissiveness of their children. There was an apparent need for the illness by the mothers as a means of demonstrating their concern. In all cases there was evidence of earlier emotional disturbance, feeding problems, difficulty in toilet training, temper tantrums, enuresis, etc.

The nine male patients were essentially passive, with marked inability to express their hostility or to acknowledge dependency needs. All were intensely dependent on their mothers, with achievement the key to maternal approval. The eight girls were either identified with their domineering mothers or had withdrawn into preoccupied separation in an effort to contain their anger. Many of the girls were pseudo-mature, intellectual, bland, and affectless.

In all instances the intense mother-child relationship was a major finding, and relationships with all other persons were shallow and inadequate. The hostile-dependent relationships of the child were also expressed in a sadomasochistic orientation with obsessive-compulsive defenses and a generalized constriction of the personality.

Although these findings were consistent and clear-cut, the authors emphasize that there was nothing specific which would establish a unique pattern of relationships or of personality development in ulcerative colitis. With Engel, they believe there is a constitutional or congenital base or prerequisite to the development of the particular illness. They suggest that as the child makes efforts toward independence he despairs of success and falls back on the "surrogate ego" condition of his earlier life. In this setting his resulting rage is inadmissible. The development of illness would then be a successful compromise for all members of the family, permitting dependence on the part of the child and domineering control and bodily preoccupation by the mother.

In their discussion of treatment, the authors turn to a team approach capable of recognizing and dealing with the multiple aspects of the disease. Psychotherapy is viewed as mainly supportive and encouraging of more open expression of the tremendous aggressiveness.

A more recent study (63) by McDermott and Finch describes their efforts to apply the team approach to treatment. Forty-nine children, aged two to sixteen years, were studied in much the same fashion as in the earlier study by Finch and Hess. If anything, their attitude toward psychotherapy is even more pessimistic than in the earlier study. Although "intensive psychiatric therapy" produced emotional improvement in all but four patients, "the disease continued unabated in its chronic course; 75 per cent of the youngsters hospitalized since the formation of the physician team required surgery." Again, " . . . chronic worsening of the bowel was the rule in spite of psychological improvement, and surgery was frequently decided upon as an elective measure" (63a).

Of the psychopathology itself, they state,

The innermost part of this core was a universally noted marked tendency toward depression and denial of the illness in all of these youngsters which posed a potentially dangerous problem both psychologically and physiologically; i.e., the tendency to withdraw at the time of exacerbation and to regress massively (63b).

Melitta Sperling has written an astonishing and brilliant series of articles describing her findings in psychoanalytic treatment of children with ulcerative colitis, often in association with treatment of the mother (95, 97, 98). The results of her studies of the past twenty-five years are summarized in her 1969 paper. She has treated twenty-one patients intensively, eleven less intensively, and forty-five were seen in consultation. In addition she has supervised the treatment of nineteen cases—a total of ninety-six patients who have been followed from three to twenty-three years. These patients all had at least one hospitalization; most had more than one. None developed cancer. Treatment was considered successful in terminating the course of the illness in thirty of thirty-three intensively treated cases. Sperling has treated more patients with a longer follow-up and with better results than any other author. Taking strong exception to the team approach of McDermott and Finch, she assumes full responsibility for the patient, recounting instances in which shared responsibility led to interruption of the psychoanalytic treatment. Treatment is neither supportive nor anaclitic nor simply encouraging of affective expression. With the previous authors, Sperling identifies a pathological mother-child relationship of mutual dependency, the mother promoting the child's continued dependency on her, while she, in turn, is dependent on the child for gratification of her own neurotic needs. Once established, this "psychosomatic relationship" interferes with the regular progression of subsequent developmental phases. Because this relationship is a central and continuing source of trouble in the younger children, Sperling believes it is best approached through simultaneous treatment of mother and child. With prelatency children, treatment of the mother alone may suffice. Psychoanalytic treatment of the older child is essential to success and must be differentiated from various forms of psychotherapy.

Sperling's overwhelming success, a total contrast with the lack of success reported by authors using psychotherapy, carries important implications for therapy. Further details of the treatment would be important. Sperling provides no medical documentation of the disease by pediatrician or gastroenterologist, no record of X-ray changes in the bowel, no information about concurrent medical treatment if any, and no information about results of medical examination at the time of follow-up. Perhaps later reports will supplement her psychoanalytic findings with this essential diagnostic and physical information.

## ASTHMA

Asthma is both the most common and the most studied of the major psychosomatic conditions of childhood. Nevertheless, both its pathogenesis and the optimal pattern of treatment remain controversial. Here as with other major psychosomatic conditions, dusty arguments based on a unitary concept of etiology continue to plague understanding. One need not look far to find pediatric allergists who consider psychological factors irrelevant to causation. On the other hand, psychiatrists have been known to persist in considering only psychological treatment in the face of self-perpetuating secondary changes in lung and bronchial structures.

Peshkin (72) defines asthma as "a recurring dyspnea, usually more marked in expiration and associated with wheezing." He distinguishes three stages of severity. Least severe is a stage of retrosternal oppression, without wheezing, reported by older children. Episodic wheezing and dyspnea with periods of remission occur in the second stage. The third or attack stage is characterized by an acute onset with continuation of wheezing and dyspnea for hours or days. Status asthmaticus or intractable asthma is an exaggerated third stage. Death may occur during particularly severe and intractable episodes or as a result of chronic pulmonary changes with emphysema and bronchiectasis.

Antigen-antibody reaction with the release of histamine is the classical allergic conception of asthma. Wheezing occurs as released histamine constricts bronchioles and causes edema and increased mucus secretion of the respiratory tract's lining membrane. Identification of the offending antigen is determined by introduction of dilute antigen into the skin by scratch or intradermal injection; resulting wheal formation identifies the responsible antigen. Dramatic incidents of symptom cessation with removal of a specific antigen occur, but are not frequent.

Inhalation of the suspected skin-test-positive allergens does not necessarily cause symptoms. Long et al. (59) collected house dust from the homes of eighteen asthmatic children and sprayed it into their hospital rooms without producing symptoms. Fourteen of these children had positive skin tests to house dust. Poor correlation of skin test with response to aerosolized antigen was shown by Dekker, Barendregt, and deVries (19). Lipton, Steinschneider, and Richmond suggest a "Koch's postulate" for demonstrating an allergic basis for asthmatic symptoms: "The disease must be reproduced by inhalation or ingestion of the suspected antigen without the patient's knowledge" (58a).

The repeated experience of sudden clearing of asthmatic wheezing with admission of a child to the hospital and equally sudden reappearance of wheezing as the child approaches home after hospitalization (51), as in the following case, graphically demonstrates the influence of psychological state on the appearance and disappearance of asthmatic symptoms.

For the fourth time in two months Jane S., age four years seven months, was admitted to a pediatric hospital with severe intractable asthma. Also for the fourth time it cleared completely soon after admission.

Her asthma began on her third birthday without preceding evidence of hypersensitivity disorder. Subsequently, wheezing was either totally absent or so severe that usual medications, including aminophyllin and epinephrine, were only temporarily helpful. Attacks ended as quickly as they began. Skin testing was done and desensitization started but then discontinued as Jane developed severe wheezing during each visit to the doctor's office.

Respiratory distress with cyanosis was so severe during the preceding two months that her pediatrician feared for her life and hospitalized her; each time the attack ended with hospital admission. During this fourth hospitalization, psychiatric evaluation and brief psychotherapy were provided.

Jane was the oldest of three girls; at four and a half years her mother was due to have a fourth child in four months. Her parents were young, bewildered, and emotionally drained by their growing family. Although Jane's mother loved to read and talk with her and did so whenever possible, the demands of two younger children and three pregnancies left her little opportunity for pleasant times with her oldest daughter.

Mrs. S. appeared to be a bright, happy person but was very controlling with both her husband and her children. Anger was a forbidden feeling; when expressed by Jane's mother it came in an overwhelming flood with yelling and spanking. When Jane herself had a rare temper outburst she was soundly spanked. Jane was controlling with parents and sibs, teasing in subtle ways and obtaining favors through cajolery.

Although both parents were angry and upset with their rapidly expanding family, neither could openly express such thoughts nor could they allow expressions of jealousy or dismay from Jane.

Jane herself was a bright, alert child, very controlling in her ways. She was unable to express anger openly and had precociously developed defenses of reaction-formation and denial against her many negative feelings.

Jane's parents, and especially her father, were very suspicious of psychiatric help and agreed only to a period of talks with Jane while she was in the hospital. In these discussions, often with her mother present, we drew pictures and talked about the hospital, her asthma, her mother's pregnancy, and her siblings. With her mother's permission, feelings connected with these aspects of her life were permitted and given verbal form and names. To a modest degree it became possible for her to talk about her feelings. In separate meetings with the mother these areas were explored in greater detail; the use of verbalization appealed to this intellectually oriented woman. Intense anger about the marriage and family, and guilt about Jane's asthma, limited the parents' ability to consider further assistance. After daily meetings for three weeks, Jane was discharged home. She remained totally free of asthmatic symptoms for over a year; her first attack occurred on the first birthday of her youngest sibling sixteen months later. She has had intermittent, moderate symptoms in the several years since that time, but none has required hospitalization. Further psychiatric care has not been obtained.

Many asthmatic children, like Jane, improve almost immediately with hospitalization and a large percentage of youngsters with previously intractable asthma remain free of symptoms for long periods of time without medication while living separate from their families at a convalescent hospital (76), a procedure termed "parentectomy" by Peshkin (72a). Apley makes a cogent and critical remark on this procedure:

Sending the child away from home ("parentectomy") is often and promptly effective (though the improvement may be temporary). It is at home, with persons who are loved (or at times hated) most, that emotional relationships are most intense and are most likely to produce symptoms. . . . To send a child away from home may stop his asthmatic attacks but it is unforgivable to leave the mother unsupported in her own unhappiness, to brood on her apparent misdeeds and her failure. It is unkind to her and it does not prepare the home for the child's return (9f).

Psychological assistance for both child and parents is advisable during the period of separation if the old emotional climate and renewed symptoms are to be avoided.

Rees (81) studied a random sample of 388 asthmatic children and a matched control group of accident cases for the presence and importance of allergy, infection, and psychological factors at the time of onset of asthma and in precipitating subsequent episodes of asthma. Allergy was judged by history, skin testing, inhalation tests with suspected allergens, and exposure and exclusion trials with suspected allergens. Infection was judged by history or clinical evidence of infection at the time of asthma. Psychological factors were judged grossly via history of stressful events (death of parent or relative, accident to patient, etc.) and by evidence of "emotional tension." Each of these factors was determined to be "dominant," "subsidiary," or "unimportant" in the onset and recurrence of attacks.

Allergy was unimportant in 70 percent of the 388 children, a dominant factor in 17 percent, and a subsidiary factor in 13 percent. Infection was unimportant in 28.4 percent, dominant in 41.6 percent, and subsidiary in 30 percent. Psychological factors were unimportant in 28.4 percent, dominant in 41.6 percent, and subsidiary in 30 percent. These figures are most important for the careful study and elimination of allergic factors in a majority of cases. Even with the rough psychological indicators used, psychological factors were judged to be the sole factor in onset and later precipitation of symptoms in 21 percent of the asthma patients.

Several authors present evidence for a specific psychological conflict or meaning of the wheezing. Alexander's famous statement that the wheeze is a "suppressed cry for the mother" (5) is the best known example. Knapp writes, " . . . the individual restrain(s) the scream of rage which might destroy the person whom he needs. . . ." (56). Sperling finds the asthmatic child expressing "aggression and rebellion against the controlling mother together with other forbidden and dangerous impulses" (96a) in the somatic symptoms.

As with all major psychosomatic symptoms, asthma has been linked to specific disturbances of the mother-child relationship. Abramson (1) speaks of the mother as "engulfing," Gerard (46) as "overprotective," and Mohr et al. (70) as mutually dependent with the child for gratification. Sperling (96a) finds the mother rejecting the child when he is well and striving for independence, and accepting him when he is sick and helpless.

However, there is less agreement between studies of the mother-child relationship in asthma than in ulcerative colitis and duodenal ulcer. This may only reflect the large number of studies of asthma. Garner and Werner's famous study of mother-child interaction in psychosomatic disorders (45) does not differentiate these conditions and yet arrives at a composite picture of the psychosomatic mother, a further contradiction with studies of the separate conditions. Their study describes a typical pathology of the mother-child relationship in sixteen psychosomatic children as compared with fourteen neurotic and fifteen physically ill children. Data are derived from retrospective interviews, psychological testing, and brief observation of mother with child. They see the mother-infant interaction as "a close mutually frustrating one." There is a "negative closeness" with the mother assuming either of two styles, "one is shrewd, complex and cold, well organized, and planful as the mother plays the part of a good intelligent mother. The other style is over-reactive, unstable and disorganized with the mother lacking the requisite integration to be consistent in handling the child."

Most of the studies of mother-child relationship are psychologically shallow, depending upon a few interviews, psychological testing, and brief periods of observation. Anna Freud's remark, quoted above (39), comes to mind; analytic study of these mothers would dispel many doubts about the specificity and importance of this relationship.

Furman (43b) describes the findings of extensive nursery school observation, "treatment via the mother," and long-term follow-up of three cases of asthma.

One child improved dramatically with treatment via the mother; at follow-up eleven years later there had been no recurrence of asthma. His illness began at age three and had been treated for a year with dietary restrictions and desensitization without improvement. His asthma attacks came at times when jealousy would have been appropriate; the asthma seemed linked to a specific affect. His psychological development at age four showed many defects: superego development was inadequate, object relationships were sadomasochistic interplays, anal conflicts dominated his libidinal development, and he tended to turn aggression against himself. Ego defenses were not age-appropriate and other ego functions, especially the synthetic function, were impaired. In spite of this considerable psychopathology his symptoms, which included stuttering and nightmares in addition to the asthma, had cleared at the completion of the therapeutic program.

The other two children were similarly assessed and treated and, in addition, received analytic treatment. Although the asthmatic symptoms improved, they were not eliminated in either child. Both of these youngsters had onset of symptoms prior to age six months and both had received extensive medical treatment. One child's asthma had progressed to development of emphysema prior to psychological therapy. Furman suggests that the greater tenacity of the symptom in these children as compared with the child who responded to treatment is related to the early onset, with undifferentiated psychic energy being bound in the organ itself, a concept derived from the formulations of Edith Jacobson (50a).

It is of interest that in these extensively studied cases, the mother-child relationship did not differ in type from the relationships of mothers with neurotic children.

Authors other than Furman have described variations within the population of asthmatic children which may be significant for prognosis and therapy. The best-known of these studies are those of Purcell and co-workers (76, 77, 78, 79) from the Children's Asthma Research Institute and Hospital. Children admitted to this hospital for long-term care of intractable asthma fall into three groups: those who lose their asthmatic symptoms within three months and remain free of symptoms without medication for a period of a year; an opposite extreme of those who require regular steroid therapy for relief of wheezing; and an intermediate group who require nonsteroid medication for relief of occasional wheezing. The first group tends to be older than the second group at the time of onset of symptoms, has more restrictive and autocratic parents, reports emotional precipitants of attacks more frequently, and has more neurotic symptoms. The authors suggest that these patients' asthma is more dependent on emotional factors than those who require steroids.

Block et al. (14) subdivided asthmatic children psychologically and on the basis of allergic potential. Those with low allergic potential were more conforming, pessimistic, and had low frustration tolerance as compared with those with high allergic potential. Their parents found them to be nervous, rebellious, jealous, and whiny as compared with the more allergic children. Again, the authors conclude that emotional factors seem more important in some children, allergic factors in others.

Although research on asthma is extensive, the literature is generally disappointing in its research methods concerning psychological factors in individual children. The vast bulk of these studies are retrospective; few have utilized intensive or longitudinal psychological investigation. Anterospective studies of vulnerable children and longitudinal studies would be most valuable.

## Theoretical Considerations

Three quite different traditions are presented in recent theoretical formulations concerning psychosomatic disease.

Many writers cling, perhaps unwittingly, to fragments of Freud's early and rather mechanical concepts of psychological disturbance. His early writings center upon the importance of the "damming up" of libido and of "strangulated affects" in the origin of psychological symptoms, and his early forms of psychological treatment included abreaction of these "strangulated affects" and suggestion or hypnosis (16). In these studies, Freud also attempted to link specific forms of psychological disturbance with specific experiences or conflicts. Although these concepts were either discarded entirely or greatly modified in Freud's later writings, and have been further modified with the development of ego psychology by Anna Freud, Hartmann, and others, their ghost lives on in a continued effort to ascribe somatic symptoms to "repressed hostility," "suppressed rage," and in efforts to make a personality type, a specific conflict, or a uniform object relationship the "cause" of a given symptom or disease entity. Recall, for example, the effort to establish a direct causative link between psychosomatic disease of older children and a specific abnormality of the mother-child relationship and the belief that each disordered emotional state had its own physiological syndrome (5). These descriptive, global formulations are most often found in studies based on diagnostic interviews and psychological testing of a sizable number of patients.

The second line of thought is best represented by George Engel and his Rochester coworkers, notably Schmale, Reichsman, Greene, and Prugh. Beginning with Engel's classic articles on ulcerative colitis (21, 22, 24, 29), they have written a series of outstanding papers on the clinical, laboratory, and theoretical aspects of psychosomatic disorder. The clinical emphasis has been on studying a wide range of patients in the setting of a general medical ward, their laboratory studies are predominantly of the physiological aspects of affective states, and their theoretical position has been an encompassing synthesis of physical, psychological, and sociological aspects of human health and disease (28). Prugh, in an extensive review (75), described this point of view in relation to children. He provides a compendium of findings and problems which bear upon many psychological and sociological aspects of pediatric medicine.

Engel has focused on the onset situation in organic disease. From his experience with ulcerative colitis and multiple sclerosis and experience of others with leukemia, diabetes, and cancer, he has defined a "giving up—given up" complex which is often present, not necessarily in a causative role, at the time of disease onset. He has contributed an outstanding discussion of the differentiation of conversion symptoms from psychophysiological reactions without symbolic meaning (31).

Engel's studies are a model of careful observation. His use of the laboratory, as in the famous studies of gastric secretion during affective states in a child with a gastric fistula (30, 32), set a standard for psychological-physiological research, and his careful approach to the question of "causation" is an example to those who would proceed too hastily.

Although his writings include many psychoanalytic concepts, Engel has not utilized intensive psychoanalytic study of individual patients as a research tool. Rather, he expresses disappointment in past efforts to obtain useful data via psychoanalysis, feeling that the psychophysiological processes involved are accessible to analytic study in only a limited way.

. . . analysts, frustrated by the small number and variety of somatic processes accessible for study among patients in a classical psychoanalytic framework, attempted to adapt the psychoanalytic method and apply the psychoanalytic know-how to the bedside and the laboratory. . . . One might say that in this present period patients with somatic disorders are being studied by psychoanalysts rather than by psychoanalysis (26a).

One reason for this disappointment may be the frustrated hope that correlations of physiological variables with unconscious elements would be established by analysis—efforts which have met with only very limited success. Engel also tends to sidestep the issue of psychological treatment, expressing no special interest or belief in the usefulness of analysis in such cases.

One of the strongest contributions by members of Engel's group, in relation to both children and adults, is their patient insistence upon the importance of psychological factors in physical illness and the value of teaching these principles to young physicians (25).

The third tradition is represented in the works of Fenichel, Schur, Jacobson, and Furman. The focus of interest is on the detailed psychology of the affected patient, the methodology is that of psychoanalysis, and the theoretical background is the mainstream of psychoanalytic thought.

In his article on visual disturbances (41), Freud distinguishes conversion phenomena from toxic disturbances of function secondary to increased erotogenicity of the affected organ. Toxic disturbances of function are not, according to Freud, directly accessible to psychoanalysis.

Fenichel (35a) distinguishes three types of psychosomatic phenomena: (a) affect equivalents, "the specific physical expressions of any given affect . . . without the corresponding specific mental experiences"; (b) results of changes in chemistry of an unsatisfied person; and (c) physical results of unconscious attitudes or of unconsciously determined behavior patterns. Fenichel notes, with Freud, that the change in function, having no unconscious meaning, is inaccessible to analysis. However, interferences to more adequate discharge may well be open to analytic intervention. If more normal pathways of drive expression become available through treatment, the abnormal alteration of function will cease.

Schur's articles (89, 90, 91) effectively bring ego-psychological and developmental considerations to an understanding of psychosomatic phenomena. From his psychoanalytic experience with adult patients, Schur describes the developmental process of "desomatization," the change from physiological to psychological experiencing and expression. As stated above, this change is an aspect of the development of the mind; it progresses in conjunction with the change from primary to secondary process thinking, with the greater control of motility, and with the greater use of neutralized energy in psychic functioning.

Schur separates regression in the evaluation of a danger situation from regression in the form of reaction to the danger situation. For example, a regressive evaluation of danger would occur if a child, asked to recite in school, suddenly felt himself inadequate and ridiculed as he did some years earlier when confronted by an angry parent because of a wet bed. However, the child's reaction may or may not also occur in a regressed form; in spite of his feelings of inadequacy, his anxiety may remain within manageable bounds and he may retain secondary process thought and expression. He may, in other words, retain composure and provide the answer. If the form of response also regresses, his feelings of anxiety may be overwhelming; secondary process thinking fails as he fumbles for words and cannot think out the answer. In susceptible individuals the regression may also affect somatic processes; erythema, urticaria, wheezing, gastrointestinal upset, or other symptoms may then occur. These would be examples of a regressive "resomatization." Schur finds no evidence for the various specificity theories. Neither personality configuration, conflict, or defense against specific phases of sexuality or aggression were consistent in his patients. This lack of specificity is certainly in keeping with the wide variation and endless complexity of human personality development. Nevertheless, a number of common findings were identified among these patients: widespread impairment of ego functions, tenuous object relationships, unusual amounts of early traumatization, and libido development with a prevalence of narcissistic and pregenital elements.

Repressed aggression has often been implicated in psychosomatic symptoms. Alexander (5) suggests the value of releasing pent-up aggression, believing symptoms result from the chronic pressure of autonomic components of unexpressed affect. In a concise critique, Schur brings the ego-psychological point of view to bear on this formulation. He describes a spectrum of controlled to uncontrolled aggression which parallels secondary to primary process thinking and the emergence of somatic discharge phenomena. He points out that aggression is not a simple phenomenon. In every instance questions must be asked which define both the instinctual and ego aspects of an aggressive impulse or action. Does it, for example, spring from pregenital or oedipal conflicts? What ego functions have been affected by it? Does the individual perceive his aggressive feelings as threatening? Does he evaluate these feelings in a regressed way (as applied to oedipal or pre-oedipal objects), and does he then respond in a regressed form or not? The patient who has moved successfully from his somatic symptoms to more mature levels of feeling and expression can be more effectively aggressive in his interactions with others, but often in a far less noisy and disruptive way than before. It is not that a quantity of aggression has been released, but that aggressive expression is more closely under conscious ego control and is more closely coordinated with other instinctual and reality considerations.

With other authors, Schur writes of the relevance of both hereditary and experiential factors in establishing the susceptibility of particular indi-

viduals to somatic symptomatology in regressed states. This somatic vulnerability may occur on a biological genetic basis, as a result of intrauterine
experience or as a result of postnatal experience.

Diagnostic formulations in major psychosomatic disorders have not ordinarily departed from descriptive conclusions based on historical an-
amneses from parents and children. In a significant departure, Furman (43c)
utilizes a modification of Anna Freud's developmental profile (38). His
formulation includes: (a) the organic factor, "all those aspects of the
organic phase of the disease that may have a bearing on psychological
treatment," including family history; site, severity, duration, and pattern of
the disease process; and the nature of, traumatic characteristics of, and response to, current and past medical programs; (b) the psychic factor, including an economic component (drive fusion as seen in the level of object
relations and of superego development, drive maturation of libido and aggression, and drive neutralization as reflected in sublimation potential) and an
ego aspect, an evaluation of ego functions and detailed consideration of
ego defenses; and (c) the "relationship factor," an assessment of "the
nature and degree of influence the emotional elements have on the body
processes in question," as determined by age of onset, type of emotional
factors, and correlation of emotional with organic factors. This formulation based on concepts similar to those of Schur and Jacobson appears
to be an important diagnostic advance; the interested reader is referred to
the original description for further details.

## Therapeutic Considerations

There is little agreement about the relative value of various types of
psychological therapy in major psychosomatic disease. However, the following considerations may be of value in considering therapy for children.

Direct therapy with modification of psychological factors is most likely
to be helpful (a) if the symptom derives from a transitory conflict between child and mother, for example, a conflict based on a developmental
interference or developmental disturbance, (b) if disease onset comes
after the major developments of psychological structuring have occurred,
that is, after age three to four years, (c) if exacerbation and remission of
somatic symptoms can be correlated with specific psychological factors,
(d) if therapy is provided soon after the onset of symptoms, that is,
before extensive secondary elaboration of symptom meaning has occurred,
and (e) if parental cooperation can be obtained in developing new modes
of affective discharge, as in verbalization or sublimatory activities, and in
undoing crippling defensive measures.

Purely somatic processes may extend tissue changes initiated by emotional factors. There must be no confusion; permanent tissue damage, such
as bronchiectasis with asthma or "lead pipe" gastrointestinal changes in
ulcerative colitis cannot be modified by psychological treatment. Patients

with such changes may benefit from treatment in other ways, but return to normal function is not possible.

Psychological treatment and prophylactic measures can be usefully directed toward psychologically important aspects of the illness unrelated to onset or exacerbation of symptoms. Improvement of associated personality problems, encouragement and development of ego strength in areas not directly related to the illness, prevention of psychological trauma related to medical treatment and diagnostic procedures, and modification of family or social inadequacies deserve careful attention in all patients.

The weight of evidence indicates that major psychosomatic symptoms are associated with severe regression of selected areas of psychological functioning. Schur (90a) states, "If regressive reactions which accompany affects and instinctual drives can produce symptoms, *anything* counteracting such regression should be beneficial." Various forms of psychotherapy, educational measures, and environmental changes may counteract the regression and thus be beneficial. When available, conservative analytic therapy of the latency or adolescent child is potentially curative, the criteria for its use being the same as in severe neuroses (47). Therapy in which the therapist satisfies regressive wishes (anaclitic therapy) has been suggested for adult patients (54, 60). Both anaclitic and abreactive therapies which reward regressive forms of ego functioning are contraindicated in psychosomatic disorders.

## Summary

Variation in psychosomatic disorders occurs both within developmental phases and with increasing maturity of psychological and somatic functions.

Within developmental phases, psychosomatic disorder may occur on the basis of developmental stress (i.e., colic in infancy, bodily pains with superego development), as an affect equivalent (the normal state in infancy prior to development of mental mechanisms necessary to the awareness of feeling, and as a defensive or regressive finding in older persons), or as a transitory or more permanent disturbance of innervation and tissue integrity associated with somatic vulnerability and psychological fixation or regression.

Increasing maturity of psychological and somatic functions are reflected in a changing locus of conflict (mother vs. child to intrapsychic conflict), in a changing ego capacity to counteract regressive tendencies, in "learned" somatic responses, and in altered somatic vulnerability.

Studies of psychosomatic problems have tended to blur the difference between epidemiological and descriptive studies on the one hand and in-depth studies of relevant psychological processes on the other. Continuing attempts to link a particular symptom with a given conflict, affect, or type of parent plague the field, drawing attention away from the need to understand the complex inner life of the afflicted child.

Recent studies in the modification of autonomic functions lend weight to the suggestion that many of these symptoms in older children and adults are pregenital conversion symptoms with primary and/or secondary symbolic meaning.

Psychological understanding would be advanced by utilizing Anna Freud's developmental profile in diagnostic studies, by close examination of the onset situation, by anterospective study of susceptible youngsters, and by detailed reports of analytic therapy of affected children and their parents.

# 11

## Mental Retardation

GERALD R. CLARK, M.D., AND
MARVIN ROSEN, PH.D.

*Definitions and Incidence*

Delineation of the limits for the term mental retardation has been a hazardous endeavor. Expanding and contracting to encompass more or less of an atypical population, the concept has been subject to a variety of interpretations by both educators and medical practitioners. Earlier textbooks outlined rigid boundaries for mental deficiency, limiting the term for use only with clear-cut physical handicap, intellectual deficit, and social incompetence. More recent concern with the ravages of poverty and cultural deprivation has served to broaden the boundaries of retardation to include large numbers of persons once labeled borderline or marginal. Currently it has become fashionable to partition the set of intellectually subnormal individuals into more specific disability groupings, such as "the child with learning difficulties," "the dyslexic child," "the autistic child," "the interjacent child." This ambiguity in definition of the concept has resulted in a wide range of variability in estimates of its incidence in the general population. While older textbooks were conservative in estimating between 1 and 2 percent of the population as mentally deficient, more recent estimates have varied between 3 and 4 percent with over six million Americans affected. The higher percent is likely not a function of increasing frequencies of disability; rather, it reflects a trend to include larger numbers of persons with functioning equivalent to that of many retarded individuals.

The definition of mental retardation accepted by the American Association on Mental Deficiency describes mental retardation as "sub-average general intellectual functioning which originates during the developmental period and is associated with impairment in one or more of the following: (a) Maturation, (b) Learning, and (c) Social Adjustment" (18). This definition is broad enough to include large numbers of mentally subnormal persons limited by psychological factors, genetic endowment, or physical impairment of the central nervous system. The terms "mental retardation" and "mental subnormality" have assumed a generic connotation and refer, in the broadest sense, to all instances of subaverage intellectual functioning including academic deficiencies, provided the deficiencies have existed since childhood and cannot be directly attributed to emotional disturbance. The terms "mental deficiency," "oligophrenia," "amentia," and the less fashionable "feeblemindedness" are becoming increasingly associated only with more severe retardation, directly attributable to some physical or external source.

Limits for the term "mental retardation" have sometimes been strained and have resulted in apparent paradoxes of circularity by attempting to include concepts of irreversibility or prognosis. Confusion arose, for example, in the interpretation of diagnosis of those persons initially incapable of social adjustment who later achieve some measure of adjustment, either as a direct result of training or by other circumstance. Earlier authorities in the field coined the terms "Pseudoretardation" or "Pseudofeeblemindedness" to handle the case of the individual who shows intellectual growth spurts from so-called retarded to nonretarded levels or who makes a more favorable social adjustment at some later time in his life. The implication of the term "Pseudoretardation" was that the initial diagnosis represented an error in evaluation. Either the assessment techniques were considered unreliable or some external factors such as a sensory impairment or emotional disturbance prevented the individual's true potential from being judged. This type of thinking was probably a result of faulty and distorted understanding of the nature of intelligence testing. If the IQ is assumed to represent native ability and to be constant throughout the life of the individual, then IQ changes, when observed, require special explanation. Psychologists and educators today are in agreement that IQs do change and that, to a certain extent, they can be influenced by environmental conditions. Instead of a device measuring intellectual "capacity," the intelligence test represents a tool for evaluating intellectual functioning at one point in time with reference to a standardization sample of equivalent age peers. It seems reasonable to adopt this thinking to the concept of mental retardation. The mentally retarded child can be seen as a child functioning below age level on intellectual tests and academic grade and to be socially maladapted to his home or school environment. Except for cases of severe deficit or those with known clinical syndromes, such as Down's Syndrome, the term need not have prognostic implications with regard to future intellectual or social functioning. With this understanding of intelligence test results, the term "Pseudoretardation" serves no useful function other than a form of hindsight with no prognostic significance. According to the manual on terminology and classification in mental retardation of the American Association on Mental Deficiency,

an individual may meet the criteria of mental retardation at one time and not another. A person may change status as a result of changes in social standards or conditions or as a result of change in efficiency of intellectual functioning with level of efficiency always being determined in relation to the behavioral standards and norms for the individual's chronological age group (18a).

## Classification and Differential Diagnosis

### CLASSIFICATION SYSTEM

Classification of mental retardation can be made according to intellectual-social, clinical, or etiological considerations.

*Intellectual-social.* Intellectual levels usually associated with mental retardation are generally based upon psychometric testing with either the Stanford-Binet Intelligence Scale or the Wechsler Intelligence Scales. While it is typically accepted that an IQ below 70 is classified as mental retardation, actual differences between retarded and nonretarded categories would not be evident in persons differing by only a few IQ points. Indeed, the standard error of these two scales (3–4 IQ points) is such that an IQ distinction between retardation and so-called "normal" functioning may be within the margin of error for the test. In practice the classification as to level of retardation—Mild, Moderate, Severe, or Profound—represents the number of standard deviations from the mean of the test; slight differences in accepted classification limits arise because of differences in the standard deviation of the respective test. The convention adopted by the American Association on Mental Deficiency (18a) also uses a numerical designation from I to IV to specify level of adaptive behavior in three areas—maturation and development, training and education, and social and vocational adequacy. Thus there is an increasing trend toward assessing social as well as intellectual functioning in the diagnosis of mental retardation. These conventions are specified in Tables 11–1 and 11–2.

*Clinical.* Clinical classification is based upon known clinical syndromes, such as Down's Syndrome, cretinism, or microcephaly. This system of classification follows a medical diagnostic system with focus upon etiological considerations. Typically the mentally retarded are divided into two broad classifications of endogenous vs. exogenous groupings. A traditional system is illustrated by that of Tredgold and Soddy (41), in which endogenous retardation (or "primary amentia") encompasses all those cases without some known external causative agent. It includes cases of familial mental retardation, where there is a high incidence of sibling retardation and traceable historical origins of the deficit, as well as the cases of known genetic determination. Instances of retardation transmitted by a single dominant gene are typically associated with neural and ecotodermal involvement, such as tubero sclerosis. Retardation transmitted by recessive genes usually involves metabolic disturbance, as in galactosemia and phenylketonuria. In these cases dietary changes may produce remediation provided the treatment is initiated shortly after birth. Probably the more recently discovered chromosome disorders should also be classified as endogenous retardation. Thus Down's Syndrome or mongolism, which

## TABLE 11-1
### Classification in Mental Retardation

| Classification | IQ Limits Stanford-Binet | IQ Limits WAIS or WISC | MA | Old Terminology | Estimated Percentage of Retarded | Anticipated Academic Achievement Grade | Standard Deviation Levels from Mean |
|---|---|---|---|---|---|---|---|
| Borderline | 83–68 | 84–70 | 13–15 | | | Fifth | –1.01 to –2.00 |
| Mild (Educable) | 67–52 | 69–55 | 8–12 | Moron | 85 | Third–Fourth | –2.01 to –3.00 |
| Moderate (Trainable) | 51–36 | 54–40 | 3–7 | Imbecile | 11 | First–Second | –3.01 to –4.00 |
| Severe (Dependent) | 35–20 | Below 40 | 1–2 | Imbecile | 2 | Below First | –4.01 to –5.00 |
| Profound (Dependent) | Below 20 | | Below 1 | Idiot | 2 | | > –5.01 |

Source: Heber, R. (ed.). *A Manual on Terminology and Classification in Mental Retardation*, Monograph Supplement, *American Journal of Mental Deficiency* (1961), p. 59. Modified by permission of the American Association on Mental Deficiency.

## TABLE 11–2
### Adaptive Behavior

| | Preschool Age<br>0–5<br>Maturation and<br>Development | School Age<br>6–21<br>Training and<br>Education | Adult<br>21<br>Social and Vocational<br>Adequacy |
|---|---|---|---|
| Level I | Gross retardation; minimal capacity for functioning in sensori-motor areas; needs nursing care. | Some motor development present; cannot profit from training in self-help; needs total care. | Some motor and speech development; totally incapable of self-maintenance; needs complete care and supervision. |
| Level II | Poor motor development; speech is minimal; generally unable to profit from training in self-help; little or no communication skills. | Can talk or learn to communicate; can be trained in elemental health habits; cannot learn functional academic skills; profits from systematic habit training. ("Trainable") | Can contribute partially to self-support under complete supervision; can develop self-protection skills to a minimal useful level in controlled environment. |
| Level III | Can talk or learn to communicate; poor social awareness; fair motor development; may profit from self-help; can be managed with moderate supervision. | Can learn functional academic skills to approximately 4th grade level by late teens if given special education. ("Educable") | Capable of self-maintenance in un-skilled or semi-skilled occupations; needs supervision and guidance when under mild social or economic stress. |
| Level IV | Can develop social and communication skills; minimal retardation in sensori-motor areas; rarely distinguished from normal until later age. | Can learn academic skills to approximately 6th grade level by late teens. Cannot learn general high school subjects. Needs special education particularly at secondary school age levels. ("Educable") | Capable of social and vocational adequacy with proper education and training. Frequently needs supervision and guidance under serious social or economic stress. |

Source: Heber, R. (ed.). *A Manual on Terminology and Classification in Mental Retardation*, Monograph Supplement, *American Journal of Mental Deficiency* (1961), p. 63. Used by permission of the American Association on Mental Deficiency.

is related to the presence of an extra chromosome, would fall under this heading as would disorders of the sex chromosomes, such as the Kline-felter Syndrome (XXY), the Turner's (XO) female, and the Super female (XXX: XXXX). Such disorders involve an abnormal number of chromosomes as a result of errors during reduction division (meiosis).

The second major clinical classification—exogenous mental deficiencies —are so labeled because of a known external causative agent. These are further subdivided into those cases attributed to infective causation (e.g., congenital syphillis, rubella, etc.); toxic causation (e.g., lead poisoning, X-radiation or atomic radiation, thalidomide); those associated with endocrine disturbances (e.g., hypothyroidism or cretinism), or traumatic causation (e.g., as by anoxia, hemorrhage); the deprivative mental deficiencies associated with deprivation of nutritional elements (e.g., vitamin deficiencies) or even psychological factors. Presumably this would also include those suffering retardation on the basis of cultural deprivation.

*Etiological.* Because of the difficulties that sometimes arise in distinguishing between endogenous and exogenous classifications, particularly in subclinical varieties of retardation, an alternative system is often employed. An etiological classification into genetic, prenatal, neonatal, and postnatal causation has been proposed and appears in more recent texts (4). Thus cases of known dominant or recessive patterns of inheritance are included under genetic etiology, as are cases of milder retardation where we are unaware of the number of genes involved or the mode of transmission but there is a presumed interaction of multiple gene inheritance and environment. Adverse prenatal factors affecting the unborn child include infection, trauma, anoxia, nutrition, chronic illness, drug ingestion, prematurity, blood incompatibilities, toxemia of pregnancy, and possibly even emotional distress. The essential elements affecting the neonatal period are the mother's health, the process of labor and delivery, and the infant's condition at birth. The effects of physical handicaps, emotional problems, cultural deprivation, as well as those conditions listed earlier that are usually associated with brain damage, all stand out as significant postnatal factors causing retardation.

Hopefully, with increasing commitment to research into etiological agents in retardation, cases of unknown etiology will diminish in frequency. Retardation on the basis of maternal PKU during pregnancy, for example, may be extremely difficult to diagnose in children since they do not test positive for the disorder. It is possible that similar conditions exist for other amino acid ureas, still undiscovered as causes of retardation.

## QUALITATIVE VS. QUANTITATIVE DISTINCTIONS

Many authors have emphasized the qualitative distinction between the more severe defective and the bulk of the retarded, consisting of perhaps 89 percent of the total, who have no known qualitative differences in physiological or behavioral functioning. Zigler (43) has made this point most succinctly in pointing out the bi-modal distribution of the IQ score. Rather than precisely following the Gaussian bell-shaped curve, IQs demonstrate a bi-modal distribution with a slight peak at the lower IQ levels. Zigler reasons that this second accumulation of cases represents a distinct population of the retarded, qualitatively different from milder retardation. The bulk of the retarded are made up primarily of those familial and culturally deprived persons who represent the lower end of the normal distribution curve of intelligence rather than a qualitatively different population.

## LEVELS OF RETARDATION

There is considerably less tendency today to attribute the same degree of prognostic significance to a labeled retardation level than was true in previous eras. Advances in educational programming and behavior control of the mentally retarded, while offering no panacea for undoing or ameliorating retardation, at least suggest the possibility that many of the limitations and behaviors once considered pathognomonic for retardation can be modified by appropriate environmental manipulations. Nevertheless it is sometimes useful to enumerate the behavioral characteristics typically associated with varying degrees of retardation, with the understanding that variations within the levels exist and designations represent levels of function rather than necessarily unalterable prognoses. Test characteristics, estimated percentages, and academic expectations are summarized in Table 11–1.

The behavioral repertoires of the Profoundly retarded are usually so deficient that meaningful responses cannot be elicited from them on standard IQ tests. These persons may show, as adults, less intellectual ability than the average one-year-old. They are often nonambulatory and may populate the back wards of institutions as "crib cases" their entire lives. Since they cannot talk or communicate, they may be deprived of all but the barest rudiments of social stimulation. This state of affairs, when it exists, is unjustifiable in light of gains which have been demonstrated when social stimulation is provided. Even the Profoundly retarded have been shown capable of responding to systematic conditioning techniques designed to manipulate motor behaviors. With appropriate attention and skillful programming of primary and social rewards, many Profoundly retarded have been taught to become at least partially ambulatory and to become more socially appropriate. Thus, even at this most severe level of intellectual deficit, there is evidence that behavioral inadequacy is as much reflective of a failure of the environment to provide opportunities and conditions for learning as it is a necessary characteristic of the syndrome.

Less severe degrees of retardation show increasingly greater potential for self-help and coping behaviors contingent both upon their capacity for learning and the training provided. The Severely retarded may be trained to care for basic needs, but typically require a dependent relationship with adults. The Moderately retarded can learn to function in a semi-self-sufficient manner in Sheltered Workshops or at simple unskilled occupations. The Mildly retarded, less likely to be handicapped by physical stigmata, can usually benefit from vocational training in unskilled or semi-skilled occupations and achieve a self-supporting status in the community, working in competitive employment situations. Equipped with some vocational skills and third- to fourth-grade academic achievement, they can usually function at repetitive tasks when there is little demand for independent decision making or response to novel situations.

The occurrence of Severe retardation is comparatively consistent throughout the population, striking without regard for ethnic groups or socio-economic level. It is judged that the more severe the intellectual limitation the greater the likelihood of organic brain damage. Mild retardation occurs unevenly, with highest frequency among parents of low socio-economic level. An increased prevalence of mild retardation is associated with lack of prenatal care, prematurity, and high infant death rates. About 200,000 of the mentally retarded are residents of institutions (33). An increasing portion of those admitted to state institutions are Severely retarded or multiple handicapped.

## DIAGNOSIS

Diagnosis of mental retardation is typically accomplished by an interdisciplinary evaluation team which may include psychiatrist, social worker, psychologist, pediatric neurologist, biochemist, and geneticist. It would be usual for the child to be referred by a pediatrician when there has been ambiguity concerning the interpretation of delayed development in speech or motor areas. Retardation is diagnosed most frequently immediately after birth or during the early school years. In cases of Severe retardation, there is often sufficient symptomatology or stigmata to identify the problem at birth. Curves for the incidence of recognition of retardation show the highest peak at age six to ten, presumably when academic demands become sufficient to identify children with the milder intellectual deficits. The pediatric neurologist is in a good position to evaluate neurological and physical signs in the context of his background with normal children. The social worker contributes in gathering background information and the family history of retardation. The psychologist contributes a psychometric evaluation of intellectual and social functioning and may aid in differential diagnosis in distinguishing between the emotionally disturbed and the mentally retarded child. The psychologist may also assist in diagnostic testing of special perceptual or cognitive abilities or language functions to aid in educational prescriptions. Psychiatric participation in the diagnostic team is especially helpful when emotional disturbance is a contributing factor.

The most difficult problems for a diagnostic team are the differentiation between developmental lags within the range of normality and lags which are indicative of retardation. Intelligence testing below the age of three has often proven unreliable because of the reliance upon motor skills which have not, except in extreme cases of deficit, proved to be good predictors of later intellectual development. Of greater value in making prognostic statements have been the development of speech and language functions and the appearance of a social response to adults. There is increasing realization that retarded children may develop emotional problems as secondary to their intellectual deficits, so that an either/or type of diagnosis is seldom valid. Syndromes, such as infantile autism, once interpreted as primarily functional in nature are now believed to involve a constitutional defect with associated behavioral disorder. Since it is often difficult to distinguish between deafness and retardation in young children, the services of a competent audiologist are often required. Biochemical studies and genetic studies are also increasingly used in the diagnostic process. Because of the need for broad, multidisciplinary services for diagnosis, community evaluation centers are in the best position to assist the local practitioner. School administrators and teachers are also being made increasingly aware of retardation as a problem and are becoming involved in the diagnostic process. Community mental health centers concerned with retardation have worked in schools in providing in-service training to teachers and in making clear the resources for referral of children identified as slow learners or retarded by the schools. Parents are also more aware of retardation and sensitive to developmental delay because of efforts of concerned groups such as the National Association of Retarded Children.

## Education

A goal, however elusive, for education of the mentally retarded has been to devise an academic situation which would provide individual remedial help for each child. Theoretically it should be possible to so thoroughly evaluate each child according to his capabilities and limtiations that the educational programming would be ideally suited to his individual needs. Present-day educational technology still falls short of this goal. The methods available are deficient on at least two counts:

First, diagnostic procedures for educational skills are not sufficiently well developed to the degree that we would consider desirable. The tests of specialized perceptual or language abilities, such as the Frostig (14) or the Illinois Test of Psycholinguistic Abilities (29) are noteworthy attempts to pinpoint a specific perceptual or cognitive area and to devise curricula for remediation of these areas where deficits exist. However, the tests themselves have not been developed properly as psychometric instruments to the same degree as more traditional intelligence tests. Furthermore, the diagnostic process involves a certain degree of circularity. Children referred for a specific problem, such as reading, may demonstrate perceptual-motor or cognitive deficits using these procedures and be placed in remedial programs to teach the specific handicap. The problem has been a failure of the proponents of these tests to demonstrate a strong relation between the areas of handicap as identified by the test procedures and the educational deficiency such as reading or to indicate that improvement in these areas by special remedial treatment will also affect academic level. Specific procedures for educating the retarded or the brain-damaged child have grown to become cults in themselves without scientifically validated effectiveness.

Second, the teaching methods themselves have not progressed to the point where universally accepted educational techniques can be applied with confidence to specific deficits when identified. Evidence indicates that retarded children in classrooms make relatively small academic gains even by special education procedures. Presently, education for the retarded consists of a "smorgasbord" of teaching techniques, procedures, and curricula, all with their enthusiastic proponents and research backing. Even the effect of special vs. regular class placement, a controversy that traces back to the 1930s, remains unresolved with little empirical evidence to demonstrate clear-cut benefits of special class placement. Sociometric studies in the past two decades have been consistent in demonstrating that retarded children in regular classrooms are rejected by their normal IQ classmates and remain in the position of social isolates (17, 21, 28, 40). Even within retarded groups sociometric status and popularity are directly related to measured intelligence (10). These findings have been used as justification for grouping retarded children into remedial classrooms, thereby removing them from interaction with children of normal intelligence. More recently the pendulum may be swinging back in the other direction. While placement in special classes may make it easier to program with the use of specialized techniques, it is difficult to evaluate the effect upon personality as a result of so stigmatizing a child as to place him in a remedial educable class. The resolution of this problem may be found with individualized teaching programs and special resource rooms staffed by remedial teachers and therapists, without removing the child from the interaction of the normal classroom.

Kirk's (25) review of research in education indicates little in the way of solid experimental support for the effectiveness of any particular teaching method. In reading instruction, for example, phonic methods have generated considerable support, while sight and other methods of teaching have an equal number of supportive studies. Kirk finds that mentally retarded children in special classes do not read up to their mental-age–reading-grade expectancy, and that special class teachers tend to de-emphasize academic learning since their interest is in the reduction of frustration and in the social and emotional development of the children. In special classes in the community, as well as within institutions, it is probably more the norm than the exception to find children recycled to the same academic material year in and year out with little change in achievement level. Research studies, examining one teaching method or another, typically find that retarded children progress upon initial involvement in such programs until their achievement reaches their mental-age–grade expectancy; as they approach this level, their progress tends to taper off. The existence of this state of affairs indicates the need for two types of activity: the development of innovative techniques for teaching the retarded, possibly by the use of other professional research disciplines for generating testable hypotheses about teaching, and the development of evaluative-controlled studies for assessing the effectiveness of new techniques.

The ultimate solutions for educational problems may come from more sophisticated use of individualized, programmed instruction materials or computer-assisted instruction (1). The evidence for both of these techniques suggests that the individualized programming has its best results with the below average student. The computer offers the potential for providing truly individualized instruction for both rote drill and the teaching of new concepts.

## Education Programs for the Retarded

Perhaps the most needed educational service for retarded children is the preschool program designed as a readiness class to evaluate and prepare retarded children for entrance into special education classes. Unfortunately, few preschool level programs for the retarded are presently in existence. Despite the current emphasis on early identification of the retarded child, the parents of these children find little in the way of community resources to help them in educational programming. Except for nursery classes for the retarded, few schools provide educational programs before the age of five or six. Yet the need for programming seems self-evident at a time when initial learning, language concepts, socialization, and management skills may be delayed or lacking. The need is greatest for a structured educational program, as well as help for parents in implementing educational activities at home. Preschool classes, when they are available, for children from ages two to five should stress basic areas of personal management, speech and language, physical and recreational activities, perceptual motor training, the development of visual and auditory attention skills, the development of body imagery, socialization, and behavior control.

In the past few years there has also been an increased awareness of the value of operant conditioning techniques for eliciting speech and "shaping" verbal expression as well as the attainment of language concepts. Operant conditioning programs for promoting language are conducted on an individual basis using primary rewards, such as food, or social rewards such as praise and attention, to "reinforce" speech. Such programs are expensive because of the individual attention required. However, therapists can be trained even though they lack a basic background in education or psychology. Typically, parents are also trained to use these techniques, so that the program can be extended into the home. The value of preschool education for the retarded has been well documented (24, 36).

Classrooms for trainables are relatively rare. Many public school systems still exclude the trainable child, often using the IQ as a criterion for exclusion from the educational program. Where trainable classes exist, the program must be flexible enough to house and manage children who are hyperactive and lack the necessary attention skills, so that they cannot be seated or contained in even a special education classroom. Programs for the trainable child should focus primarily on basic problems in self-help and management, obeying commands, psychosensory training, and communication skills. Trainable children must be taught to respond to simple commands, such as "come," "sit," "line up," and to understand basic concepts, such as "yes," "no," "home," "animals," "clothing," "food." For the trainable child education becomes a practical home- and community-oriented instruction in toileting, washing, care of teeth, dressing and undressing, combing and brushing, and eating. Programs also include ample opportunity for developing physical skills in the gross motor activities, such as the use of mats to develop crawling, creeping, tumbling, and jumping skills. Simple musical instruments are used to develop basic sounds and rhythms. Drawing, painting, pasting, cutting are also a part of the trainable program. While for many children the trainable programs represent the terminal level of progress, the goal of these programs should be to prepare the child to enter the educable track.

Educational programs for the retarded are geared toward the Mildly retarded child who is able to be contained in small classroom situations and demonstrates sufficient self-control and self-maintenance behavior so that these areas do not have to be stressed in the programs. Ideally, the curriculum is geared toward practical goals and knowledge that would be necessary for functioning within the community. It is imperative that the curriculum, in community schools as well as within institutions, be designed to foster the social and academic skills needed to prepare the individual for independent living. For children who have spent any portion of their lives within an institutional setting, it is especially important that their learning experience counteract the inherent conditions of residential living and ameliorate the special problems fostered by the shelter of the institution. Many school programs have been developed for the educable child, but there has been little attempt to develop a curriculum which would be universally acceptable. Reviews of the area have commented on the present poorly organized state of the field of special education. Sparks and Blackman (38), for example, comment, "Proof must be forthcoming that there is something more special about special education than the children assigned to these classes."

Typically, the educational curriculum should include such topics as monetary skills, newspaper skills, and the use of community resources and recreational activities. Programming for basic academic subjects is usually de-emphasized in favor of this more practical type of teaching. Remedial work in reading and numerical skills may often have to be accomplished by individual tutoring for progress to be demonstrated. Classroom teaching should ideally be supplemented with as many community trips as are feasible. Special materials for the retarded are available with emphasis on community skills. Textbooks and readers must be written to combine a low level of reading difficulty with areas of high interest value to retarded children.

For adolescent educable retarded, the school curriculum frequently involves a work-study program. The vocationally oriented classroom can be supplemented with vocational training and on-the-job experience. Various programs have been developed with students spending part of their day in each setting or alternating assignments between the classroom and the job. This program serves as a transition between school and vocational training for the retarded. When the school is limited in resources for providing vocational training, jobs in the community can be used for the vocational training assignment. Also during this period it is advantageous to refer the student to the state rehabilitation agency to begin planning realistically for his future. The success of the work-study program depends upon the coordination between the two phases of the program. Classroom teaching must be used to supplement the work and community experiences of the student and academic training is further de-emphasized in favor of practical concrete work and community oriented skills.

Ancillary services should be available in school programs for the retarded throughout the school history of the child. Only very specialized facilities, however, would typically be staffed with the physical therapist, speech therapist, and other specialists and consultants who would be needed for the multiple handicapped child. Children with special disabilities associated with retardation, such as the cerebral palsied child or the blind or deaf retarded child, would usually need an extremely specialized facility if they are to receive an educational program. Children suffering retardation as a result of German measles in the mother during the first trimester of pregnancy may have very severe visual and auditory handicaps. The rubella epidemic of 1964 produced thousands of retarded children, now of school age, with such severe handicaps that few educational programs are available to meet their needs. Because many retarded children have additional handicaps, special education teachers for the retarded need to be extremely flexible in their orientation and broad in their skills.

## Vocational and Social Rehabilitation

Ideally, rehabilitation programs are organized along a continuum of training experiences with the ultimate goal being independent community living. Any student may begin at the lowest level in the continuum or at a level commensurate with his ability to progress through a graduated series of vocational assignments of increasing complexity. The programming is also sequenced so that increasing social demands are made upon the individual. Typically, a rehabilitation program involves vocational training and adult education instruction in areas judged important for community functioning. A diagnostic evaluation unit designed to assess vocational skills, capacities, and interests is used to assign students to their appropriate level. In addition to traditional vocationally oriented tests, such as the Minnesota Rate of Manipulation and Purdue Pegboard, specialized scales of vocational potential have been developed at various facilities. Attempts have also been made to develop interest tests for occupations suitable for the mentally retarded. Unfortunately, many of the vocational aptitude tests that are suitable for individuals in the regular schools or work settings do not have a sufficiently developed set of standardized norms for the low IQ subjects. It is not unusual to find all students functioning within the first or second percentile of the standardized tests and therefore to be unable to make adequate discriminations between individual students. For this reason, work sample types of evaluations have been developed at individual facilities where norms developed are specific for that facility or the population being studied.

The vocational programs may start at the lowest level with an occupational therapy classroom. Within institutions this is often intended for the most severely retarded or elderly students. A Sheltered Workship is an essential part of a vocational training program for the retarded. The Workshop provides unskilled work in tasks, such as assembly and packaging. This work is contracted by private industry and usually involves tasks which are too seasonal or monotonous and unattractive for the companies' regular factory workers. Workshops are able to handle these jobs by using large numbers of workers and organizing the job to the special skills of the retarded. Workers may work on an hourly or piece-rate basis. The Workshop conforms to minimum wage requirements by prorating the worker's salary according to his estimated degree of disability. Although better methods for improving productivity in Sheltered Workshops for the retarded still need to be developed, present-day Workshops provide employment for many individuals who might otherwise be denied any meaningful activity. The Sheltered Workshop may be the highest level of work adjustment for a retarded worker, particularly those in severely or moderately retarded categories. It may also provide initial training in work skills and work adjustment to serve as prerequisite for more advanced vocational trade training assignments for higher level retarded. Workshops may be located within community settings or within an institution for the retarded.

For the individual who has learned minimal work skills at a Workshop level and has satisfactory attitudes toward work, and perseverance, more advanced vocational trade training is appropriate. Occupations found most suitable for the retarded have included those primarily in unskilled or semi-skilled levels, especially in service or custodial occupations. Retarded workers have been found to make successful adjustments as custodians and janitors, food service workers in preparation or cleanup, and unskilled factory workers. In certain cases, retarded workers have been trained as keypunch operators or as helpers and assistants in the manual trades as well as in print shops. It is important that training be given only in areas where there is a reasonable likelihood that the retarded individual will be able to obtain employment. He should, as much as possible, be allowed to express his own preferences for an occupation, and it is sometimes advisable to utilize a period of exploratory placement in several occupations, so as to form a basis for a choice. Regional differences in occupations should also be considered in training programs. Occupations such as farming, shoe repair, gardening, and nursery work, once considered appropriate for training the retarded, are no longer considered beneficial in urban areas because of the lack of demand for such workers or the seasonal nature of the work. In one rehabilitation facility for the retarded, the most frequent occupations used for training are custodial and janitorial work, kitchen work, and hospital orderly assignments for males; kitchen work, nurse's aide, and housekeeping work are used most frequently for females. Other training, such as power sewing, business education, printer's apprentice, electricians, carpenters, and plumber's helper may also be valuable, but are usually restricted to upper grade retarded.

It is essential that an active educational program be used to complement the vocational training well beyond the school-age years. This program may have to function during the evenings for students receiving vocational training during normal work hours. Adult education classes are used to provide three services: (a) basic remedial work in academic skills considered essential for functioning on the job or in the community; (b) instruction in utilizing community services; (c) counseling for problems encountered by students in their job or community experiences.

The problem of deciding which areas need to be taught during adult education classes is still ambiguous. Common sense judgments are used to develop a curriculum which typically includes courses in money handling and banking, transportation, post office skills, employment application procedures, and use of leisure time activities. Basic social sight vocabularies teaching the recognition of vital words are also included. However, there is a lack of necessary information as to what skills are absolutely essential for training the retarded to function in the community. The completion of job application blanks, for example, is often a skill which is very difficult to teach retarded students and may actually not be required in unskilled jobs as part of the application procedure. Counseling may be accomplished by group or individual approaches and is usually very practical in nature and related to real-life situations. More traditional types of counseling and therapy with the retarded may not prove effective.

Following the vocational training phase of the rehabilitation program, a community-based, halfway house experience as a transition to independent living may be beneficial. For institutionalized retarded being trained to return to the community, it is usually considered essential. The halfway house provides a less structured setting than the institution where the individual may work in a job in the community and still receive some shelter and support. The halfway house may be provided with rehabilitation services for adult education and counseling and may function as a social club for retarded persons living in the community. It offers the advantages of being separated from the institution and free from institutional rules and regulations which sometimes operate as a detriment to rehabilitation programs stressing independent functioning. It may also be possible to introduce certain types of programming, such as sex education, in a community-based halfway house facility, when it is not feasible within an institution or school setting.

Follow-up studies of retarded persons identified during their school years or while they were residents of institutions have been performed with some regularity over the past several decades (2, 6, 42). The results are consistent in documenting the relatively good community adjustment of upper grade retarded. Whether the persons studied were first identified in public schools or within institutions, the results indicate that they are generally capable of independent community functioning. They have been able to maintain employment in competitive work situations at their level and to maintain themselves socially so as to avoid legal difficulty. Many have married and had children. As a group they have performed less well than control subjects of normal intelligence along many criteria of functioning, but cannot be distinguished from normal intelligence groups of comparable socio-economic background (23). This opinion, while still controversial, has gained acceptance among most workers with the retarded. Ambiguity in interpretation of these results arises because of the absence of solid criteria of adjustment along which to judge retarded in the community and it is difficult to arrive at a percentage of successes vs. failure cases in the community to use as a standard. For example, if a rehabilitation program within an institution for the retarded reports 75 percent of its discharged subjects are able to maintain themselves over a five-year period without need for reinstitutionalization or serious social difficulties, is this sufficient justification for the program? There is no easy way to balance the 25 percent of the cases who may have had serious problems against the larger percentage of successful graduates of the program. The only resolution is the development of more refined prognostic indices of later community adjustment, so as to increase the accuracy of selection for discharge.

## Therapies

The major responsibility for treatment of the retarded rests with educational and rehabilitation programs. However, there are many medical, physical, or psychological therapies which may be required at some point during the life span of the retarded individual. Often a retarded individual may be maintained on a dosage of a given drug to make him more amenable to other treatments. Medication is applied not as specific to mental deficiency, but to certain behavioral problems or symptomatology. Thus anticonvulsant drugs are used when seizures are a problem, tranquilizing medication for aggressive or behavioral disturbance, and antidepressant medication where appropriate. Naturally, the physician would be called upon to care for the physical illnesses as they develop in the retarded person all during the course of his life.

Physical therapists work with orthopedic and gross motor deficits usually within educational or rehabilitation settings. Many of the techniques of the physical therapist have proven valuable in teaching retarded children to walk and in helping them develop better motor control.

Psychological therapies with the retarded are probably somewhat less varied than with normal intelligence groups. However, many techniques have been developed. In general, the higher frequency of speech deficits and communication problems in the retarded may make the verbal therapies less useful. Most retarded persons have the capacity to relate emotionally to a therapist and the relationship may prove effective in producing therapeutic outcomes. Goals of therapy are directed less toward insight and more toward the modification of inappropriate behaviors and the learning of appropriate ways of reacting to others. Counseling relationships have been most successful when they have focused on job or community problems most relevant to the retarded individual's immediate situation. Therapeutic efforts are directed toward ego development and body imagery more so than with other disability groups. Acceptance of one's limitations, understanding the nature of the handicap, and the setting of realistic levels of aspiration and expectancies are very real problems in counseling or therapy with the mentally retarded. Retarded children and adults have typically been subject to a much greater degree of rejection and failure experience than other groups and levels of self-esteem may be unrealistically low. Unrealistically high expectancies of success may also develop in retarded who have been overprotected within the home or have been placed in dependent and sheltered relationships within residential institutions. As with other groups, therapy with retarded children has often needed to involve parents. Counseling for the families of retarded groups is especially important in dealing with patterns of guilt and infantilization which may occur. It is often necessary to teach parents to react appropriately to the retarded and to encourage them to develop traits of independence in their children.

A major innovation in treatment of mentally retarded over the past decade has been the introduction of behavior modification techniques of control and teaching. These techniques, based upon the psychology of learning, have proven particularly effective in cottage programs, especially for those low level children for whom very little exists in the way of education or training. The most useful techniques have been derived from operant conditioning procedures based upon the work of B. F. Skinner. The general principle applied, labeled "reinforcement," is based on the findings that a response followed by a state of affairs which is pleasing or gratifying to the individual will increase its probability of recurrence. Operant conditioning techniques systematically apply reinforcement to appropriate responses and withdraw reinforcement of inappropriate responses (extinction). Operant conditioning programs have been used to teach self-help skills, such as dressing, washing, and toileting, to groups of retarded children by imposing rigidly enforced reinforcement systems for behavior. Typically, attendant staff are trained to dispense a conditioned reinforcer, such as a poker chip or token, of successive approximations to desired behavior. These tokens are later exchangeable for material rewards, such as food or toys. The conditioning process (shaping) initially involves the reinforcement of behaviors which are only approximations of the desired terminal behavior. Gradually demands for behavior are increased before reinforcement is applied. In-service training programs are used to provide the attendant staff with a theoretical basis for the procedure and to train them in the actual techniques. Textbooks are also available for this purpose (19, 31).

Individually applied operant conditioning techniques have also been useful in teaching retarded or autistic children to speak. With this technique food or social reinforcement is given for very small approximations of a desired vocal response. Initially any vocalization is reinforced. Later reinforcement is given only for imitation or partial imitation of a sound. Words, phrases, and sentences are built up piecemeal, and the ultimate goal is functional and conversational speech. This technique is vividly illustrated in the film *Reinforcement Therapy* (37).

With severe behavior disorders, such as self-mutilation or violently aggressive behavior, it is sometimes possible to achieve behavior control by the use of aversive conditioning. Punishment such as the word "No" paired with a sharp slap or electric shock stimulation applied to the arm or leg has been effective in controlling such behavior. Aversive stimulation can be used in three ways: (a) an aversive stimulus can be applied directly following some inappropriate response; (b) termination of an aversive stimulus can be made contingent upon some socially appropriate response; (c) termination of the aversive stimulus can be paired with some previously neutral stimulus to make it become more positive. This last technique has been used to condition autistic children to respond more appropriately to their parents (27).

Speech therapy has been applied to the retarded, primarily for dealing with articulation problems and stuttering. As contrasted with operant conditioning, the intent has been to apply knowledge of the voice and speech mechanisms and structures, rather than the application of principles of learning. Because of the limited intellectual skills of the retarded child or adult with speech problems, techniques effective with other handicapped populations have not been as successful with the mentally retarded.

Recreational activities have also been used as therapy for the retarded. Under this broad heading can be included such diverse activities as music therapy, which uses rhythms and melody to encourage vocalization and emotional expression; corrective gymnastics used as an adjunct to physical therapy; and a wide variety of organized games and sports activities which may have educational value while providing exercise and fun for the retarded. Specific techniques for recreating the retarded have been developed and geared toward the intellectual and physical limitations of the child. The use of such activities as swimming, bowling, roller skating, miniature golf, and movies has the additional advantage of introducing the retarded person to these activities with the intent of making them more available to him as a source of recreation outside the institution or school. Because many retarded individuals are reluctant to try new activities, it is essential that they have the opportunity to sample as many different forms of recreation as possible during their training years.

## Impact upon Families

Physical and emotional rejection of the mentally retarded can occur at many levels. Many families are emotionally ill equipped to deal with the trauma of a retarded child, especially when the retardation is severe and physical stigmata are apparent. In such cases, the psychological health of the parents, especially the mother, can be maintained only by immediate placement of the child in a suitable residential facility. The tragedy of bearing a severely defective child and the disruptive effect upon the family can be truly appreciated only by those who have had this experience. In many cases these wounds heal only with the death of the retarded child. Yet modern-day medical care and medication now make it possible to maintain even profoundly retarded individuals into adulthood. The greatest tragedy, however, is not with the profoundly retarded child who is placed at birth into a residential facility, but with those who are less limited and able to perceive parental rejection. State and private residential facilities are filled with many abandoned children. The phenomenon of the retarded child within an institution, futilely watching other parents arrive on visitors' day, is all too common. Frequently such children cling to fantasies about their natural parents or even some professional person, such as a social worker, who has had only fleeting responsibility in the placement process.

Also common is a degree of more subtle emotional rejection which may exist for a child with intellectual handicaps. Often parents are unconscious of the extent of their feelings toward the child who has failed to live up to their expectations intellectually. Parental reactions are often accurately perceived and reflected in the behavior of normal siblings. Rejection may be expressed by communications to the child of expectations for him that are below his actual capacity. In one Mildly retarded, brain-damaged child, who at seven was still not toilet trained, parents despaired of his ever being able to assume normal bowel functions. It was only after professional help was applied and the child was trained that parents were able to recognize their own feelings for the boy as something "less than human." An even more insidious form of rejection is expressed as a smothering infantilization of the child, reinforcing his dependent behavior and limiting his potential for emotional growth and maturity. This type of behavior is usually fostered by parental guilt; parents act out their fantasy that the child cannot exist except when being continuously monitored and controlled by them. It is not uncommon that mentally retarded persons are kept in the home and denied appropriate schooling or vocational training experiences until these are no longer feasible. Eventually these persons find their way into institutions when their parents become too old to provide further care.

Other parents of the retarded may deny any problem exists. Elaborate intellectual defenses are erected to explain away the slowness of language and motor development. Unrealistic demands are continually placed upon the child. One parent of a Mildly retarded girl, for example, reportedly chided her for failure to keep up in her French, so that she might apply to college.

It is possible for parents of the retarded to accept the child's disability without rejection, infantilization, or denial. Such parents are able to accept the individual for what he is, to find the appropriate programs geared both to assets and limitations of the child, to react to him naturally without either guilt or excessive sympathy, to be able to apply consistent methods of discipline, punishment, and control when necessary, and to encourage the retarded individual to attempt new tasks to the utmost of his potential. The retarded child growing up in this atmosphere often seems markedly superior in his general adjustment and development as compared to children growing up under more adverse circumstances. The role of the professional must be one of support for the family of a retarded child. He must communicate by all his behaviors toward the parents that a mentally retarded child is a worthwhile individual with special needs for acceptance and education.

## Residential Programs

In many cases the decision to institutionalize a retarded child is made by a state agency, such as the Department of Public Welfare or Public Assistance. In such cases children are sometimes referred more because of social inadequacies than because of their intellectual limitations. Children referred by this means have often suffered from parental abuse or may have inadequate or disinterested parents. They may also have been referred by the courts because of delinquent behavior. When a child is referred to a residential program by the parents, the decision is often painful. There are no hard and fast rules for indicating when such referral is necessary. The decision is an individual one which must rest upon the nature of the disability and the availability of education or training resources outside of the institution. The trend toward more community involvement with the mentally retarded, in the public schools and through community workshops and training centers, has made institutionalization unnecessary for many retarded. The functioning of the family of the retarded child is also a consideration. Many retarded children are maintained in the home at a considerable expense to other siblings. Generally, the more severe the retardation, the more likely it will be that institutionalization will be necessary at some point in the individual's life. Assuming that parents are not rejecting of the child and are emotionally mature enough to deal with the reality of his disability, it is usually assumed that placement in a residential setting should not occur before the school-age years. Even when the individual is so placed, family involvement with the child through visits, letters, and telephone calls is encouraged. This is in marked contrast to attitudes which were prevalent as recently as ten years ago; it was not atypical for parents of institutionalized retarded children to be discouraged from maintaining contact with the child because of a "disrupting" influence. Ideally, the modern institution for the retarded should serve as a school and rehabilitation facility. The dichotomy between home and residential settings should not be maintained. The programming in the institution can extend into the home through parental counseling; parents can contribute by providing the institution with the proper understanding of the child's background and development and by extending treatment and education programs into the home.

Unfortunately, this ideal is seldom achieved at institutions. For children who have been separated from parents at an early age and who spend major portions of their lives within the institutional setting, our public institutions have been described as dehumanizing environments with devastating effects upon personality development (16, 26). We are only now beginning to understand the large gaps in social repertoires of children brought up in institutions. Many deficits in adult retarded relate more closely to their institutional upbringing than to the original effects of mental subnormality. Inadequate numbers of attendant staff and indifference of professional staff to problems in wards and dormitories often leave residential programs largely custodial. Attendant staff, with little training or support, are left largely to their own devices to deal with severe behavioral problems. Homosexual behavior, for example, fostered by close confinement and the absence of appropriate outlets for sexual impulse, is a problem in every institution for the retarded. Yet in many implicit ways the institution communicates to the child that such behavior is both expected and condoned. Even in more modern institutions with progressive education and rehabilitation programs, residence units often lag far behind the progressive philosophy of other aspects of the programs. The greatest need is for a structured social learning experience within the residence units. Residential programs, typically the special province of nursing or "cottage life" departments, need to be managed by teaching and professional staff versed in social engineering principles and the ecology of institutions. Residences must be viewed as laboratories for the academic program, and teachers, like other professional staff, should be flexible enough to leave the safety of their classrooms to deal with the real problems of residential living in their natural setting. The therapeutic milieu approach within institutions for the retarded is still a rare phenomenon. With the retarded this concept means more than just inculcating an understanding or permissive attitude among the nonprofessional attendant staff. Indeed, the use of in-service training approaches with attendant staff for the retarded can often have a detrimental effect. By conveying to staff the attitude that early environmental influence or physical factors can cause retardation, it may also suggest little can be done about the problem. A "nominalistic fallacy" can easily develop with the mistaken assumption that labeling a phenomenon is the same as understanding it. The therapeutic milieu for retarded persons in residential settings must involve appropriate measures for behavior control and for fostering independent functioning.

## Cognitive Functioning

The quest for some psychological factor which would differentiate the mentally retarded from "normal" populations has been as intense as the search for physical, neurological, biochemical, and genetic factors. Unfortunately, the results have not been as productive except in terms of theoretical approaches offered, which are numerous. Major theoreticians of learning in the mentally retarded are split into two opposing orientations. Yale psychologist Edward Zigler (43) has labeled this split the "defect vs. developmental" orientation. Those taking a defect position attribute learning and performance deficits in the mentally retarded to some structural or organic handicap. Thus Denny (9) describes an inhibition deficit in the retarded, Ellis (13) finds evidence for short-term memory deficits, and Spitz (39) sees evidence of a defect in cortical satiation processes.

As an alternative to structural approaches to deficits in retardation, an opposing school of thought attributes learning and performance deficits, at least in upper grade retardates, primarily to motivational lags stemming from cultural-social phenomena. According to this "developmental" orientation, the familial retardate's cognitive development differs from that of the normal individual only with respect to its rate and upper limit. Low intelligence of the familial retardate is viewed as a particular manifestation of the general developmental process. Zigler has been the most outspoken proponent of the effect of motivational and emotional factors influencing the environmental histories of retardates. Zigler points to the greater amount of failure experience of the retardate, and his history of greater social deprivation. "Factors thought to be of particular importance in the behavior of the retardate are social deprivation and the positive-and-negative-reaction tendencies to which such deprivation gives rise; the high number of failure experiences and the particular approach to problem-solving which they generate; and atypical reinforcer hierarchies" (43a). This same general position has been proposed by Cromwell (8) in a series of studies reflecting the higher expectancy of failure of retardates. Cromwell suggests that the retardate is more highly motivated to avoid failure than to achieve success.

A position somewhat between the structural or "defect" approach and "developmental" approaches has been offered by Bijou (5). Bijou has argued against viewing the cause of psychological retardation as a theoretical construct such as mentality, or as a biological phenomenon such as impairment of the brain. Instead, he suggests that retardation be conceived simply as failures of coordination between stimulus and response functions. Quoting Kantor (22), Bijou argues,

In such cases as have been traditionally called idiocy, imbecility, and moronity, the basic principle is the failure of the individual to build up response equipment to certain things. There is a failure to coordinate certain stimulus-response functions.

In other words, a retarded individual is one who has a limited repertory of behavior evolving from interactions of the individual with his environmental context which constitutes his history . . . From this point of view, the task of behavioral research is to investigate the observable . . . conditions which produce retarded behavior, not retarded mentality (5a).

The conditions subjected to investigation are the biological, physical, and social interactions past and current. It is contended that retarded development is generated by variations in biological, physical, and social factors. This point of view provides an adequate integration of the defect and developmental positions. Inadequate reinforcement histories, which may be expected to occur in many social situations, would be expected to limit repertoires in self-care, "manners," emotional-social reactions, and pre-academic and academic skills.

Denny's (9) review of the learning and performance literature in mental retardation lists four ways in which a mentally retarded person appears to learn or perform inadequately:

1. An inhibition deficit as manifested by increased resistance to extinction in classical conditioning, difficulty in discrimination learning, and special susceptibility to disinhibition or distraction.
2. Defect in complex learning as exhibited in poor performance on learning set, delayed reaction, and double alternation problems.
3. Difficulty in verbal learning as reflected in poor performance on verbal rote learning and abstraction tasks.
4. A lack of verbal control of the motor sphere as shown in poor semantic conditioning, difficulty in following verbal instructions, lack of verbalization, and discrimination reversal.

On the other hand, there are also positive characteristics:

1. As compared with normals of the same chronological age, retardates initially do very poorly at motor skill tasks, but with continued practice, show a rapid rate of improvement. If a task is not too difficult, they might even catch up with the normals.
2. In rote learning, if familiar nonverbal material is used, an association seems to be established as quickly and retained about as well as in the normals.
3. There is little evidence of an appreciable retention deficit in any motor performance area.
4. The retardate can learn to use verbal mediators when specifically trained to do so, although they do not seem to use them spontaneously.

Denny concludes:

The outlook for the mentally retarded is surprisingly optimistic—at least theoretically. It should be possible to develop appropriate motivational procedures and special training techniques to overcome an appreciable portion of the retardates' difficulties, at least to the extent that they relate to closely connected deficits in incidental learning, attention, and verbal control. These defects might be amenable to correction by (a) long-term training to attend or orient to stimuli, especially verbal stimuli; and (b) motivating retarded children sufficiently and building in what they failed to learn incidentally during the early years, as, for example, with specially designed and programmed teaching machines (9a).

## Social and Emotional Functioning

The evaluation of social and emotional factors affecting personality of the mentally retarded can proceed in two directions. Analysis can be made by psychological or psychiatric assessment of individuals or groups. It is also possible to make judgments about emotional and social functioning by the study of behaviors of known retarded populations. Both procedures have their pitfalls. Retarded persons as a group are relatively nonverbal and inarticulate. Therefore it is easy to infer a lack of well-differentiated emotional development or personality structure from the absence of verbal response. Projective testing with retarded populations is frequently an unproductive procedure for just this reason. Often a large percentage of responses on projective tests can be attributed to intellectual rather than personality or emotional factors. Experimental procedures in the laboratory have been used to provide more direct evidence of emotional responsiveness and subjective reactions. Simple laboratory procedures, such as the level of aspiration technique, used with retarded populations have led to the conclusion of Cromwell (8) and others that retarded children have a lower generalized expectancy of success than normals as a result of having had fewer successes in past situations. Evidence exists demonstrating differential effects, in normals and retarded subjects, of failure in experimental situations. Residential care for the retarded seems to be more conducive to optimism and self-confidence than is nonsheltered school and community experience. This suggests that optimism and self-esteem are related to competence in meeting the demands of one's social situation. Institutions for the retarded, like those for the mentally ill, provide a set of demands and expectations that differ from those provided by a non-institutional environment. Protection, encouragement, training, more realistic standards for performance, and more realistic conditions of competition may well serve to heighten optimism and self-evaluation.

Perhaps the most relevant information about social functioning of the retarded derives from controlled observations of their behavior in schools and institutions and as a result of follow-up investigations of retarded persons in the community. Since the largest groupings of retarded persons are within institutions, it is natural that most of our understanding of the retarded has come from this source. Unfortunately, it is extremely difficult to separate the effects of retardation from those of institutional living. It is a widely accepted belief, for example, that the child with Down's Syndrome is a placid, happy, easily managed, and cooperative child. This is often the case, but aggressive, hyperactive, and even psychotic mongoloid children can also be observed. Thus individual differences are as prevalent among retarded individuals as among normal populations.

One of the unfortunate consequences of living in an institution may be analogous to what has been described as "conditioned helplessness" (35) in animals. When dogs are exposed to a noncontingent electric shock, the result is a chronically constricted and passive behavior. After a conditioning procedure consisting of many trials of unpredictable shock, which the animal cannot avoid or escape, he develops a helpless "cowering" behavior which extends into later trials even where escape from the shock is possible. Institutional experience at an early age may also impose many noncontingent aversive situations upon the retarded individual over which he has little or no control. Passivity, dependency, and the lack of initiative may be the end product of such learning. Other retarded persons who were institutionalized as children may never outgrow a rebellious, defiant disrespect for authority which can distort social perceptions and handicap interpersonal relationships long after the institutional experience is over.

Retarded adults in the community usually demonstrate at least the minimal social skills and behaviors to maintain independent existence. However, their social judgment may continue to be poor, their decision-making processes of marginal quality, and their susceptibility to deception or fraud can be quite high. Older ideas about moral degeneracy in certain retarded are no longer seriously believed. However, retarded persons of higher level, functioning in the community, may be more susceptible to social problems because of poor judgment and gullibility. This may be especially true in females who can be taken advantage of both economically and sexually. These instances among one previously institutionalized population now living in the community, though relatively rare, were frequent enough to be of concern to the institution. The problems are no longer considered the result of personality deviation of genetic or constitutional origin, but a function of the absence of sound emotional and interpersonal experiences in growth and development. It also may be possible that better training programs of sex education and contraception would be effective in generating more successful adjustment.

The link between crime and delinquency and mental retardation has also been the subject of a considerable amount of investigation, with a gradual liberalizing of professional attitudes toward this problem. Studies of families such as the Jukes (12) and the Kallikaks (15) around the turn of the century were instrumental in influencing public opinion about the link between mental retardation and all the social ills of our society. Goddard's study of the Kallikaks traced two lineages of descendants, both by the same individual. One lineage was the result of an illegitimate relationship with a "feebleminded" girl; the other was the descendants of his later marriage with a normal, "respectable girl of good family." Through several generations the first lineage produced a high frequency of mental deficiency, mental illness, crime, prostitution, and alcholism. There were few instances of this deriving from the second lineage. This study seems extremely unsophisticated in light of today's insistence on appropriate controls in scientific investigations. The most obvious criticism of the study is the failure to control for environmental conditions as significant determinants of delinquent behavior in the Kallikak family.

Similar conclusions about the link between mental deficiency and crime were drawn from studies of prison populations which reported high incidences of IQs below 70. These studies demonstrated one aspect of a correlation between IQ and prison record, but they failed to investigate the entire relationship. While the studies indicate that there is a higher probability of low IQ persons in prison populations, they do not examine the frequency of having a prison record as a function of being retarded. When such studies are performed, the demonstrated relationship between criminal behavior and retardation is very small.

A recently published follow-up study conducted at Elwyn Institute (7) described the postinstitutional adjustment of sixty-five persons discharged from the institution who were orphaned or who had families that were inadequate or unwilling to accept them after discharge from the institution. All of these persons had been diagnosed as "feebleminded" or mentally retarded upon their admission to Elwyn and their average length of institutionalization was fifteen years.

After six to twelve months in the community, the group was making a satisfactory vocational, economic, and social adjustment. They were able to maintain their jobs, which were primarily in unskilled or semiskilled occupations, in personal, food, or building services, or as operatives, laborers, stock and factory workers. They were doing an adequate job in housekeeping, had purchased furniture and other possessions, had established savings accounts, were paying their bills, acquiring driver's licenses, purchasing automobiles, paying income tax, avoiding excessive debts, purchasing life insurance, marrying, bearing children, and avoiding legal difficulties or social welfare rosters. On the negative side their salaries were fairly low and they showed a certain degree of dissatisfaction with their salary levels and their relatively low status on the job.

In general, the sample showed more work dissatisfaction than normal (nonretarded) workers, but could not be differentiated from handicapped (nonretarded) workers. The most promising predictors of criteria of community adjustment were derived from tests and behavioral ratings completed during the subjects' institutional training experience. These consisted of perceptual-motor tests and ratings of work behaviors and work potential. Tests of verbal intelligence and academic achievement showed almost no significant relationships with criteria. Interestingly, although vocational supervisors were able to predict, with some accuracy, the students who would make the best adjustment in the community, staff members concerned with social functioning, discipline, and general behavior in the residence units were unable to make successful predictions. It may be that social conformity within the institution is not a reliable index of later social adjustment in the community.

The question of marriage for the mentally deficient is still a controversial issue. Marriage for the "weak-minded" is forbidden by the law in three states and possibly fifteen others depending upon the interpretation of the state statutes. It is generally accepted that an IQ of 50 represents approximately the lower IQ limit of people who have been able to support themselves independently in the community, so that the question of marriage for Moderately and Severely retarded seldom arises. Some writers (3) have taken the position that marriage for the retarded can be beneficial provided the marriage remains childless. Those advocating marriage under these conditions believe that if the partners agree to sterilization, marriage will contribute to the general well-being and psychological health of the mental defective by providing a stabilizing influence and an opportunity for satisfaction of close interpersonal needs. It is felt that the retarded have sufficient difficulty in making the adjustment of independent living and that the additional burden of child-rearing may be overwhelming. Since there is not a sufficient amount of available data about the child-rearing abilities of the mentally retarded, the question remains unanswered. It is still the exception, rather than the norm, for institutions or public schools to provide the retarded with sex education courses and information about contraception. Some institutions are pioneering in working with organizations such as the Planned Parenthood Association in helping discharged graduates of the rehabilitation program obtain contraceptive advice or sterilization if they so desire.

## Prospects for the Future

It is difficult to predict future trends in the field of mental retardation without a sound appreciation of the history of the field and its recent developments. How far have we really come since Itard (20) undertook the education of Victor, the wild boy of Aveyron? In many areas certainly, the first hundred years in the history of retardation were disappointing. The development and growth of our large public institutions for the retarded, which are, in many cases, warehouses for mentally deficient persons, represent little improvement over previous conditions. Gone also, perhaps, is the unbridled optimism of the early physician-teachers of the retarded—Itard (20), Seguin (34), Descoeurdes (11), Pestalozzi (32), and Montessori (30). In its place, however, is a more realistic concern with scientifically validated methods for teaching the retarded and for developing educational technology.

The future for retardation promises further thrusts in biochemical and genetic understanding of the causes of retardation. Discovery of the relation between PKU and mental deficiency promises further breakthroughs since other amino acid ureas may have similar effects. Improved methods of chromosome study may lead to further insight about genetic disorders related to retardation and a firmer basis for genetic counseling. The new sciences of Dentochronology and Odontoglyphics provide a detailed history of brain damage recorded in the morphological structure of the teeth. Further research will discover ways of distinguishing between organic defect, genetic deficiency, and mere backwardness and, hopefully, the development of differential programs for each condition. It should help us to understand and control prematurity and the enzymatic disorders as major causes which are susceptible to prevention. Educational programs for the retarded will need to be improved to keep pace with diagnostic improvements and advances in the application of learning theory to teaching programs. Public school education will need to provide more classes for all categories of retardation. The latest educational technology, such as computer assisted instruction (CAI), will have to be tried with the retarded and judged as to its merits for providing a truly individualized form of instruction. The most important changes will undoubtedly be in residential programs and institutions for the retarded. The development of community services with social activities, recreational outlets, Sheltered Workshops, and supervised employment will gradually change the population of institutions. Increasing numbers of upper grade, educable retarded will receive sufficient vocational and social rehabilitation to return to independent or semi-sheltered community living situations. Many will never have to be institutionalized.

Institutions, in turn, will show gradual increases in the number of severely retarded, brain injured, and geriatric retarded. They will serve as a special education facility for the multiple handicapped retarded, such as those with severe visual or hearing handicaps. Within institutions a major thrust will have to be extended into the residence units themselves to apply innovations in education and training. Operant conditioning techniques are becoming increasingly useful within institutions, particularly in residential programs, and this trend should continue. With time will come the disappearance of the overcrowded ward or dormitory, typical in many residential facilities. These units, filled with half-clothed Severely and Profoundly retarded persons, often lack even the slightest hint of toys or educational materials and are ignored by professional personnel, teachers, and educational training programs. Instead building programs will come to be considered a practical applied laboratory for extending teaching and rehabilitation programs into the living situation of the retarded. Parental groups which have become a powerful lobby for better federal and state programs for the retarded should increase in their effectiveness. Small privately operated homes and schools may be needed to take up the slack and reduce the long waiting lists for state institutions. Finally, it seems evident that society's increasing awareness of and determination to provide for the poor and the underprivileged of our country will do much toward alleviating the causes of the largest percentage of mental retardation, by providing better prenatal care, a better understanding of nutrition, better medical facilities for children, and more intensive educational services at preschool age levels to culturally deprived populations. Viewed in this light the elimination of familial retardation and cultural deprivation may be largely a function of scientifically managed social engineering programs drawing from a wide range of professional disciplines.

# 12

## The Displaced Child:
## Problems of the Adopted Child,
## Single-Parent Child, and Stepchild

RALPH A. LUCE, M.D.

With the increased number of illegitimate children in the United States and the accelerated rate of family disruption occasioned by separation, divorce, and remarriage, there has been an astronomical increase in the number of displaced children, of children raised by adoptive parents or by single parents, of children who have suffered the loss, permanent or temporary, of one or both natural parents at critical stages of development, of children who have had to adapt abruptly to adoptive or step-parents with or without siblings and step-siblings in new surroundings at times unfavorable for such changes. It is our purpose to examine the more important problems inherent in what we shall call "the displaced child syndrome." We shall attempt to develop a dynamic understanding of the intrapsychic elements both within the child and within the parent or parent substitute and also, insofar as possible, to elucidate the family interaction patterns seen most commonly in clinical practice.

### The Problems of Adoption

#### THE PHENOMENOLOGY OF THE ADOPTED CHILD

The circumstances of life place the adopted child in a unique position in the world. He is condemned to rootlessness, a biological anomie, born of ignorance. He can never know or ever be sure of the forebears whose genes he carries. He can only speculate and imagine, which is to say, project, his own, real, idealized, or depreciated attitudes and attributes on a blank ancestral screen. He is permanently suspended in a state of not-knowing, yet forced by the circumstances of life to assume an attitude toward those whom he does not know. When he becomes fully aware of the meaning of adoption, he finds himself in a state of contradiction. Rejected by his biological parents but especially chosen by his adoptive parents, he must work through the fantasies and ideas of not knowing and not being loved by his "real" parents. Was he unworthy of being loved? Were they too evil, or perhaps too sick, to love him? His adoptive parents indirectly may encourage him to feel anger toward his biological parents who rejected him and gratitude toward those who chose him, but in reality he may feel neither or the opposite. What he may detect is the undercurrent of conflicting feelings in the adoptive parents related to their latent rather than professed motives for adopting him. If he was adopted at birth, the degree to which he feels rejected by his adoptive parents will depend upon the amount of conflict between them and the extent to which they have not resolved their ambivalence toward him. If the child is not adopted at birth, the degree of rejection he feels from nurturing figures is compounded by the amount of maternal deprivation or mistreatment he may have suffered in a hospital, orphanage, or unsuitable home environment prior to the adoption. A child adopted at birth and truly loved by his adoptive parents undoubtedly is much less adversely affected by his adopted status and may even feel particularly favored by it.

Although it is generally conceded that adopted children have a higher incidence of emotional problems than children raised by biological parents, the reasons are poorly understood and the statistics are woefully inadequate. Undoubtedly many factors play a part in creating emotional difficulties in the adopted child. Only a few of the more important will be mentioned. It is generally agreed that maternal deprivation, frequent changes of nurturing figures with lack of consistency, and even relatively short separations from mothering figures in early infancy can be permanently damaging to the healthy emotional development of the child. The consensus of opinion is described by Bowlby (2) as follows:

For the present, therefore, it may be recorded that deprivation occurring in the second half of the first year of life is agreed by all students of the subject to be of great significance and that many believe this to be true also of deprivation occurring in the first half, especially from three to six months. The balance of opinion, indeed, is that considerable damage to mental health can be done by deprivation in these months, a view which is unquestionably supported by the direct observations, already described, of the immediately harmful effects of deprivation on babies of this age.

The question which naturally follows is to what extent the damage can be undone when good mothering is provided later. Bowlby (2) speaks of this, as follows:

The comparative success of many babies adopted between six and nine months who have spent their first half-year in conditions of deprivation makes it virtually certain that, for many babies at least, provided they receive good mothering in time, the effects of early damage can be greatly reduced. What Dr. Goldfarb's work demonstrates without any doubt is that such mothering is almost useless if delayed until after the age of two and a half years. In actual fact this upper age limit for most babies is probably before twelve months. But the probable existence of a safety limit should not give rise to complacency: the fact that it may be possible to make good some of the damage done by deprivation in the early months is no excuse for permitting it to be inflicted in the first place.

The age at which a child learns about his adoption and the way in which he is told are considered important by most clinicians. The general practice among adoption agencies is to recommend that the child be told between the ages of two and four or when he first begins to ask questions about where he came from. Spock's book *Baby and Child Care*, the child-rearing Bible for millions of mothers, offers similar advice. Spock (16) says,

Let's say that a child around 3 hears his mother explaining to a new acquaintance that he is adopted and asks, "What's adopted, Mommy?" She might answer, "A long time ago I wanted very much to have a little baby boy to love and take care of. So I went to a place where there were a lot of babies, and I told the lady, "I want a little boy with brown hair and brown eyes." So she brought me a baby, and it was you. And I said, 'Oh this is just exactly the baby that I want. I want to adopt him and take him home to keep forever.' And that's how I adopted you."

This makes a good beginning because it emphasizes the positive side of the adoption, the fact that the mother received just what she wanted. The story will delight him, and he will want to hear it many times. Later on in the same chapter Spock advises that when the child begins asking more detailed biological questions such as whether he grew inside the mother's abdomen, the adopting mother should explain simply and casually that he grew inside another mother before he was adopted. Spock (16) admits that this may confuse the child for a while, but it will be cleared up later. It is apparent that either too much talk about being adopted, or keeping the adoption a secret, is unhealthy. L. Peller (11, 12) feels that early and repeated telling about the adopted status is confusing and destructive to the child. She feels that the standard procedure of telling a child about adoption between the ages of two to four is incompatible with analytic knowledge of the young child's needs. Peller (11, 12) further asserts that it is impossible to tell a very young child the story of his adoption without implying at the same time the cruelty of desertion and rejection, or at least unintentionally providing all the elements for such a fantasy. She states, as do other authors, that out of this fantasy the child creates a longing for the original parent which according to Schechter (14) and his coworkers leads during late adolescence and early adulthood to overtly searching for the natural parents. The likelihood is that a loving adoptive parent will use good judgment in deciding when and how much to tell the child, shaping the explanation to the framework of the child's needs rather than being driven by his own neurotic compulsion, sadistic need, or the shame that he may feel if the situation originates from his own sexual inadequacy.

Even though a child may be told about his adoption very early, the emotional impact may not occur until much later. Adopted children may react to the fact of their adoption only during what Blos (1) calls "the second individuation process of adolescence." An example is a fifteen-year-old adopted boy referred for "huffing" aerosol paint as well as defiant and threatening behavior toward parents and teachers. His father gave the following information at the time of intake, "From the beginning we followed what we believed was the best approach and told him that we had adopted him. We didn't want this information to come as a sudden shock to him later in life and to learn that we had been misleading him over a number of years. He accepted the information in his younger years as a matter of course and didn't make much of it. However, about a year or two ago there was an article in the Sunday magazine section written by a mother who several years before had given up a child for adoption because she was unwed at the time. She made no excuses for what she had done, but expressed her best wishes and love for the child wherever he might be and her hope that he would have a wonderful life with his new parents and would be successful in whatever he did. It was a beautiful piece from a parent's point of view, or a woman's for that matter. As such my wife saved and later showed it to Jim. The results were disastrous. For the first time he really became aware of the possibility of the illegitimacy of his birth. He felt degraded. He was mad at his natural mother and father for what they had done to cause him to be born under such circumstances, and he was mad at us for making him aware of this. I don't think to this date he has fully recovered from this experience."

Much has been written about how young children attempt to handle their ambivalence toward their parents by imagining that they are not their real parents and that they, themselves, are the children of royalty. This fantasy can occur with adopted children also, particularly if they are feeling especially negative toward their adoptive parents, but it is relatively infrequent. According to Simon and Centuria (15), in the patients they treated, fantasies describe the biologic parents as bad, prostitutes, drunks, etc., sometimes physically attractive but bad. It seemed to them that such fantasies were efforts to explain why they were abandoned. The identification with the "bad" biological parents is strong. These fantasies reinforce the projected hostility from the adoptive parents and the self-concept then takes on even more negative content. Simon and Centuria (15) believe that there is a depressive core behind what they describe as sociopathic pathology. The fantasy of reunion with the biologic parents appears, in their opinion, to be an effort to deal with the depression that grows out of fantasies around abandonment. In other words, children who have been adopted and who have a low self-esteem often will project the badness which they feel about themselves onto their biological parents, whose real nature they do not know. This theme has been explored further by Schechter (14) and others who believe that the awareness of the presence of two sets of parents makes it more difficult to fuse the intrapsychic "good" and "bad" parent images of infantile object relations into a workable, more realistic identification. In such persons a splitting of the ego and fixation at an ambivalent level is maintained by the very nature of the adoptive child's life situation. It may be that this latter also helps to explain the increased incidence of the aggressive and sociopathic behavior described by Menlove (8) and others.

It is the observation of this writer that adopted children may have a more turbulent adolescence than others, partly because of their identity diffusion derived from the split between identification with adoptive parents and imagined real parents, and partly also because of some very real factors that have to do with hereditary differences between adoptive parents and adoptive children. The latter increases the need to be emancipated from adopted parents, to separate the self from characteristics that are experienced as not one's own despite what appear to be long established patterns of identification that have functioned smoothly over many years. If there are very real differences between the adopted child and the adoptive parents in terms of intelligence, talent, manual skills, academic ability, etc., the adopted adolescent has a very difficult time in separating himself from the values and goals of the adoptive parents and establishing his own appropriate and unique identity. This process can be a very real problem for adopted adolescents who live in a family who have also had natural siblings who follow the goals outlined by the adoptive parents. It means that the adopted child in a sense becomes the black sheep of the family if he decides his direction must diverge from the expectations of the parents who often think of the adopted child in the same terms as they do their own natural children.

In clinical practice, the adolescent boys who seem to have the greatest difficulty are those who have adoptive fathers who are either very weak or adoptive fathers who are highly authoritative. In the family with the weak father, the adoptive mother is usually the dominating influence, and the boy must struggle to disentangle himself from the emotional bonds to her. Often such bonds are erotic as well as dependent, because the dominating mother may have acted seductively toward the boy, using him for her affectional needs when and if the father has been unloving or sexually inadequate. Sexual feelings between adopted children and adoptive parents may be more problematical because of the weakening of the incest taboo, in which case seductive behavior may be more conflict-producing. By contrast, the highly authoritative father who demands submission from the adopted son is in essence telling the boy that he can not become himself but must follow a path established by the father. The boy instinctively knows that this is wrong, that he must find his own path because of the inherent differences between himself and his adoptive father. Such boys often go through severe turmoil, bordering on schizophrenic and paranoid states with much acting out of aggression in the home and community. In those children with depressive trends, suicide threats and attempts are common. Although the problems of the adopted boy have been emphasized, it seems unlikely that the problems of the adopted girl are significantly different in a psychodynamic sense. It is well known that the problem of low self-esteem in the adolescent girl often manifests itself in a pattern of sexual promiscuity, shoplifting, prevarication, and/or dramatic suicidal attempts. The taking of hallucinogenic and narcotic drugs has recently been added as a manifestation of rebellious or disturbed behavior in both sexes. Academic underachievement, though more common in boys, can occur in girls who are locked in a passive-aggressive struggle with parents. Of crucial importance to any girl but more so to the adopted girl is the quality of relationship she has with her adoptive mother. It may be slightly easier for an adopted girl to accept identification with mother and mother's goals since in our culture these tend to have less variability than do the widespread choices and possibilities open to men. However, this is speculative and open to question with the rapidly changing attitudes and relationships between the sexes.

## THE PHENOMENOLOGY OF THE ADOPTIVE PARENT

The reasons for adopting children are varied. Aside from the healthy wish to be a parent by raising a child, there is often the need to own a thing or display a symbol of sexual adequacy or fertility. Paradoxically, the adopted child may symbolize the father's impotence or the mother's sterility, an ever-present reminder of the failure of one or both parents to fulfill their individual and mutual biological needs. Depending on adoptive parental values, the child may have been adopted to cover a feeling of shame for "not being like everybody else," to hold together a faltering marriage, to compete with siblings who are fertile, or for an object-oriented couple, as a gift from one to the other. In the latter instance, the child is experienced as a thing, an object rather than a person. When one parent is potent or fertile and the other is not, the resentment felt toward the defective spouse may be unconsciously projected onto the adopted child. Similarly, an adoptive parent may see a child of the same sex as a rival for the attention and affection of the spouse. In such a family, the envy and competition between father and son or mother and daughter usually becomes greatly intensified during puberty and adolescence.

In addition to the family that adopts a child and later has one or more natural children of their own, there is the family that begins with a natural child only to adopt other children later when they find themselves unable to have additional children. One such family in my practice, a couple who were highly intelligent and creative, had one natural child, a daughter who was a brilliant artist. Because the mother had a debilitating disease and was unable to have additional children, the couple later adopted a boy who proved to be of only average intelligence and ability. During adolescence this boy was in such extreme conflict with his over-demanding, highly critical, and authoritarian, adoptive father that it was necessary for him to go to a special boarding school. Prior to leaving home this boy exhibited extreme paranoid rages in which he would threaten his parents and break furniture. His principal means of maintaining a tenuous and largely negative identity was by being excessively negativistic and oppositional. During family interviews it was apparent that the father would not let the boy speak and would then speak for him. By not acknowledging his son's right to a separate and independent existence, he held the boy in a double-bind that was psychologically castrating and from which the boy could extricate himself only by violent and regressive behavior which had all the appearances of a paranoid schizophrenic reaction. However, once away from home, this boy improved rapidly and is currently doing quite well in a small Southern college. It might be added that the natural daughter in this family solved the father problem by identifying with him and fulfilling goals that he had originally set for himself. She also left home abruptly during her third year in art school, much to the consternation of the parents who could not appreciate her need for emancipation. The parents themselves had a symbiotic marriage in which the mother played a passive-submissive role and the father, an active-domineering one. In addition to living together, they shared a business which brought them into continuous, close contact throughout the working hours. In solving the problem of becoming independent people, their children had been able to solve a problem that the parents had left unresolved.

In the family just described an argument can be made to the effect that the parents fitted the expected stereotypes of masculine and feminine roles. The adopted son's conflict revolved around submission to the father vs. emancipation from him. His paranoid symptomatology reflected the underlying libidinal component. I will now describe another family where the parental roles were reversed and wherein the emancipation struggle during adolescence was between the mother and the adopted son. The boy is the same "Jim" previously described in the quotation by the father about the traumatic effect of being confronted with the possibility of having been an illegitimate child. Jim's adopted parents were unable to have children because the mother had myasthenia gravis. Two children were adopted: Jim and a younger sister who was brilliant but deaf and resided most of the year in a special boarding school. Because mother considered father impotent and inadequate, she turned most of her attention and affection to Jim. In addition mother controlled the family with an iron hand with the father being cast in the role of a passive little boy for whom his son had nothing but contempt. The father also had a large, latent homosexual component with some apparent feminine characteristics which made the boy's identification with him even more difficult.

It appeared that Jim's repeated aerosol paint "huffing" was an attempt to escape from a repressive home environment which he described as being like a funeral parlor. His choice of a passive means of escape would tend to confirm his mother attachment. However, one effect of the paint huffing was to release the otherwise repressed aggressive component to the extent that the boy experienced a radical personality change akin to pathological intoxication. While under the influence of paint fumes he would be extremely belligerent, threatening both parents with violence and breaking various objects in the home. He frequently would leave the house at odd hours of the night and sleep in the nearby woods. He was unable to adjust in various school settings and was eventually arrested for the possession of narcotic drugs. Following a period of hospitalization, he seemed improved at home for about three weeks and then began again to huff paint. He is currently serving an indefinite period of time in a state forestry camp.

Raised in a home with a seductive but controlling mother and a weak, passive father, Jim underwent a particularly turbulent period in that phase of his adolescence where emancipation from parental domination and the establishment of an independent identity were necessary for his maturation. Unfortunately, there was a large element of negative identity which contributed to the self-destructive way in which he attempted to free himself. Not only was the paint huffing physically damaging, but it also represented a regressive mode on an oral level to resolve his early attachment to mother. It has been my observation that those adolescents who have serious difficulty in navigating the drug scene are those whose mothers have been the only or the dominating parent. The attempt to emancipate involves an oral regressive method which substitutes one dependency for another in a way that is physically debilitating and psychologically destructive. The lack of a strong father creates a deficit in the willingness or ability to deal with reality problems, or, to say the same thing in a different way, to tolerate the frustration inherent in the process of a progressive working through of life's difficulties. The mother-attached adolescent castrates himself with drugs, meanwhile projecting hostility on those father figures who make demands of him, such as teachers, police, or other impersonal authority figures who represent impoverished and obviously imperfect symbols of the father identification he has failed to internalize. Boys like Jim can often be helped in a structured situation like a special school, forestry camp, military service, or other father-oriented situation where the boy is able to identify with male figures in an environment where each must suffer the consequences of his own actions. Under such circumstances the feminine superego wherein the child is accepted and loved but nothing is expected of him is modified by more realistic expectations of personal integrity, responsibility, and competence of performance.

A third family will be described briefly to illustrate still another possible complication of the adopted child syndrome. Mother was unable to conceive because of an infantile uterus. Both parents came from large families and all of the adult siblings had several children of their own. It was of great concern to this couple that their brothers and sisters all had children but that they could not conceive. As a result, they adopted four children, the oldest being a boy. When he was three a sister was adopted. Five years later an infant brother was adopted. When the older boy was first seen at the age of fourteen, it was apparent that his adoptive father had rejected him. The father readily admitted that he did not like the boy. Further probing revealed that the boy was a symbol of the father's inability to have children. Also as the boy developed sexually, the father was envious of the boy's youth and sexuality. As a result of the father's rejection, and an envy of the younger sister who had displaced him at a crucial time, the boy was beset with fantasies of having his brain removed and replaced with a female brain. He had concluded that it would be more desirable to be a girl, that in that way he might acquire the parental love that had been denied him. In early adolescence he showed a sexual interest in very young girls, a situation which distressed his parents greatly. With psychiatric help this boy was able to accept a more adult masculine posture, give up his fantasies of becoming female, and transfer his interest in young girls to activities appropriate to his age.

Although many other variations of the adopted child syndrome could be cited, this will be deferred in favor of summarizing what seem to be a few of the more important dynamics. It should be apparent to any careful observer that the problems of the adopted child stem from a combination of factors related both to the fact of being adopted and to the psychodynamic factors within the adoptive parents, some of which were pertinent in the adoption process and many of which were not. It perhaps can be said that the problems specific to the adoption are grafted onto the preexisting pathology within the family.

### SUMMARY OF SIGNIFICANT DYNAMIC FACTORS FREQUENTLY OCCURRING IN ADOPTED CHILDREN AND ADOPTIVE PARENTS

To maintain the illusion of identity between parent and child there is a denial of real differences between adoptive parents and adopted children. Such denial is of greater significance if the disparity between parent and child is greater with relation to characteristics that are inherited such as intellectual ability and special talents.

The split between good and bad parental images which exists in all children becomes a special problem for adopted children. The adopted child tends to split the good and bad images between the adoptive parents and the imagined, biological parents. Such splitting often results in a fixation at a primitive level of thinking where projection, lack of internalization, and aggressive behavior may be persistent problems until the end of adolescence.

Because the adopted child usually projects the bad parental image on the imagined, biological parents, he tends to incorporate this within himself as negative identity. He becomes the unwanted or illegitimate child whose "real" parents were criminals, prostitutes, or alcoholics. He feels guilty toward and unworthy of the parents who especially chose him. His hostility toward them may be repressed and turned against himself, only to explode later during adolescence.

Lack of knowledge and relationship to biological parents contributes to identity diffusion in the adopted child and makes his emancipation from adoptive parents during adolescence more turbulent and the establishment of a mature identity more difficult.

Because of the foregoing, the adopted child tends to react in an exaggerated fashion to conflicts within the family and to developmental crises within himself.

## Problems of the Single-Parent Child Relationship

### THE PHENOMENOLOGY OF THE SINGLE-PARENT CHILD

The child who lives with two healthy parents can afford to be ambivalent. He can experience both intense love and intense hate without fearing for his survival. He can make the choice of loving one parent and hating the other, of being terribly angry at one parent while taking refuge with the other. He can alternate feelings in such a way that he knows it is possible to love one parent at a certain moment and hate the same parent at some other time without harming either himself or the parent. He can experiment with his feelings and test them out within the bounds of real relationship. Ultimately, such experience will enable him to resolve his ambivalence more readily because he has no reason to repress either positive or negative feelings. The ego defense of denial should not be prominent in a child raised by parents who encourage honest expression of feelings.

The single-parent child is not so fortunate. All of his feelings must be played out in relation to one parent upon whom he is totally dependent, or projected in fantasy on the absent parent whose presence cannot correct the child's distortion. If he alienates the remaining parent, the child knows his own survival may be jeopardized. His concern for the welfare of the remaining parent will be increased if he has already lost one parent about whom he had ambivalent feelings, a loss which he may attribute to his own omnipotent wish to be rid of the lost parent during a moment of anger. In such a situation angry feelings and death wishes toward the remaining parent are usually repressed, but may be dealt with by projection, reaction-formation, or the development of obsessive-compulsive or phobic symptoms. When ambivalence cannot be resolved, the child is caught in a passive-dependent relationship from which it may take him many years to extricate himself. The repression of hostility toward the remaining parent together with the associated passive-dependency constitute the most important dynamic factors found in the single-parent child relationship.

The child's reaction to the loss or absence of a parent depends upon which parent is lost, at what age it happens, and what the relationship is to the child at the time of loss. How the loss occurs may also be important depending on its suddenness, whether it was expected, and whether it was due to accident, divorce, acute or terminal illness. The loss of the mother in infancy was touched on in the previous section. Neubauer (9) characterizes its importance as follows:

Bowlby [2] summarized the number of variables on which the effect of early maternal deprivation depends: the age at which it occurs, the length and degree of deprivation, the quality of the previous mother-child relationship, and the availability of mother substitutes. Other yet barely measured variables, such as the varying cultural demands on individuals, and the constitutional "object-seeking" strength of the child himself, may play a part. Nevertheless, one may conclude that ego development will be jeopardized if the psychobiological unity of mother and child is seriously disturbed in the first year of life, because of the consequent interference with drive satisfaction.

If the loss of the mother occurs beyond infancy but in the pre-oedipal period, the child may remain fixated to the mother substitute at a pre-oedipal level of development. Loss of the mother is always serious but may be less crucial during latency or late adolescence. Loss of the mother at puberty, especially for the pre-adolescent girl who had intensely negative feelings toward mother at that time, may fixate her in the latency period because she feels it is safer to be a child than a woman. Not only are the incestuous feelings toward the father increased by the loss of the mother at a time when the sexual drive is increasing, but the absence of the mother leaves the girl bereft of the help she needs in learning how to become a woman. The loss of a parent at any age creates an environmental deficiency that interferes with the emotional development of the child and has serious repercussions for ego maturation.

If a child loses his father before he is born or shortly thereafter, the effect may be felt only indirectly through the mother's reaction or by the awareness that develops much later that he is different from other children by the absence of his father. If a father substitute is not available, the child may develop idealized fantasies about the lost father. The observations of fatherless children in wartime conducted by Anna Freud (4) and Burlingham are well known. According to Neubauer, the intense and persistent attachments to a fantasied father which these children constructed out of even the most meager relationships to any man, or even in the absence of any father experience at all, state the case in reverse: they seem to indicate that children in the oedipal phase are compelled to create in fantasy what does not exist in fact. In an extension of this point, Nunberg (1955) views the idealized fantasy of missing fathers as a bridge to an attachment to a real man, through whom some children may achieve oedipal and superego development. He points out, though, that other children who grow up without fathers are full of resentment, behave ruthlessly, as if they had no guilt, and thus take revenge on the world for not having a father.

The effect of the consistent lack of a father during childhood on the behaviors and attitudes of the child is described by Ostrovsky (10) as follows:

This lack manifested itself generally in a misorientation toward, or an insufficient acquaintance with the male role, or an uncertainty in behavior toward, or a series of conflicting attitudes with regard to, man. We also find that there existed a somewhat unbalanced concept of the functions and traits of men, which attributed to them only limited properties and isolated characteristics, thus distorting their image in the mind of the child. This distortion resulted in an inverse misorientation concerning the role of the female adult: Many of the functions which the father might have fulfilled, and those attributes not ascribed to him, were projected onto the mother, and she was often made a spokesman for the father. In addition, we have seen that the mother was sometimes the person who interpreted the functions of the father's role to the child, thereby creating his image as seen through her eyes. This image, being only seldom challenged or modified by the actual presence of the father, did not give the child much opportunity to clarify his own concept of the paternal role through everyday contact and a constant sharing of experience with the father.

Ostrovsky believes that the consequences of the distortion of the male role, as well as those of the unevenly distributed parental influence, are such as to create several resulting disturbances within the child. His observations confirm that the first of these is a general limitation of experience, which prevents the child from utilizing his potential to the fullest extent. Such limitation of experience permits the child only a narrow perspective and relatively inhibits the use of his full powers. Ostrovsky (10) believes that this limitation is such that it will affect, directly or indirectly, all areas of the child's behavior and consequently weaken his ability to cope with his environment, or tend to make him approach new situations with a habitual set of limiting values. This could result, according to Ostrovsky (10), in an uncertainty about himself and others, or in a desire to exclude the forces which challenge his pattern of values.

Lederer (7) has contributed significantly to our understanding of the importance of the father throughout development, but especially during adolescence. As he says, "the 'dreaded father of reality' is not just really dreadful, he is also really protective—and not just as a fantasy beast. The identification with such a father, his eventual introjection, does therefore include more than his prohibitive aspect; it includes, optimally, also his aggressiveness, his assertiveness, his effectiveness as a man." He is particularly concerned about the symptoms produced by superego agenesis or dysgenesis where a strong father or father substitute is lacking:

No one grows up without either father or father substitute; where there is no father from the beginning, mother, or a relative, or an institution takes over and provides the superego model. But grave difficulties arise in those instances in which a father, or father substitute, once accepted by the child, then fails or vanishes. It is well known how the disappearance of a father during the oedipal period can lead to various distortions in the psychological development of the child. These are formative years of the superego; but the further maturation of the superego during adolescence is equally important, and a failure of father at that time can be equally damaging.

The writings of Blos (1) also confirm adolescence as a time when the person has a second chance to individuate, to resolve previously unresolved infantile problems through a necessary regression in the service of future growth. Blos (1) believes that this period is critical for character formation, which makes the presence of two reasonably healthy parents extremely important at that time.

Of greatest concern to the single-parent is whether the child brought up exclusively by him or her will be sexually normal. It is now generally believed among a psychologically sophisticated public that homosexuality, expecially in males, may be attributed to an unhealthy closeness to mother in childhood. Freud (5) himself stated, "The early loss of one of their parents, whether by death, divorce, or separation, with the result that the remaining parent absorbs the whole of the child's love, determines the sex of the person who is later to be chosen as a sexual object and may thus open the way to permanent inversion." Other investigators have concluded that homosexuality can develop in this way but that it need not if the remaining parent is mature enough to establish a new life apart from the child after the loss of the spouse. However, when the mother-child relationship is sufficiently pathological, homosexuality can develop in either sex. Eisendorfer (3) described the development in two women under the combined conditions of an early, abnormally intensified mother-child relationship and an absent father: an increased primary homosexual attachment to the mother occurred, with oral fixations, an immature ego structure, and repression of aggression against the mother which was then inevitably turned inward. Most such cases, as noted by Neubauer (9), include early processes of maternal narcissistic seduction, oral fixation, retarded ego controls, and repressed pregenital aggression. Annie Reich (13) expressed it as follows:

When early identifications with unsublimated sexual behavior have taken place and sexual characteristics as such remain an ego ideal, a fixation on or regression to primitive, aggressive, pregenital levels is frequent, which leads to a persistence of particular, cruel superego forerunners. The combination of opposite factors—of megalomaniac, sexualized ideals and of particular, sadistic superego elements—must lead to a type of superego which cannot possibly be lived up to in reality.

Isaacs (6) described a young boy who defended himself against early maternal seduction by the idealization of a dead father:

His secret hatred and resentment against a mother who had demanded not only his exclusive devotion, but that he share her hatred of the dead father as well, made it too dangerous for him to love another woman, lest this new love bring with it the same fear and hatred as the old. Never daring to withdraw love from his mother lest the hatred escape, he turned instead to idealized and sadistic love relationships with men, reflecting his secret, chronically disappointed search for his idealized absent father.

Despite the lack of any unique clustering of symptoms, Neubauer (9) indicates that there is a characteristic pathology of phallic fixations, whether the parent of the same or opposite sex is absent, which leads to homosexuality and superego disturbances, expressed by either a too severe superego with the sadistic features of a harsh, pre-oedipal quality, or a deficient superego which allows incestuous acting out.

It can be anticipated that a child who has lost a parent in infancy or in the pre-oedipal period will find it extremely difficult to individuate in adolescence. Additional clinical information is needed before any conclusions can be drawn about the possibilities of a child who did not reach an oedipal level early in life, arriving at such a level during adolescence and "individuating" not for a second, but for a first time. Under ideal circumstances, such growth should be possible, particularly if the family has been reconstituted and if both parent and step-parent understand the meaning of regressive and disturbed behavior on the part of a child who is striving to move away from infantile patterns. In contrast to the fixated child, the child who has lost a parent at some time after the oedipal period will in all likelihood have regressed to a pre-oedipal attachment to the remaining parent. His struggle to extricate himself during adolescence may be exceedingly turbulent but it should not be as difficult a task, since he has already traveled part of the way before.

The necessity for regression in adolescence to resolve infantile ties has been stressed by Blos (1). Parental pressure to achieve, as well as the academic pressure of the secondary school system in America where everyone who wishes to succeed is expected to go to college, leaves little opportunity for legitimate regression on the part of the adolescent. In recent years the use of drugs has become particularly prominent as the preferred mode of regression. Those adolescents who seem most prone to drug abuse and addiction are those who are pre-oedipally fixated. One important motive for the drug experience, according to Wieder and Kaplan (17), is the attempt to restore the lost object. Hence it can be concluded that the single-parent child is particularly vulnerable, particularly when his rationalizations for drug-taking and peer pressures mask his regressive motivations.

## THE PHENOMENOLOGY OF THE SINGLE-PARENT

The single-parent who has lost a spouse through separation, divorce, or death must be responsible for the child but also tends to expect him to act more like an adult. Such a parent will often burden him with adult demands, and try to depend on him emotionally as a husband or wife substitute. Frequently the emotional demands made on the child are excessive because of the remaining parent's need. Because this occurs at a time when the child himself is feeling the loss of the absent parent, he is usually less able to respond to even normative demands. The frustration of the single-parent is thereby compounded, tempting him to project onto the child his mounting resentment. If the child has a strong resemblance to the absent parent, the lack of responsiveness may be attributed to a similarity to the absent one. Such a child may be blamed unjustifiably for being "just like his father," which means having all the negative characteristics of the absent parent who is often thought of as totally bad. The child is placed in the position of having to deny, hide, or feel shame for his identification with the missing parent, a person for whom he may have largely positive and highly idealized feelings. The single-parent may try to ally the child with him in his hatred for the missing parent or he may think that the child frustrates him in the same way that the absent parent did or does, simply by not being there when needed.

The remaining parent is often in a state of psychological regression following the loss of the spouse and may experience strong depressive, paranoid, and ambivalent feelings. The wife whose husband has left by separation, divorce, or death may be intensely angry at him for abandoning her. Such anger may be short-lived or, depending on circumstances, it may persist for many years. Because the previously shared responsibility, the child, becomes the remaining parent's exclusive responsibility, he may become the object of the abandoned parent's anger. However, most single-parents tend to repress their resentment toward the child because of guilt feelings and because they know intellectually that the child does not deserve it. If there has been a separation or divorce, the remaining parent may feel responsible for depriving the child of the other parent. Single-parents often feel guilty because they so intensely resent the child's dependency on them which keeps them from being free to enjoy the manifold possibilities of making a new life for themselves. They may see the child as an impossible financial burden, particularly if financial security deteriorates as a result of the loss of the working parent. The single-parent usually feels overburdened and deprived both emotionally and materially. The single-parent often must try to be both father and mother as well as provider and homemaker. This undertaking occurs during the time when the single-parent is attempting to work through the effects of a narcissistic injury resulting from rejection, when there may be little or any family to support dependency needs, and when the reactions of family, friends, and community may produce intense feelings of shame and humiliation. A marriage failure is usually experienced by both partners as a personal failure regardless of extenuating circumstances.

Although separation and divorce are extremely common in contemporary society, opposition to it for moralistic reasons is prevalent. The shame and humiliation which single-parents feel as a result of the personal failure and changed circumstances of separation and divorce are often aggravated by the reactions of friends, neighbors, and relatives who feign understanding but indirectly condemn the divorced person as immoral or irresponsible. The adverse judgment of friends who themselves have endured unsatisfactory marriages "because of the children," for fear of alienating relatives, for fear of jeopardizing business or social status, or for other reasons is another difficulty to which divorced, single-parents are subjected. An understanding that such friends may be unconsciously jealous of the single-parent's ability to solve problems, albeit through divorce, may somewhat reduce the sting of their condemnatory attitude. However, most single-parents find that they are no longer welcome in many social situations where previously they felt comfortable. Such social ostracism, for whatever reason it occurs, contributes significantly to the feelings of rejection and deprivation suffered by the single-parent.

The single-parent, usually the father, who lives apart from the child may feel guilty as well as deprived both emotionally and materially. He may feel that it is unjust for him to lose the privilege of being a full-time parent because he and his wife were incompatible. Also if, in case of a divorce, he has been left with only enough money to live a marginal existence in a rented room or small apartment where, in addition to supporting himself and his absent family, he must also tend to his own personal needs, he may feel that he is being punished for a situation for which he is only partially or perhaps not at all responsible. The latter is felt particularly strongly in those instances where the wife has deserted the husband but kept custody of the children. Because American courts almost invariably and regardless of circumstances favor the mother, the father may lose all faith in legal process, particularly if he feels his children are suffering as a result. The inability of the father to gain custody even when he is the more responsible parent and may have remarried is not unusual. The archaic and arbitrary nature of American legal process must accept its responsibility for aggravating the suffering of many children when there can be no arbitration about custody.

Although there are many instances where visitation with the absent parent and return to the usual living situation can be accomplished without emotional turmoil for all concerned, such visits are often disruptive. Because the parent who has custody is also the parent who disciplines the child, the visiting parent is frequently resented as the one who indulges the child but does not take real responsibility. The child may play into this by making unfavorable comparisons between the custodial parent and the visiting parent. The visiting parent, because of his guilt, may indeed indulge the child, overdo the giving of gifts, and avoid disciplining the child even when it is needed. Such a parent may be warding off the child's hostility to him, and attempting to buy the child's love. It is incumbent upon both parents in the divided situation to be aware of their own conflicts concerning the child as well as the problems that the child is having in relation to each of them.

It is particularly important for those interested in the problems of the single-parent child relationship to be aware of the nuclear relationship that develops over a period of time between mother and child. As previously described, the child is fixated or regresses to a pre-oedipal level where his hostility toward the mother is, to a large extent, repressed. Because of her guilt feelings, need for the child's love, etc., the mother also denies or represses hostile feelings toward the child, often using the child as a narcissistic extension of herself. She may become overprotective of the child or overconcerned due to her tendencies toward reaction-formation, thus initiating behavior which further infantilizes the child. The child's passivity further confirms the mother's need to overdo for the child and a vicious circle is established which is often impossible to break even when remarriage occurs. A serious problem in many remarriages is the continuing nuclear relationship between mother and child which prevents the consolidation of the new relationship between the partners. The child is always in between, appears preferred by the original parent, and places the new spouse in a secondary position which he may have difficulty in either accepting or resolving, particularly if neither spouse is especially insightful as to what is occurring. Although the child may appear to welcome a new parent, even be relieved by his presence, he will bitterly resent what he considers being displaced by him in his relationship to mother.

## SUMMARY OF CLINICAL MATERIAL

Four adolescent patients from single-parent homes will be described briefly to illustrate some of the points made earlier.

When first seen, T. was a fourteen-year-old girl, the younger of two siblings, living with a working mother who had separated from T.'s father three months before. Referral was made following a serious suicidal attempt from an overdose of tranquilizers. Initially, it appeared that T. felt caught in between mother and father, not wishing to choose between them but being forced by mother's extreme hostility to father to ally herself with mother. Her rage toward mother at being placed in an unfair position was repressed, turned on herself, and expressed through the suicidal attempt. Later, when the conflict between the parents subsided and T.'s dependence on mother became primary, she developed a closeness to mother characteristic of a pre-oedipal attachment. When father reappeared and attempted a reconciliation, T. opposed it, feeling that her closeness to mother was too valuable to renounce for a normative, two-parent relationship. With the help of a positive father transference, T. was able to become more accepting of her negative feelings toward mother, despite a continuing strong need to avoid and deny.

At the time of referral J. was a fifteen-year-old boy, the youngest of three siblings, living with his mother and a seventeen-year-old sister. The father, a very authoritarian person who was a minister, had died two years previously. The reasons for referral were that J. had run away from a military boarding school one day after enrollment, was disobedient and rebellious at home, and had become involved in smoking marijuana and taking hallucinogenic drugs. Family evaluation revealed that mother was still mourning the death of the father and was emotionally unavailable to the children. J., also still grieving for the father, had allied himself with a "hippy" group in the community and was resorting with increasing frequency to marijuana, LSD–25, and other black-marketed drugs. With the help of special school placement and psychotherapy for both J. and mother, J. improved from a borderline state until he was able to function well in school and to renounce drug usage. With the death of his father, J. essentially lost both parents inasmuch as mother was no longer available to him for emotional support. During various LSD–25 "trips" J. reported hallucinating a variety of archetypal father figures. His drug usage is seen as an attempt to escape an oppressive relationship with mother, to resolve depressive feelings of his own, and regressively, to restore the lost object, the father.

The third patient was a sixteen-year-old boy, the older of two male siblings, who at the time of referral was living with his father. D. was seven when his mother died. Six months later father made an unsuccessful attempt at remarriage which ended in divorce when D. was eleven. Although the boy was referred for academic underachievement, it was apparent that his main problem was his relationship to his father. The father, who was extremely critical and controlling in a highly intellectual way, had placed D. in the role of wife substitute, demanding complete submission and primary loyalty. When D. became seriously interested in a girl, father was extremely jealous and did everything he could to restrict the relationship and make D. feel guilty about it for "betraying" father. In group therapy D.'s identification with father was very apparent in the vicious but highly intellectual way in which he attacked the female members of the group. His inability to accept the feminine part of himself, related to his ungratified need for mothering, eventually became conscious. Through therapy he became better able to handle the unrealistic demands of father, to solve his school problems, and to move toward a more healthy heterosexual orientation.

Our fourth vignette is concerned with K. who, at the time of referral, was a fifteen-year-old girl, the oldest and only girl of three siblings. She was living with mother who had separated from father, an alcoholic, eight months previously. The chief complaints were that K. had taken money from her mother's purse, was smoking marijuana, had slashed her wrists, and taken an overdose of sleeping pills. K. was an aggressive, somewhat masculine girl who was also failing in school. Following the separation and unbeknownst to mother, K. had taken LSD–25 on numerous occasions. When a friend of hers died from a "hot shot" of heroin, K. temporarily renounced drugs but sporadically returned to them in the early part of therapy. In spite of continuing therapy, it appears that the relationship between K. and mother is largely a pre-oedipal one. Following the separation, mother allied K. with her in "putting father down" in every possible way. Once in therapy, K. was able to express some of her repressed hostility to mother at which point communication between mother and daughter improved considerably and K. became less depressed. At the present time, K. is drug free but continues to fail in school.

SUMMARY OF DYNAMICS

To summarize both the foregoing theoretical and clinical material, it appears that the most important dynamic factors in the single-parent child syndrome are as follows: A nuclear relationship develops between parent and child which is almost symbiotic in character. This relationship results from an intertwining of dependency and libidinal needs modified and distorted by conscious guilt and the repressive use of defenses. The child, most commonly, is fixated or regresses to a pre-oedipal level of attachment to the parent, usually mother. The exclusiveness of the relationship causes the child to repress his hostility to the parent upon whom he is dependent. Such repression of hostility often leads to a turning against the self which may be manifested by serious suicidal attempts, a phenomenon that is most common in adolescent girls. Because of the intensity of the nuclear relationship, the single-parent child can be expected, almost universally, to oppose the remarriage of his parent on an emotional level. Such opposition occurs because the child views the remarriage as an intrusion of a rival between mother and himself. Where remarriage occurs, the oedipal problem is activated or reactivated, and must be reworked before there can be any harmony in the family. Such reworking may occur only in adolescence. The single-parent child has the greatest opportunity for emotional health if the remaining parent is able to make a new life for himself soon after the loss of the first spouse.

## Problems of the Step-Parent Child Relationship

### THE PHENOMENOLOGY OF THE STEPCHILD

The realities of daily living in a new family with one original parent and a step-parent are usually quite different for the child than were the idealized fantasies experienced in anticipation. The stepchild pictures himself as the primary interest of the new parent, only to find that he is competing with his own parent for attention and affection, and perhaps also with other children with whom the step-parent has a prior relationship. Intense feelings of jealousy may be provoked by the discovery that his own parent is more preoccupied with the new marital partner and with his children than she is with him. If the step-parent's children from a former marriage accompany him into the new home, the stepchild finds himself immediately and permanently displaced from the center of interest. If the step-parent's children do not live in the home but are regular visitors, the stepchild finds himself displaced periodically and abruptly, often perhaps when he is just beginning to feel that he does have a special relationship with the step-parent. In addition, he is under considerable pressure to give up his nuclear or pre-oedipal relationship to his original parent, usually the mother. Although he may realize intellectually that it is healthier to have two parents and thus be relieved of the unreasonable demands that may have been made upon him to behave more like an adult or even to act as a husband or wife substitute, he bitterly resents the intrusion of a third person between mother and himself. The hostility that he has repressed toward the remaining parent or that he harbors for the missing parent often is projected onto the step-parent. The step-parent becomes the final common pathway for the flood of resentment which frequently has been dammed up for years. Because the step-parent is being unfairly treated by a child who may seem sullen and recalcitrant, his reaction is likely to be retaliation by overdisciplining the child or by expecting him to have the same degree of maturity that a child who has not been deprived of a parent might be expected to have. A vicious cycle can develop in which the child provokes the step-parent either by continued passive resistance to reasonable demands, by rejection of attempts to establish relationship on the part of the step-parent, or by continued aggressive defiance under similar circumstances.

Although lack of warmth by either child or step-parent can limit the relationship, it appears most frequently that the child's inability to accept the step-parent leads the step-parent to develop a primarily disciplinary relationship with the child. In psychoanalytic terms, the child's unresolved ambivalence leads to a sadomasochistic struggle with the step-parent. The child may refuse to participate in activities that reflect the step-parent's interests and may refuse to allow the step-parent to participate with him in interests of his own. In addition to these difficulties, the natural parent may be severely disappointed by the inability of her child to relate to the step-parent and blame the step-parent for rejecting the child when, in reality, the opposite may be true. Often the child is delighted if he sees mother in conflict with stepfather because this, temporarily at least, restores his closeness to mother. If both parents do not understand what the child is experiencing, they may find themselves victimized by the child's systematic attempts to sabotage their marriage. In such circumstances the stepfather may feel abused not only by the stepchild but also by his new wife who accuses him of neglect when he actually has taken upon himself an additional and quite ungratifying burden. If he expects and perhaps deserves appreciation but receives only criticism and lack of understanding, his willingness to remain in the new marriage may be limited. Many second marriages break up over the inability of the new spouses to resolve the difficulties arising over the attempt to integrate children from two families into a new family unit. Each spouse may feel that the other is giving preferential treatment to his own children while neglecting or even rejecting the stepchildren.

The child who has lost one parent by death or divorce and who feels he has lost another parent by remarriage may feel defeated by life. His narcissistic hurt may reflect itself in a permanent, negative self-image. He may want to avoid relationships with adults whom he may see as only hurting him. He may feel that growing up is undesirable and may retreat into a regressive and ineffectual fantasy world of dependency and revenge. By rejecting those who he thinks rejected him, he may deny himself the identification figures necessary for his emergence from the world of childhood into adult life. Lacking sustained interest and unable to develop competence in any area of life, such a child demeans the success of his peers, opposes established social values, and remains fixated at an infantile level. If he avoids depressive feelings by projecting the blame for his shortcomings on others, he also avoids taking responsibility for himself and finding a way out of his dilemma. When the traumatic events occur in early childhood, the pattern of social and school failure is usually apparent toward the end of the elementary school years or early in junior high school. The child who has lacked a father in the latency years enters adolescence without the masculine identification and the ego strength necessary to succeed in the highly competitive public school system. He lacks self-discipline; his ability to concentrate is usually limited; his negative self-image encourages a pattern of failure which feeds on itself. The most common defense of such a child is to maintain himself in a compensatory world of narcissistic omnipotence where he "knows everything" and believes no one can teach him anything. His rejection of the authority or father figure, whether in the guise of the overdisciplining step-parent, the teacher, or the police, may be virtually complete. He feels superior to all and maintains his position by contempt and rationalizations about the "irrelevancy of the system." Frequently his attitudes are reinforced during the high school years by association with a coterie of similarly minded compatriots. If, for some reason, his private system of defense breaks down, such a person may make a suicidal attempt, become psychotic, addicted, or act out in a variety of antisocial ways. The use of alcohol or drugs may weaken an already weak ego sufficiently to precipitate an acute episode of impulsive, self-destructive, or antisocial behavior. Referral for psychiatric evaluation and treatment most commonly occurs in the adolescent years following a runaway, suicidal, alcoholic, drug-taking, or delinquent episode precipitated by a buildup of pressure intolerable to a weak ego.

Somewhat like the adopted child, the stepchild may hold onto a fragmentary identification with a lost parent whom he has either idealized or with whom he did have a relationship at an earlier period in his life. Often the identification with the lost parent, especially if the parent was lost by divorce and if the remaining parent has attempted to alienate the feelings of the child toward the lost parent, is clung to tenaciously no matter how negative or destructive such clinging may be. Even an alcoholic or criminal father who failed in school and never succeeded in life may become the ego ideal of a boy who feels that if father succeeded in being a failure, why shouldn't he? The repetition compulsion to repeat parental patterns is strong in all people, and, thus paradoxically, a negative self-image can represent a positive identification. In a child who has lost a parent, such narcissistic identification may never be outgrown. In the exceptional case where it is outgrown, the change usually does not manifest itself until late adolescence and only then if there have been consistent, mature parent surrogates of both sexes available as models for healthy identification. Depending on the age of the child at the time of the parent's remarriage, the stepchild's capacity to identify with the stepparent is an essential ingredient for the continuing emotional growth of the child. The relinquishing of old and undesirable identifications may be slow but can be accomplished if the parents are understanding and patient enough. Obviously an overly permissive or an overly punitive parental approach can be damaging to a child who is trying to overcome the effects of early traumatic experiences.

In contrast to the child who chooses the regressive mode is the child who seems to progress too fast. Although pseudomaturity in adolescents may be the result of premature physiological changes, many such young people appear to mature early socially because of the wide variety of emotional stresses to which they have been subject. For example, some single-parent children and stepchildren who have experienced an unusual number of family changes, including frequent moves and school transfers, may appear much more mature and sophisticated than children not so affected.

The pseudomaturity syndrome in the emotionally deprived ghetto child is well known. In recent years the pseudomature, middle-class child who is failing in school but knowledgeable about sex, drugs, and the ways of the world has become a common sight in the psychiatrist's office. Such young people are often victimized by a state law which requires school attendance at least until the age of sixteen. If they cannot learn in an academic school program, the pattern of failure may be so ingrained by the age of sixteen that they are unable to succeed in a work situation. Such people often do best in vocational training programs which allow them to work and experience tangible success with a minimum of frustration. A work program may be indicated in some adolescents as early as thirteen; to keep such a child in an academic program is not only inappropriate but destructive. Often the psychiatrist can do little more than understand the origin of the problem and suggest practical measures to relieve the person of the responsibility of long periods of concentration in an academic program which is meaningless to him. It is the child who suffers most not only from family disruption, but also from incredibly outmoded laws pertaining to divorce, custody, and obligatory school attendance. In the United States in 1970 the number of children living with only one parent exceeds 15 percent of the entire child population. An understanding of the complex problems such children experience, and the unsatisfactory conditions they endure, is long overdue.

Among other things, the problematic outgrowths of the broken family system emphasize the inadequacy of our diagnostic classification system for the emotional disturbances of childhood and adolescence. In the foregoing, I have mentioned two common and distinct syndromes that are readily observable in clinical practice: (a) the complex of symptoms seen in the pre-oedipally fixated child who is able to maintain with parental consent and participation a nuclear relationship with mother. This child refuses to grow up and is constantly seduced by any encouragement or sanction to regress. Perhaps the term "regressive nuclear syndrome" would appropriately describe the condition; (b) the complex of symptoms seen in the pseudomature child who denies his dependency needs by developing a veneer of social sophistication. This child often seems to grow up all at once but frequently cannot function in an academic learning situation. The pre-oedipal fixation shifts from unsatisfactory parent objects to dependency on drugs, sexual indulgence, peer group approval, etc. In some ways this syndrome is the polar opposite of (a). It might best be termed pseudomaturity syndrome.

## THE PHENOMENOLOGY OF THE STEP-PARENT

Few men or women marry or remarry for the express purpose of raising someone else's child or children. Most such marriages occur in spite of the stepchildren involved or, at best, if both spouses bring children into the marriage, to provide a two-parent home for all the children concerned. Such an arrangement is a compromise in which both partners agree to assume additional burdens for the sake of each other and for the benefit of the children. What neither partner can anticipate is the degree of hostility that is likely to greet him when the child sees him as inferior to the lost real parent and as the rival who is displacing his jealously guarded position with the remaining parent. If the original loss occurred through divorce, the child may blame the step-parent for taking "Daddy away from Mommy" or vice versa. Also neither partner in the new marriage can anticipate how the children from two previous marriages will meld with each other. The latter is complicated by such obvious factors as the pre-existing relationships between siblings, age and sex differences, differences in intelligence, temperament, and emotional maturity. The oldest child in one family may suddenly find himself to be the youngest or the middle in the new family. Managing the many unexpected reactions and possibilities arising from the new family meld invariably tests the resources and maturity of the new husband and wife. Any unresolved infantile conflicts which they bring with them into the new marriage are apt to further complicate the resolution of problems. Not infrequently such parents discover problems within themselves which they never knew existed. That a majority of second marriages succeed is a tribute to the problem-solving capacity and the pertinacity of the participants.

The step-parent who is on the receiving end of much undeserved hostility has to find ways of assuaging his injured narcissism. The step-parent who, after years of concerted effort, finds that his stepchild still refuses all possibility of identification with him must find ways of managing his disappointment and frustration. Many times the child has been too severely traumatized in early life and cannot relate. The pre-oedipal attachment to mother may be too subtle and have been maintained too long to be broken; the new parent may have arrived too late. A myriad of factors may militate against the undoing of old mistakes, and often step-parents must be grateful for minuscule results from Herculean efforts. Much has been written about the mean step-parent but very little about the sacrificial one. An understanding of the often unrewarded efforts of the conscientious step-parent is past due. He is often blamed for problems that are not of his creation and not within his power to resolve. Both partners in a new marriage need compassion for each other, for each must suffer the consequences of the other's mistakes and often the mistakes of original parents no longer present.

Perhaps the greatest tragedy is the second marriage where one or both partners blindly repeat past mistakes, or where one or both deny full step-parenthood to the other partner by maintaining the nuclear relationship to their child that pre-existed the marriage. In clinical practice it is not unusual to see a second marriage in which two sets of children live together but essentially have only one parent, the remaining real parent denying the step-parent access to her child. The idiosyncratic arrangements of the nuclear arrangement persist and the child remains insulated from the new parent with whom he may need to identify or from whom he may need reasonable discipline, particularly if the real mother is over-indulgent and permissive. The mother who binds her ambivalence in a nuclear relationship to the child will often offer her child for treatment but refuse to participate in a way that will allow resolution of the nuclear relationship. It becomes the responsibility of the child to grow and break the bond which he may attempt to do by erratic, impulsive behavior such as running away, serious drug involvement, or antisocial acts.

The tendency in an exposition of this kind is to emphasize the pathology and the most difficult reality problems. Obviously, many step-parent child relationships develop satisfactorily and work out for the benefit of all concerned; many difficult family melds integrate in constructive ways. Others may start with complex problems which resolve themselves over a period of years. Although no statistics are available, it seems safe to assume that the earlier in a child's life the new family forms, the greater chance there is for successful adaptation to occur. Ultimately, when children reach adolescence and begin to see significant parental figures as people rather than as idealized or demonic stereotypes who merely play the role of parent or parent surrogate, antagonisms diminish. Relationships can then be based on common interests and a discussion of differences rather than beset by withdrawal, lack of communication, and mutual resentment.

## CLINICAL EXAMPLES

Two family situations will be described in detail. Both illustrate many of the dynamics previously described, including the nuclear relationship to mother, regressive and pseudomaturity syndromes, the exclusion and lack of identification between stepson and stepfather, resulting marital conflict, etc. Both families have severe problems which have existed over a number of years and which require continuing psychiatric intervention.

The R. family consists of father and his three children from a previous marriage which was terminated by the death of the mother from cancer when the oldest child was eight and mother together with her two children from a first marriage which terminated in divorce when her oldest child was five. The R.'s marriage is now about three years old but the children are living together as if they belonged to two separate families. The conflict and division in the family has focused on the oldest child of each parent, both boys. Father's children consist of two boys and a girl, seventeen, thirteen, and eleven years of age; mother's of a boy and a girl, fifteen and thirteen years of age. Father's oldest son, E., had reacted regressively to the death of his mother and entered the new family situation with many infantile characteristics and symptoms of severe emotional disturbance, including school failure, the tearing and destruction of clothing and household items, lying, stealing of money within the home, messy eating habits, etc. Two contributing factors seemed to be that, following the mother's death, neighbors oversympathized and indiscriminately mothered him, whereas father developed an increasingly authoritarian and sadomasochistic relationship with the boy in which he employed excessive physical punishment. E.'s conflict with stepmother has been most pronounced since the advent of the new marriage. Stepmother is extremely distressed by E.'s lying, stealing, destruction of clothing, and general messiness, for which she tends to blame father's management of the boy. She, on the other hand, has maintained an exclusive relationship with her own son, M., and prevented stepfather from having anything but casual contact with him. Despite the lack of paternal discipline, M. had tended to mature in some ways beyond his chronological age. Quite early in the marriage he became a rebel, threatened to run away from home, refused to attend public school, and adopted the attitudes and attire of the hippy. Mother attempted to maintain rigid control and was able to limit the boy's use of drugs and to enlist his cooperation in returning to school. M. continues in public high school, has an older girl friend, and has developed intense interest and considerable competence in photography, which he intends to follow as a vocation. Unlike E., who is attempting to emancipate himself from family influence by immersion in a peer group involved in heavy drug-taking, M. has already partially established his separate identity. E.'s father continues to be preoccupied obsessively with the wish to send E. to a residential school but is unable to make a decision about it. E. continues to antagonize stepmother by his messy behavior and lack of discipline. Her hostility is directed not only toward E. but also toward her husband whom she blames for E.'s regressed state.

During the three years of marriage there have been several crises during which mother has threatened separation from father. Each crisis was precipitated by E.'s behavior which led father to be extremely physically punitive to E. The display of physical violence by father was intolerable to mother and each time she made specific plans to leave, and to take her two children with her. Mother is seen as an extremely controlling woman who is threatened by male strength and in considerable conflict about her own sexuality. She had been completely frigid in the marriage, allowing her husband to have relations with her only rarely and then with the attitude, "If you have to do it, go ahead and get it over with as quickly as possible but don't expect me to participate or like it." The husband has accepted the limitations of the marriage with little protest, probably because he was willing to maintain the marriage at all costs. Under threat of separation by his wife, he has refrained from physical punishment of E. for more than a year. However, he has refrained from limit-setting in other areas so that E. at the present time continues in a completely unstructured way, truanting from school, staying away until the early morning hours, etc., without receiving so much as a reprimand from father. Whereas mother used to be angry at father's punitiveness, she is now angry about his renunciation of any disciplinary role. Mother's ambivalence and father's ineffectuality combine to help perpetuate an essentially sadomasochistic marriage where unresolved conflicts between the parents have been projected onto the oldest son of each partner. Unfortunately, neither parent has been willing to invest himself sufficiently in the therapeutic process to bring about any insightful change. It is anticipated that ultimately E. will require placement outside the home, whereas M. will leave of his own accord. At that point the focus of conflict will probably shift to the younger children or intensify between mother and father to the extent that either resolution or separation will be likely to occur.

The problem in the R. family can be discussed from many points of view. E.'s loss of his mother at an early age and rejection by an obsessive and ambivalent father have resulted in an adolescent picture of regression and infantile fixation. Symptoms and behavioral reaction resulting from the latter have provoked E.'s rejection by his stepmother, a relationship which might have been crucial in his gradual recovery from earlier traumatic circumstances. What E. was unable to find in either parent he is now seeking through drugs and peer relationships. He has little sense of self and no competence in any area. Without residential placement or massive therapeutic intervention, it seems likely that he is destined to remain a dependent and infantile person for life. M., on the other hand, though pre-oedipally fixated to mother and closely identified with her, has been able to move successfully into a heterosexual mode of adjustment, has developed a sense of self with vocational goals, and has been able to transcend reasonably well the effects of previous traumatic situations while living in an extremely conflictual family situation. Although M. has had mother's love, he has been able to achieve significant progress toward maturity without any meaningful father relationship. It appears that his own wish and need to separate himself was crucial in his development toward independence.

The second family situation to be discussed is that of the S. family which consists of mother and father in their early forties, and three children, two boys and a girl. The two oldest children, R., eighteen, and B., fourteen, are the son and daughter of the mother from her first marriage which was terminated by the accidental death of her husband when R. was three and B. was in utero. The second marriage for mother and the first for father began thirteen years ago when R. was five. The youngest child, A., a son, and the only child of this marriage, is now ten years of age. Although both R. and B. were legally adopted at the time of the marriage, the problems inherent in the family are typical of the step-parent child relationship with the focus of conflict being on the oldest boy whom the mother believes is constitutionally much like his biological father, a fun-loving, self-indulgent person who never grew up. R. left home precipitously in the spring of his last year in high school. Although he did complete his high school program, he spent the next year living a borderline existence with a group of like-minded young people who were heavily involved in psychedelic drugs, hashish, and marijuana. He worked only sporadically and only long enough to pay his immediate debts, his rent, and to buy food. Much of the time he allowed others to provide for him or stayed in homes where a vacant room was provided without expense. As a way of obtaining easy money, he began dealing in psychedelic drugs and was eventually arrested for the possession of a substantial amount of hashish. Although his parents had endeavored to have him seen psychiatrically even prior to his leaving home, he had resisted, and only agreed to psychiatric evaluation following his arrest and impending trial. Psychiatric interviews and psychological testing revealed a young man almost totally lacking in frustration tolerance, essentially without a conscience, and without any significant identification with his stepfather with whom he had lived since the age of five.

Both parents in this case were highly conscientious people of an idealistic and hard-working type. Both had been successfully psychoanalyzed. It appeared that following the real father's death when R. was three, R. had been fixated at a pre-oedipal level. There was no evidence to indicate that he had reached or resolved his problems on an oedipal level despite the fact that he had done fairly well in school. Mother felt that stepfather had been hypercritical of R. from the beginning and that the relationship between R. and stepfather had been primarily disciplinary. R. denied any feeling of hostility to his stepfather and voiced the idea that they were two different people without much in common. He seemed to respect his stepfather, but to have been unable to identify with him. R. felt he could communicate better with mother but did not seem unduly attached to her either. After leaving home, R. seemed to avoid relationships with adult males and found places to stay either with contemporaries or with mothers of contemporaries who sympathized with him and made no demands on him. He did have a steady girl friend with whom he was heterosexually involved. His heavy drug usage, unwillingness or inability to work consistently, and rejection of goal-oriented, middle-class behavior were some of the manifestations of a severe character disorder of a psychopathic type. Cultural, constitutional, and early traumatic factors undoubtedly contributed to the clinical picture seen at the time of evaluation. It was difficult to determine to what extent the mother might have unconsciously excluded the stepfather from relationship with the boy, although the exclusion was not apparent in retrospect.

Following R.'s arrest, the parents were in severe turmoil. R. returned home but made little effort to conform to the family pattern of living. He had no motivation to work, stayed out with friends until the early morning hours, and then slept most of the day. Mother concluded that the best way to maintain a constructive relationship with the son in the house was to make no demands on him. The stepfather acted with considerable restraint despite the fact that his wish was to institute a program for the boy requiring that he keep regular hours, look for a job, etc. Mother blamed father for feeling only negatively toward the boy even though R. showed no indication that he wished to change his impulsive and self-indulgent style of life. It seemed likely that in the crisis situation the parents may have been re-enacting what had gone on in the home over the years in relation to R.'s upbringing. It seemed difficult for mother to realize that father's expectations were reasonable and for father to realize the depth of concern that mother felt about the possibility that the boy might again leave home in order to resume what mother believed to be a self-destructive pattern of living. In summary it appeared that R.'s lack of conscience, poor ego strength, and deficient father identification condemned him to a life of dependency on external structures which he seemed determined to reject. His poor judgment suggested that the external structure might inevitably be in the form of a penal institution.

SUMMARY OF SIGNIFICANT DYNAMICS

Because of the discrepancy between fantasy and reality, the stepchild is often disappointed in the new family situation. Repressed resentment toward his real parent and resentment at the intrusion of the step-parent between himself and his real parent tend to focus the hostility on the newcomer. The step-parent tends to become the final common pathway for the hostility of the stepchild. Many other factors such as the presence of step-siblings may exaggerate the feeling.

The stepchild is in conflict between his desire to maintain his pre-oedipal attachment to mother and to move ahead into resolution of oedipal feelings which will permit identification with the new step-parent. The two extremes of this conflict are seen in the regressive mode wherein the child maintains, often with mother's help, the nuclear relationship, and in the progressive mode, wherein the child rejects his dependency on available parental objects and exhibits behavior which can best be encompassed by the descriptive term "pseudomaturity syndrome."

The child who remains pre-oedipally fixated, despite the best efforts of all concerned, is likely to reach adulthood with a severe character disorder. Such people in contemporary American culture tend to drop out, become addicted, and follow lifelong patterns of dependency and irresponsibility.

Legal revision, alteration of school programs, and therapeutic intervention on a wider scale are desperately needed to prevent the intrenchment of failure patterns in children who have been seriously traumatized by family disruption early in life. Statistically, more than 15 percent of children in the United States live with only one biological parent. Their problems now constitute a significant portion of child and adolescent psychiatric practice.

# 13

## Learning Disabilities

JULES C. ABRAMS, PH.D.

### Introduction

The world of psychology has devoted much attention to learning disabil·
ities. For one thing, probably the single, most immediate reason for children being referred to child psychiatric clinics, child guidance clinics,
child therapists, etc., is difficulty in school. Unfortunately, all too often
the child is approached with a unitary orientation so that extremely important aspects of his unique learning disorder may very well be ignored.
There is certainly no one single etiology for all learning disabilities.
Rather, learning problems can be caused by any number of a multiplicity
of factors, all of which may be highly interrelated.

When a child experiences difficulty in school, his problems are all too
often exacerbated by a number of other factors. Constant failure and
frustration may lead to strong feelings of inferiority, which, in turn, may
intensify the initial learning deficiencies. Under the impact of continued
failure, the child may withdraw or may act out aggressively. Interpersonal
relationships may be severely affected, while the child, too, may displace
many of his problems onto the home situation. All of this suggests the
importance of the child's school experiences and his ability to make most
efficient utilization of his thinking processes in his ultimate adaptation to
the world around him.

Psychologists have long recognized that social and emotional maladjustment occur in conjunction with learning difficulty. Much of the controversy in this area has raged around the "chicken or the egg" proposition
—i.e., which is cause and which is effect? Although many have taken the
view that personality factors constitute a primary cause of learning disability, many other investigators are of the opinion that the disturbed and
deviate behavior of many children suffering with learning problems stems
directly from the tensions, anxieties, and conflicts associated with the
failure.

While a psychoanalytic orientation enables us to understand the etiology
of neurotic learning disabilities and to offer proper therapy for these cases,
it is not the approach to be preferred for all. Gates (10) states that emotional maladjustment is sometimes the cause of learning disability, sometimes the effect, and sometimes the concomitant factor. Betts (2) seems
to favor the "effect" point of view as is evidenced by his feeling that in

most cases of reading retardation the frustration in the learning activity has clearly produced adjustment problems.

Fernald (6) indicates that emotional instability may be the predisposing cause of some learning disability, or the reverse might be true. Robinson (24) suggests that emotional difficulties may cause reading disability in the beginning, and that this disability may in turn result in frustration, which further blocks learning and again intensifies the frustration. She describes the interaction and intensification as a vicious circle leading to intense emotional maladjustment and complete failure to progress in learning.

Yet the psychoanalyst has made a strong argument for the role of unconscious conflict in effecting learning disorder. In *The Problem of Anxiety*, Freud says: "The ego function of an organ is impaired whenever its erogeneity, its sexual significance is increased . . . the ego renounces those functions proper to it in order not to have to undertake a fresh effort of repression, in order to avoid a conflict with the id" (7).

Other inhibitions evidently subserve a desire for self-punishment.

The ego dares not do certain things because they would bring an advantage which the strict superego has forbidden. . . . The more general inhibitions of the ego follow a simple mechanism of another character. When the ego is occupied with a psychic task of special difficulty . . . as by the necessity for holding constantly mounting sexual fantasies in check, it becomes so impoverished with respect to the energy available to it, that it is driven to restrict its expenditure in many places at the same time (7).

Blanchard's main thesis is that there is a need on the part of the retarded reader to inflict self-punishment to relieve anxiety and guilt feelings. In many instances the reading disability is a disguised expression of hidden motives, satisfying the need for punishment and relieving guilt by exposing the child to a situation of failure in school and to criticism. Blanchard elaborates on her point still further, attributing many reading disabilities to difficulties in establishing masculine identification and in handling aggressive impulses, together with excessive anxiety and guilt of a destructive, hostile nature and sadistic feelings. The signs of emotional conflict appear chiefly in the educational disability and overactive fantasy life (3).

Pearson (20) discusses disorders of the learning process in terms of two major classifications: (a) when the learning process *is not* involved in the neurotic conflict, and (b) when the learning process *is* involved in the learning conflict. Such factors as sibling rivalry, feelings of guilt or dread of castration, learning impotence, and repudiation of learning because it is associated with masculinity or femininity make up a large part of his conceptual framework.

Klein (18) speaks of the bright pupil's narcissistic maintenance of his status in his need to succeed without further effort or study. Some whose narcissism has been fed throughout childhood by the realization that they are so bright they do not need to work experience a great blow when this is no longer true. The inability to endure relative failure with subsequent restriction of ego activity is not due to narcissistic factors alone. Klein also discusses in detail failure in learning resulting from intense castration anxiety. Other narcissistic children withdraw from competition because they cannot bear to have their performance compare unfavorably with someone else's. Some children experience learning difficulties because of a fear of their own curiosity which inhibits them from exploring the environment and accumulating knowledge.

Clinical experience has alerted this author to the possible effects of a personality problem in the etiology and development of a learning disorder. On the other hand, if the child is constantly exposed to a milieu in which he cannot compete successfully with his peers in relation to learning activities, then it will not be surprising that the child develops intense feelings of insecurity and inadequacy. A child who is tense, worried, fearful, etc., cannot focus his mind on intellectual pursuits any more than can an adult who is consumed with anxiety and worry. What we have is a continuing series of interactions between the insecurity generated by the lack of success in learning on the one hand and any emotional instability which may be independent of the learning failure on the other.

Our approach, then, to the area of learning disorders is found in the tenets of psychoanalytic ego psychology. The center of attention will be on the ego functioning of the disabled youngster. In line with the pioneer efforts of Hartman, Kris, and Loewenstein (14), the basic functions of the developing personality are referred to as the functions of the developing ego. It is apparent that all these functions play a crucial role in the individual's adaptation to life. In fact, they are the very essence of psychological life—perception, memory, cognition, thinking, action, postponement of gratification, repression, anxiety, integration, and synthesis. As Pearson (20) has pointed out, anything which interferes with the development of the ego and any of its functions will undoubtedly influence the child's adaptation to life, including one very particular adaptation, namely, the child's capacity for learning.

## Definition, Causation, and Description

### DISORDERS OF THE CENTRAL NERVOUS SYSTEM

When a child suffers brain damage, prenatally, perinatally, or shortly after birth, he has experienced an insult to the very matrix of the crucial organ of learning, the brain, and its sensory and motor systems. There is a defect in the primary ego apparatuses (23). These apparatuses consist of such basic skills as perception, concept formation, motility, and language development. In the normal child, these primary ego skills represent a potentiality for development—a potentiality which, through a process of maturation and experience, ultimately develops into the secondary ego functions that are so vital to the learning process—sublimation, delay of impulse, reality testing, synthesis, analysis, integration, etc.

On the other hand, an early insult to the central nervous system constitutes a severe threat to the integrity of the organism and may bring about deficiencies in the primary ego apparatuses which, in turn, interfere with the child's ability to interact with his environment in an adaptive manner. However, it is important to note that more recent research has suggested that the defects to the ego apparatus in some cases may result solely from a situation where the child is completely deprived of intellectual and/or emotional stimulation. In any event, in order for the ego to develop properly, there are two basic requirements: (a) the intactness of the primary apparatus, that is, the neurological substrata of the ego, the central nervous system, and (b) the proper degree of stimulation in the environment.

Let us consider the four basic skills that we have mentioned above in the light of disrupted ego functioning. For the sake of brevity let us consider perception and concept-formation under the broader heading of inadequate integrative functions. We are now talking about the child who is able to take in stimuli, but who has trouble fitting them appropriately into things he already knows. For example, a child may learn how to climb on a jungle gym, but when he is out in the woods and faced with the possibility of climbing a tree, it might not occur to him that the climbing skills he has learned in one area can be applied to another. This is illustrative of the child's tremendous difficulty in making any kind of generalization. It is as if he can deal with that which is specific and concrete; he cannot engage in the kind of active mental manipulation that is such an essential aspect of abstract conceptualization or generalization.

We are thinking also of the child who has trouble pulling out of his storehouse of knowledge things that are related to something that is introduced in a class discussion. This is illustrative of the child's disorder in the cognitive processes. Although he may be able to deal successfully with that which is rote and represents simply an acquisition of information, he has difficulty in applying that information to functional situations. It is no surprise that his score on a test assessing his judgment is often far inferior to his score on a test which measures his fund of general knowledge. To apply information requires the kind of mental manipulation and freedom of psychic energies which is so antithetical to the type of ego functioning so characteristic of this disability.

We are thinking of the youngster who might be very accurate in handling numbers when these numbers are related to some aspect of himself, but who cannot make the simplest computations when the numbers do not deal with him directly. We are thinking of the child who persistently and consistently makes letter and word reversals long past what might be considered a part of a developmental stage. We are thinking, too, of the child who has a distorted idea of his own self, his own body, how big he is, how he is shaped, and the relationship of the body parts to one another. Problems in laterality and directionality are very common.

These children also have a great deal of difficulty in manipulating verbal concepts. If they are asked how a peach and a plum are alike, they may very well deny that there is any similarity whatsoever. If they are given the aid of external structuring, they will most likely respond in terms of functional or concrete properties of objects. This is illustrative of their disturbance in concept-formation and abstract function. This kind of youngster finds it virtually impossible to make generalizations from one specific learning situation to another.

A second area of disruptive ego functioning is that of inadequate impulse control or the control of ideas and feelings. It is well known that these youngsters tend to be highly narcissistic, disinhibited, hyperdistractible, hyperactive, and to experience severe problems in impulse control. These symptoms should, at all times, be related to the deficiencies in normal ego development since there is no conclusive evidence that hyperactivity or distractibility are related to defective neural transmission or specific brain cell malfunction. All the symptoms mentioned above represent rather the ego's method of defending the rest of the personality from awareness of its defects. Thus the child who has had a basic deficiency in the primary ego apparatus of perception or motility has been hampered in his ability to explore his environment adaptively, and cannot acquire a sense of mastery or a feeling that he is "one who can" rather than "one who cannot."

We know that the normal child is given a tremendous impetus toward achievement of separateness, individuation, and independence by the experience of locomotion. If, as part of the total syndrome of ego malfunctioning, motility is inadequate, the child is further robbed of the gratification of mastering new functions, which interferes with the development of self-esteem. Thus the child has difficulty staying in a chair, not because he wants to get up and destroy the class, but because it really is almost impossible for him to keep himself in one place. This is illustrative of the child's difficulty in acquiring adaptive secondary ego functioning. He has not learned to tolerate the anxiety he would feel by the necessity of delaying immediate gratification.

The child, too, has tremendous difficulty paying attention not because he is really inattentive, but because he is overly attentive to far too many stimuli. This illustrates the child's inability to discriminate and choose among the many stimuli which are constantly impinging upon him. Not only must he deal with the external stimuli, but he must also learn to cope with the bombardment of his own internal stimulation.

We would like to consider the defensive maneuvers on the part of the ego in coping with the anxiety brought on by the very intense feelings of inadequacy and defectiveness. The child who has experienced early insult to the central nervous system feels a severe threat to the integrity of his organism. He feels helpless in the face of his own intense handicap, and when he feels this way, he becomes more frightened and anxious. As a result, he tends to be more aggressive, more hostile, or sometimes withdrawn. He also becomes highly egocentric and shows feelings of omnipotence which, of course, represent his defense against his strong feelings of defectiveness. His egocentricity reveals itself in his need to relate all objects to himself before he can relate them to others. (Perhaps this plays an important role in his difficulty in generalizing.)

This child finds it extremely difficult to understand that he cannot control the world around him. He sees himself as the center of the universe. He is also angry that other people in his environment are not experiencing the same problems that he must strive to overcome. It is almost as if he is saying, "I am damaged, and I want to get even, to even up the score." He retreats into his omnipotence and sets up a condition in which his mental energies become involved in dealing with his own anxieties and fears. He must avoid any challenging situation at whatever cost to himself. He must retreat from learning because any possibility of failure represents a severe threat of further wounding his pride and self-esteem. As a result, the synthetic and analytic functions of the ego are greatly impaired. This is a vicious circle because it accentuates learning difficulty and ultimately exacerbates the intense feelings of inadequacy and inferiority.

The hostility which these children experience often leads to a kind of power struggle both at home and in school. These youngsters become "dependent despots"; they use their dependency to control. They try in manifold ways to control the teacher and to control their parents.

One cannot ignore, too, the probability of this child's being a real disappointment to his parents who inevitably must respond differently to him than they would to a normal offspring who would be a wished-for extension of themselves. The mother, particularly, may turn away from the child because of her own feeling of depression and narcissistic wounding. Unconsciously she may ask herself why she has been given the "bad product." If, as part of her own personality, she is experiencing a great deal of guilt, she may view the child as punishment for real or imagined transgressions. She may experience hostility, a feeling of anger which is intolerable, because she basically loves the child. As a result, she may tend to become overly protective or overly indulgent in order to compensate for the underlying hostility to the child.

## MATURATIONAL AND DEVELOPMENTAL PROBLEMS

Even when no specific insult to the central nervous system has occurred, disturbances can arise from some interference with or delay in the maturation or development of the ego apparatus and its functions which are necessary for formal academic learning. Certainly there are some children who, for one reason or another, are not prepared for formal learning at the usual age in our culture. It must be emphasized that just because a neurological or biological difficulty exists in a child, it does not necessarily indicate that the child will develop a serious learning problem. It may well be that in order for a youngster to develop into a so-called remedial-type case he must have this predisposition; but simply because the tendency is present, it does not mean that he must develop the disorder.

Most teachers today recognize the fact that some children are maturationally unprepared for learning to read when they are first introduced to the printed symbol. A small percent of these children may not have mastered certain ego functions which are basic to reading. These functions include perception, concept-formation, and, specifically in the reading area, associative learning ability. This kind of child experiences real difficulty in the association of common experiences and the symbols (words) which represent them. Since reading, in the last analysis, is a process of association, difficulty in this area presents a major problem for the student. He tends to have less difficulty in association when both the visual and auditory sensory pathways are involved as compared to the making of strictly visual associations. In other words, he is better able to associate when he is using both the visual and auditory sensory mechanisms.

This youngster often evidences definite interferences in memory span. As opposed to many neurotic children who evidence interference in attention span, this kind of child does not have the ability to summon up the resources within himself to focus attention; that is, he cannot concentrate.

When this child is initiated into reading at a time when his ego deficiencies do not allow him to profit from the normal methods of teaching reading, he almost inevitably experiences failure. It is no wonder that a secondary emotional problem may then ensue with great discouragement on the part of the child and a negative attitude toward reading.

This negative attitude may account for many of those symptoms which are associated with the remedial child. It is no mere coincidence that this child has difficulty with concentration in dealing with only word-like or school-like material. The memory span of these children, when dealing with visual objects rather than letters, is quite superior. Their ability to make visual-visual associations is more than adequate when the stimuli are geometric rather than word-like. It is true that they most characteristically show better achievement in the nonverbal area of an intelligence test than in the verbal area. Nevertheless, an analysis of their responses indicates that their poor performance in the verbal area is directly attributable to inability to concentrate on abstract stimuli. Concentration on concrete stimuli is superior even to that of achieving readers.

## EDUCATIONAL FACTORS

Many children experience learning disorders simply because they have been exposed to adverse educational situations. Probably the greatest cause for the milder learning problems is to be found in the group of conditions which might be classified as educational. The vast majority of reading problems are brought about by ineffective teaching or some other deficiency in the educational situation. Once the child has begun to have some problem in school, his deficiencies are exacerbated because he does not have the skills to acquire new learning. In turn, as pointed out above, he feels inadequate and frustrated, which interferes with his ability to attend and to concentrate and increases the probability that he will not learn.

Probably the chief educational factor behind learning deficiency is the all too frequent circumstance in which a child is not taught at his true instructional level. For one thing, many teachers are not equipped to evaluate the child's instructional needs and to appraise his proper level of functioning. If, for example, a teacher relies solely upon a standardized test of reading achievement to determine the instructional level in reading, many children will be placed one to three levels above their true instructional level. Frustrated by material which is much too difficult for him, the child, not surprisingly, loses his interest in reading and often withdraws from the reading process.

We have spoken previously about the fact that some children simply are not ready to learn at the time they start school. An appreciable number of children who arrive at the first grade are not ready to read in the typical program. Many of these children require an extensive period of reading readiness before they have sufficient skills to cope with the requirements involved in learning to read. If a child is introduced to reading activities prior to the time that he is ready physically, intellectually, socially, and emotionally, he is not likely to experience success in classroom reading activities.

The importance of effective teaching cannot be overestimated in the etiology of the milder learning disorders. Many factors can contribute to an unsatisfactory teaching experience. Sometimes the teacher herself is improperly trained or only gives lip service to the factor of individual differences. Surprising as it may seem, there are still many classes in which children are all taught at the same reading level. Sometimes there is an undue emphasis upon the mechanics of reading to the neglect of the major purpose of reading, that is, reading for meaning. In other situations, the administrative policies may either prevent adjustment of instruction to individual differences or not give the teacher sufficient time to provide proper readiness for learning.

## ENVIRONMENTAL AND REACTIVE PROBLEMS

Of course, the major environmental situation affecting the child's progress in learning is the school environment which has been discussed above. However, there may be disturbances in the child's current home situation which may have a devastating effect upon his learning ability. Harris (12) has pointed out that the best assurance a boy may have of being properly equipped and motivated to get the most from our educational system is the possession of parents and grandparents of a socio-economic group that places a high value on education. In his study he found that differences in social class prove to be one of the few general factors distinguishing the entire learner group from the entire nonlearner group. The reasons for the relationship were considered to be that lower-class parents place a lesser value on formal education and provide less intellectual stimulation because their time and interest are taken up principally with the problems of practical existence.

It should be pointed out, nevertheless, that the child from a low socio-economic environment often does not have an adult model with whom he can identify and who appears to be cathected to learning. Most children want to emulate adults who command power, status, and prestige. Children desire these intangible goals but often do not know how to obtain them. The child from a low socio-economic environment often does not see his parent as someone who values intellectual mastery. Thus there is little motivation on the part of the child to achieve intellectual competence since he does not see the attainment of these skills as a necessary prerequisite for the adult resources of power and competence that he wishes to possess.

Some children experience difficulty in learning because of inadequate cognitive stimulation during the early years. The culturally deprived child does not experience the same impetus to ego development as is experienced by the child from a more stimulating environment. On the whole, this child has had limited contact with the "outside world." He has experienced less opportunity to listen to the kind of complex speech that will enhance his own vocabulary development. His conceptual repertoire is quite limited. In many cases, he develops a language which is extraordinarily different from the language that he is exposed to in the average school. As a result, he performs less well on the verbal measures which are characteristically used in a typical school situation.

In addition to the limited conceptual background, children from culturally deprived areas are often not prepared for the kind of learning attitude which is necessary for success in the classroom. There is little motivation on their part to conform to the rules and regulations which are so foreign to their own upbringing. They tend to react to this unnatural situation with disdain, suspiciousness, and an unwillingness to sublimate their own impulses. The deficiencies in language further hamper the ego's efforts to mediate and delay instinctual drives. In addition, there is often little external support from the parent to bolster the ego in its efforts to adapt to the learning situation. Many of these children come from homes where there is no father or an inadequate father figure. In a sense, there is no ego ideal or even an ego ally to help reinforce the child's own efforts to mediate his impulses.

Reactive problems, however, are not limited by any means to those children from an impoverished background of experience. As has been pointed out above, in order for a child to learn, he must be able to attend to and to concentrate upon what is to be learned. Pearson (20) has pointed out that the

centering of the attention on the academic subjects to be learned and the inhibition of the deflection of the attention to other internal or external situations is necessary for a successful learning process. This interferes with the potential that is drawn to other external situations which the child finds important because they can serve as a means of gratification for some pressing instinctual desire or because certain instinctual desires are forcibly attracting the child's attention to themselves.

If a child, for example, is concerned with the home situation, with the possibility of parental separation or divorce, with intrafamilial conflict, exposure to seduction or threatened seduction, etc., it is not likely that he will be able to focus his attention on learning activities in a meaningful fashion.

The attitudes of the parental figures toward the child play an extremely influential role in determining his receptivity to the learning process. We have spoken above about the youngster who is not motivated to learn simply because there is no adequate ego ideal with whom to identify. On the other hand, there are families in which an undue emphasis has been placed upon the necessity for school achievement. The child very early in life learns that it is extremely important for him to achieve in order to maintain an adequate relationship with the mother figure. When a child begins to despair of ever completely gaining his parents' approval, he may withdraw from the struggle. It is as if he feels that his parents are simply too hard to please and that no matter what he does, he will only meet with criticism from them.

## NEUROTIC FACTORS

When the child's conflicts have become internalized and are either entirely, or in part, outside of conscious awareness, his learning disorder most likely will be directly involved with the conflictual factors inherent in the neurosis. For example, some children avoid thinking things through because they are afraid of what might be revealed. We are reminded of a female adolescent patient who was quite successful in reading activities as long as she merely had to communicate back in parrot fashion what the teacher had given or what she had read. At no time could she engage in inferential thinking, or organize her communications around her own experiences, or draw conclusions, or generalize. This was much too threatening for her because bringing in her own experience involved the possible arousal of unacceptable ideas and feelings which she necessarily had to repress. It was only after her own conflicts concerning her fear of growing up and assuming the adult female sexual role were worked out that she could really become actively involved in the learning situation.

Some children unconsciously use learning, or rather not learning, as a weapon to express resentment toward the parental figures. It is an effective weapon and one over which the child maintains complete control. Nobody can make him learn if he does not want to. The older child who is angry at his parents may use nonlearning as a two-edged sword—he punishes his parents and also himself. He feels so guilty because of his resentment toward the parents that he must appease his guilt through self-punishment.

An overly harsh superego can lead to a restriction of the ego and abandoning of one activity after another. In one little girl of eight, it was learned through psychotherapy that she had a good deal of hostility concerning her feelings of emotional deprivation. She was a child with good creative potential, sensitive and warm, but she felt emotionally starved. However, she could not aim the hostility outwardly as she felt it, but instead had to masochistically turn the hostility on herself. One aspect of her hostility was her wish to flout authoritarian dictates. The only way she could achieve that without risking further rejection or emotional deprivation was through her own inadequacy. That is, when an authority figure told her to succeed, and instead she was inadequate, she was flouting that authority. This is akin to the intrapunitive themes mentioned earlier.

## Diagnosis

The diagnosis is primarily concerned with the accurate identification of the constellation of presenting and causal factors which appear in a case of learning disability. However, diagnosis, to be effective, must also result in accurate communication to the remedial clinician, the therapist, the school, and the parent of sufficient information about the problem so that a profitable program of rehabilitation will result. If the only resultant in a thorough diagnostic procedure is an explanation of the difficulty, the process has been next to useless. For the child, the home, and the school the problem is still one of finding a *solution* to the inadequate forms of adjustment which were the precipitating reasons for the referral in the first place.

To provide the basis for planning an effective program of rehabilitation, the diagnostician must obtain information in four major areas. First, a detailed history is needed to provide the basis for understanding and interpreting all of the remaining clinical data to be obtained—the "cognitive ways" upon which all other factors are to be overlaid. Second, a careful analysis of the child's current *physical-social-emotional status* should be made. Third, an individually obtained assessment of the client's *general capacity for learning* is required. Finally, the presenting picture with *respect* to achievement in each of the academic and communication areas involved must be detailed sufficiently to clarify the specific nature of his difficulties and the resources which he has available to him in meeting any learning demands which are made upon him. In each of these four areas the information should be obtained as carefully and objectively as possible. The more data obtained, the more likely that the decisions made will be valid and related to the most appropriate solutions to the problem. There are no short cuts to be found in a valid and reliable diagnostic procedure.

## HISTORY

As already noted, the child's adjustment mechanisms employed at any particular point in time are a product of the accumulated dynamics of his interaction with his environment since conception. It is important, therefore, to gain as much insight as possible into the sequence of this behavioral development. A detailed history of his growth and development should be obtained as a first step in the diagnostic process. Through interviews with the parents and the client himself, a skillful interviewer can elicit most of the significant information desired. In many instances, especially in getting accurate data in the medical or educational history, it will be necessary to contact the physician, the hospital, or the school to verify information given or to supplement it with additional items of significance. In an occasional case, other family members and/or other professional workers who have had clinical contact with the client may need to be consulted for further data.

Basically, four highly related areas of significance bear careful objective study in obtaining the history of the development of a problem. The first of these pertains to the family constellation itself and the child's positioning within the family group. For each member of the family and others who may be living in the home, information about their age, educational experience and achievement, occupation, general health factors, interests, hobbies, normal daily schedule of activities, and general reading habits should be obtained. A general description of the home itself and the community within which it is located, recreational spaces available, library facilities, reading matter within the home, and work areas suitable for private study are recorded. A report of the handedness of the various family members and particularly of the procedures normally utilized in assigning home responsibilities and handling disciplinary matters should be taken. In other words, as complete a picture of the nature of the home environment and the normal behavior of all within it as it impinges upon the client's behavior (past and present) should be drawn.

Second, all facts pertinent to the pre- and postnatal development of the child must be obtained. Thus a complete description of the mother's pregnancy period, the child's birth and development through the pre-school years is necessary. Here, particular attention should be given to factors that may indicate insult to the central nervous system or reflect abnormality in the rate of language development. The interviewer should be alert to indications of sensory deprivation, either environmentally caused or due to delay in the detection of sensory deficit, particularly auditory and visual.

Third, a complete record of medical treatment and general health factors since birth is obtained. Accidents, illnesses, immunizations, and behavioral characteristics noted preceding and following each of these instances should be included. It is often necessary for the interviewer to follow up on a recorded medical episode by contacting the physician, etc., involved in the treatment for additional data. Therefore it is important to record the name and address of the treating physician or agency. Once again, of particular significance will be those episodes which appear to have bearing upon subsequent neurological and/or communication functioning.

Finally, since learning disability is primarily related to lack of progress in an academic environment, the client's educational record is of significant importance. A complete accounting of his educational experiences from preschool to the present should be required. His initial reaction to school, regularity of attendance, early symptoms of difficulty, what was done at that point to identify the problem and provide assistance, referrals for diagnosis, tutoring, remedial treatment, etc., all may have bearing on his current difficulties and should be carefully recorded. Contacts with the current educational setting may be advisable and information should be obtained especially from all diagnostic and/or treatment agencies or any individuals who have had contact with the child.

INTELLECTUAL FACTORS

A learning disability is represented by a significant difference between the child's measured potential level of functioning and his present achievement level in any given area of achievement. Other elements being equal, the greater this discrepancy, the more extensive or serious the disability. Thus the diagnostician generally begins his accumulation of objective test data with an individual measure of intelligence. Although a number of such instruments are available, those devised by David Wechsler are most commonly used. In cases of reading disability, they are particularly appropriate since they combine measures of both verbal and nonverbal intellectual abilities and provide a scattering of subtests which measure specific abilities which appear to be highly related to difficulties in reading. In addition to the overall intelligence score and the comparison between verbal and performance tests as a whole, those subtests related to concept-formation, perceptual abilities, memory span, and visual-motor association skills are often particularly helpful to the clinician. Weighted scores may be translated into mental age equivalent ratings which are usually more helpful when compared with achievement measures than IQs or percentile ratings. For a further discussion of the various subtests the reader is referred to David Rappaport's text, *Diagnostic Psychological Testing* (22).

Earlier, the frequent difficulty in making associations between visual and auditory stimuli and their meanings was discussed. Tests are often required to measure these difficulties more precisely. Those most frequently employed are the *Gates Associative Learning Test* and *Van Wagenen Reading Readiness Test—Word Learning Cards* (11, 27). Distinct patterns of functioning on these batteries have been clinically used to designate those children who are likely to experience extreme difficulty in learning to recognize words when the teaching modalities employed are only visual or a combination of visual-auditory. For such children, the need for a multisensory approach, as in the Fernald or V-A-K-T technique, is suggested. It should be noted that Kass (16), reporting on the performance of reading disability cases on the *Illinois Test of Psycholinguistic Abilities* (15), found more deficiencies at the automatic-sequential level than at the representational level and more problems in association than in decoding or encoding.

Similarly, we have referred to difficulties with attention, concentration, and retention as they relate to learning disability. Although some memory abilities are involved in responding to most individual test items in any area, a specific memory-span battery is helpful in identifying the nature of the child's ability to attend to and retain stimuli experienced in different modalities. The *Wechsler Memory Scale* (29) or specific memory subtests selected from the *Detroit Tests of Learning Aptitude* (5) are often employed. Tests used to measure attention and concentration should be composed of both discrete and related items as well as stimuli presented in various modalities (visual, auditory, or a combination of these). Stauffer's (26) findings suggested that the more severe learning disability cases in reading will present significant abnormal performances on tests of this nature. Orton (19) noted that severe difficulties in visual memory are almost always identified in children with learning disability and Pearson (21) has shown that a lowered attention span was characteristic of such cases.

Perceptual-motor abilities, while measured to some extent in certain subtests of the Wechsler scales, bear further specific evaluation. The *Bender Visual-Motor-Gestalt Test* (1) is, perhaps, the most frequently used, although a number of other instruments are available and yield similar findings. Several variations of the original procedure for administration and scoring this instrument have been developed.

Although much has been written about lateral dominance and its influence on children with learning disability, the importance of measurement in this area is still unclear. The *Harris Tests of Lateral Dominance* (13) or those techniques described by Linda Smith (25) utilizing the *Van Riper Form Board* may be included to measure peripheral and central dominance. However, it is a moot question whether modification of a child's dominance patterns will improve or, in fact, impair his current behavioral patterns. Nevertheless, until more is known about the influence of dominance upon motor and language behavior, some appraisal of the child's current laterality status is advisable.

The *Frostig Developmental Test of Visual Perception* (8) assesses five areas which may be related to academic skills: figure-ground relationships, eye-hand coordination, form constancy, position in space, and spatial relationships. Motor skills are necessary for adequate performance in each subtest. The DTVP yields a "perceptual quotient" with norms for children from ages four to seven.

Several assumptions have been made about the interrelationship between visual perception and motor ability. Some have indicated that visual perception is dependent upon learning gross motor skills. This implies that disorders in gross motor skills should be corrected before training in visual perception is undertaken. If, for example, a child, during his early years, was handicapped in the development of motility because of inadequate ego apparatuses, he would not be likely to develop a sense of mastery which would also contribute to a sense of identity. In any event, some kind of evaluation should be made of the child's motor development. Kephart (17) has outlined in great detail procedures to be used in assessing the motoric skills of brain-injured children.

### PERSONALITY FACTORS

A clinical evaluation of the child can be of inestimable aid in understanding the child's strengths and weaknesses relevant to his emotional status. Specifically, the diagnostician, in this area, is concerned with the child's ego strength, that is, with the child's ability to see things as other people see them, his capacity to relate to other persons, and his effectiveness in dealing with his ideas and feelings in an adaptive manner. The psychiatrist or psychologist attempts to learn how the child copes with disturbing emotions. He attempts to discern the maneuvers the child employs to bring about desired reactions from others; he also studies the particular defense mechanisms that the child utilizes which may facilitate or impede educational progress. He assesses the anxiety level of the child and looks for the presence of neurotic or psychosomatic symptoms.

The clinician also gives much of his attention to the child's perception of important people in his environment. He is concerned with the child's attitude toward his parents, toward other authority figures including teachers, and toward his own peers. The perception of the child may not necessarily coincide with reality. The child can see the teacher as frightening because of displacement of anxiety. In essence, the diagnostician, through the clinical evaluation of the child, attempts to acquire a clear-cut picture of the important factors that would either be etiological or sustaining to the learning disability.

In addition to the clinical observations of the child, psychological testing may make an important contribution in understanding the nature of the learning problem. For example, the psychologist must determine if there is any significant discrepancy between the child's functioning intelligence level and his potential capacity. Through a careful quantitative and qualitative analysis of inter- and intratest variability, as well as the verbalizations of the child, the psychologist searches for any significant interference to the thinking processes. Since all effective learning involves the ability to engage in random, passive attending, as well as the ability to focus one's attention—that is, to concentrate—the relationship between these two factors is studied extensively.

As pointed out above, perceptual and conceptual skills must be investigated. Deficiencies in these areas may have a direct influence upon reading ability, but more likely they influence the child's general learning efficiency. Responses are judged as to the breadth and quality of conceptual thinking. Inadequate or loosely defined concepts must be evaluated to determine whether they represent simply an educational deficiency or are symptomatic of a more serious disorder. For example, an inability to engage in analytic-synthetic thinking might be the result of some underlying organic involvement, or might just as well derive from the child's tremendous anxiety and his basic need to keep things hidden from himself.

In addition to the formal evaluation of the thinking processes, the psychological assessment will usually include projective testing. The child, in responding to relatively unstructured materials, will project his own ideas and feelings, his conflicts and anxieties, on these stimuli and thereby furnish a kind of X-ray of the personality. By carefully interpreting the results of projective tests, the psychologist may gain very important clues as to the child's general effectiveness in a learning situation.

More specifically, the psychological evaluation will be aimed at assessing the child's ability to organize and synthesize life experience into meaningful, goal-directed patterns. It will explore the child's ability to differentiate between what is constructively aggressive and what is destructively aggressive. If this ability is lacking, for example, then the child will not be able to be assertive in the learning situation and will not be able to compete.

The psychological evaluation will also be directed to evaluate the child's attitudes toward dependency, his feelings about anger and rage, his need to inflict punishment upon himself, his level of aspiration, his motivation, and his self-concept. In essence, the psychological evaluation should help to determine whether there is truly a psychogenic etiology to the learning disability or if symptoms of emotional maladjustment result from continued frustration and failure in school.

### VISUAL-AUDITORY-NEUROLOGICAL FACTORS

There are many kinds of visual defects, some of which appear to have more etiological significance in connection with learning problems than others. Visual problems which are particularly important in terms of their relevancy to reading disability are those which involve the accommodative-convergence relationship, that is, the ability of the child to see clearly at all working distances, to see singly at all working distances, and to do so in a comfortable, harmonious fashion. Most of the problems in the visual area which are either etiological or exacerbating to the reading failure represent some disturbance in the accommodative-convergence relationship.

When an individual is experiencing real difficulty in the coordinate functioning of the eyes, he may attempt to compensate (just as the ego attempts to defend against stress). He may overcome his fusion problem through sheer effort (ultimately resulting in eye fatigue, headaches, etc.). He may engage in suppression of vision in one eye, which temporarily alleviates the problem since he no longer needs to converge. Or, if he is experiencing a breakdown in the accommodative-convergence relationship, he may very well withdraw from those activities which have produced the stress—namely, near-point activities such as reading.

A thorough diagnosis of learning disability should include visual screenings designed to evaluate the coordinate functioning of the eyes. Specifically, the screening should be directed to detect problems of visual efficiency, that is, accommodation, convergence, and the relationship established between accommodation and convergence. The diagnosis and treatment of a visual problem rightly belongs in the realm of the vision specialist who is trained to handle such problems. But the diagnostician of the learning disability should be equipped to screen out visual difficulties that may affect the child's ability to learn. The *Massachusetts Vision Test* and the *Keystone Telebinocular* are two good examples of simple tests which can be utilized to detect visual anomalies.

Hearing problems may play a role in the etiology of learning disabilities. Since reading is taught in most schools as a process whereby the child associates printed symbols with speech sounds, the student having a hearing loss readily is confused. Some children do not experience any difficulty in auditory acuity, but are unable to discriminate between sounds which are similar (auditory discrimination). Assessment of auditory acuity for children typically includes an audiometric evaluation, tests of speech-sound discrimination, and informal observations.

The pediatric neurologist is concerned with the evaluation of the integrity of the nervous system and with detection of organic involvement. Observation of gait, evaluation of coordination, the study of sensory processes as well as visual-spatial motor activities, etc., constitute the major part of this examination. The emphasis, nevertheless, is not on organic factors per se. Unquestionably, there are many children who experience soft-signs and, for that matter, who definitely have some neurologic deficiencies who have no difficulty whatsoever in the learning situation. What we are concerned with here is, as always, the ego functioning. Specifically, the neurologist is interested in determining if any deficiencies in perception, concept-formation, motility, coordination, and language development interfere with the child's ability to interact with his environment in an adaptive manner.

EDUCATIONAL FACTORS

It is perhaps axiomatic that the educational evaluation of the child is of utmost importance in determining the nature of the remediation steps that will be pursued. Thus it is almost unbelievable that frequently a child with learning disability is evaluated without the benefit of an educational diagnosis.

It is the responsibility of the diagnostician to determine where the child is functioning in all aspects of language development, such as listening, speaking, reading, and writing. More specifically, he must appraise (a) how well the child's current achievement compares with his intelligence level; (b) how his performance matches up with the performance of other children of his age; (c) what level of material he can be expected to read on his own and where he will most profit from instruction (not to mention where he will be frustrated by the complexity of the material); and (d) how well he can evaluate his own performance and be aware of his own deficiencies.

For a considerable number of years now it has become generally accepted that the answers to most of the questions stated above can best be elicited by the intelligent use of informal inventories. Although the group reading inventory provides a valuable instrument for determining levels of performance, a much more thorough and diagnostic method is to appraise the performance of each pupil individually. In essence this procedure consists of having the child read orally at sight and then silently from a series of reading selections which increase in order of difficulty.

During the oral reading, the clinician makes a detailed recording of the child's performance. Such things as omissions, substitutions, insertions, repetitions, etc., are duly noted. In addition, the clinician should be alerted to the phrasing of the reader, the voice control, possible speech defects, etc.

As the child reads silently, the clinician notes any evidence of lip movement, subvocalization, etc., as well as recording the rate of reading. Since reading is never simply a matter of recognizing words, comprehension of both the oral and silent reading selections are checked by means of factual, inferential, and vocabulary-type questions. Finally, the ability of the child to locate information and to improve the quality of his oral reading performance after initial silent reading is appraised.

While there is a great deal of information which can be acquired by employing this inventory, probably the most important knowledge obtained is that of the different achievement levels. For example, in reading it is extremely important that the clinician distinguish between the child's *independent* level—where he is able to read on his own—and his *instructional* level—where he can profit most from instruction. At the *independent level* the child is expected to make no more than one error in 100 running words, and to maintain a comprehension score of 90 percent or better. At the *instructional level* the child should make no more than one error in 20 running words, and maintain a comprehension of at least 75 percent. The child will be considered to be at his frustration level when his word recognition drops below 90 percent (more than one error in every ten running words) or his comprehension is less than 50 percent.

The *hearing comprehension* or *capacity level* of the child can be appraised as part of this inventory by reading selections to the child and then checking his comprehension. The child is considered to have adequate capacity for reading at a particular level if his hearing comprehension score is 75 percent or better, and if his oral language level is comparable to the language level of the material. By then comparing the child's instructional level with his capacity level, we are able to get at least an approximate estimate of the amount of retardation in reading, or to put it slightly differently, how his current achievement compares with his potential level.

Informal inventories, although very diagnostic, are dependent to some extent upon the experience and competence of the examiner. In addition, they only indirectly yield information as to how the performance of the child compares with other children of his age. This then becomes the major purpose of the standardized test—to compare the achievement of one child with his peers, or, more accurately, to compare a class' level with the national norm.

The educational diagnostician also studies the patterning of the child's attention-span capacities. Certain relationships have been established which help to differentiate the child who is experiencing specific learning disability from the child who has difficulty in concentrating based upon some psychogenic etiology. It is also important to determine whether there is impairment of the functioning of any of the sensory modalities. The focus of the educational aspect of the evaluation is always upon its practical value to the person who is going to teach the child. Diagnosis and labels per se have no real significance; what the teacher requires is specific suggestions as to the techniques that may be employed to overcome weaknesses in any area.

## Treatment

Our basic orientation to the study of learning disorders is on the ego functioning of the disabled youngster. It has been pointed out above that learning problems can be caused by any number of a multiplicity of factors, all of which may be highly interrelated. The tendency of each professional discipline to view the entire problem "through its own window of specialization" often obscures vital factors which may contribute to, or at least exacerbate, the basic difficulty. It is just as invalid to conceive of one cure, one panacea, applied randomly to all types of learning disorders. Not every learning disabled youngster requires a special school, or psychotherapy, or kinesthetic techniques, or perceptual-motor training, or, for that matter, regression to crawling along the floor!

### EDUCATIONAL CONSIDERATIONS

When a child experiences a severe learning disability, it may become necessary to consider a special school placement. There are undoubtedly many reasons why a child with severe learning problems may require the setting of a special school. Some of the advantages he encounters in such a setting include smaller classes and more realistic instructional levels. There is usually more teacher personnel with increased sophistication and tolerance for disruptive behavior. The class is generally grouped in such a way that the child with difficulties does not stand out in such great relief as he formerly had in his regular school.

In setting up such a program, the necessity for structure must be kept in mind. The brain-injured child, in particular, may be disturbed by changes in routine and by unexpected situations. Proper structuring of the child's environment will go far in reducing the child's anxiety level and alleviating the basic tendency to be hyperactive, hyperdistractible, and disinhibited. By a structured environment, we are not talking about a situation characterized by extreme rigidity. Warmth and concern for the child can exist in a setting of structure where the youngster is not overly stimulated. The teacher must be comfortable with structure, be able to establish limitations, and be able to maintain limitations. The manner in which firm limits are applied is extremely important.

It is perhaps trite to say that the child with neurologic handicap needs lots of praise and reassurance. Although these children show much bravado and feelings of omnipotence, this is most often a cover-up for their own felt defectiveness. They need to develop skills to cope with the external world because such skills compensate for the feelings of inferiority by giving them self-confidence and success in mastery.

Another interesting phenomenon is that of *tangential learning*. At times the teacher will attempt to teach one child a particular concept. He will withdraw, become abusive, get involved with his own idea rather than the teacher's. Yet when the teacher now shifts her energies to another child, the former one sits passively, but interestingly enough learns the concept. This again appears to be a direct effect of the child's narcissism preventing his learning while he feels openly threatened.

Teachers of children with severe learning disabilities must be selected with great care. Waldman (28) has pointed out that the predominant goal is to help the teacher become a learning therapist. Often an understanding of the child's psychodynamics can help the teacher to respond in an appropriate fashion. A major advantage to the teacher would be a more comfortable reliance on her intuition in meeting the many difficult situations that can arise during any school day. As the teacher becomes more aware of the child's psychodynamics, he would then be more attentive to stratagems that could help the child accommodate more readily to the classroom.

The teacher must expect the unexpected and take nothing for granted by way of skills. Often the children will show a skill at a high level and yet have very serious gaps of understanding at a lower level. Diagnostic teaching is imperative. When the nature of the child's specific learning disability has been adequately diagnosed, the necessary remedial procedures may then be instituted.

For example, one of the major problems exhibited by the dyslexic child is the difficulty in perceiving and retaining a detailed image of a word. This is seen clinically when a child recognizes a word on one line and is unable to recognize it, or incorrectly identifies it, on the very next line. The severe difficulties in word recognition manifested by these children seem to be attributable to a basic associative learning problem. It has been found that dyslexic children tend to have less difficulty in association when the visual and auditory sensory pathways are involved as compared to the making of strictly visual associations. They are better able to associate when they are using both the visual and auditory sensory mechanisms.

These children, then, are even more greatly assisted when the visual-auditory-kinesthetic technique (VAK) and the visual-auditory-kinesthetic-tactile technique (VAKT) are employed. These are techniques which provide additional sensory reinforcement. Writing or even tracing the word is useful not only because of possible kinesthetic-tactile facilitation of memory but, more important, because the child's attention is called to the word. The very nature of the kinesthetic-tactile approach is one which forces concentration and attention. If we postulate that one of the factors interfering with concentration and attention is the child's own anxiety and narcissism, then any technique that will force concentration will be helpful.

By having the child write and read or dictate and read stories which represent his present interests and his past experiences, we are making certain that he is always dealing with concepts with which he is already familiar. Any words which he learns in these stories he should always encounter again in new and different contexts, so that there is a great deal of reinforcement. As the child finds that he can learn and retain words through the use of VAK and VAKT, and as he sees that he is successful in the reading tasks prepared especially for him, greater satisfaction comes from trying than from evading.

The improved attention and concentration usually occur not only within the word learning situations but in other areas as well. Even in listening activities, concentration becomes more important, more worthy of expenditure of energy, because the child is actually concerned about the ideas he can get through concentrating on materials read to him. In reading, the material commands attention because he can get meaning from it, something that may not have been true in the past.

## ADJUNCTIVE CONSIDERATIONS

Although the learning therapist (teacher) is unquestionably the major instrument in correcting the problems of the child with learning disability, ancillary personnel may also be used to advantage. A means of giving aid to child and teacher separately, as well as in their interaction, is to employ a psychotherapist within the school setting. Quite often the child with emotional and social difficulties is unable to tolerate the pressures created by his efforts to master academic skills. In the course of his school day he can act out his strained feelings in various disruptive and aggressive ways. At these times the psychotherapist in the school setting can be of inestimable value by intervening in specific crises. In conjunction with other staff personnel, he might underscore those factors which need to be dealt with immediately and get the child ready for learning again.

The psychotherapist will occasionally see some of the children in individual therapy. If, however, the child is ego-disturbed, some modifications in traditional clinical practice are warranted. The nature of the child with ego disturbance does not allow him to adapt to the usual approaches employed in psychotherapy as it is traditionally practiced. Rappaport (23) has excellently described the nature of the therapy employed with a brain-injured child.

A thorough assessment of the child's ego skills may prove fruitless if one does not consider the family constellation in which the child must function. The parents of the brain-damaged child (particularly the mother) feel extraordinary ambivalence which arouses intolerable and unacceptable guilt feelings. The anger and hostility which they almost inevitably must feel toward the child cannot be tolerated by their superego, and defenses against these impulses are erected. These take the form of overprotection, overindulgence, denial, projection, etc., all of which, in turn, rob the child of opportunities for growth and the development of adaptive secondary ego functions.

The parents then need considerable professional guidance if they are to be helped to understand their role in the sustenance of the severe learning disability. In many special school settings, parental counseling is considered to be an indispensable aspect of the total program. The problems encountered in school are often very similar to the problems that the child has experienced in the home setting. For example, the same frustration and anger that have been experienced by the parent in his relationship with the child can also be felt by the teacher, and, as with the parent, serve to bring about an inflexible approach to the child that will lessen the teacher's effectiveness. Bricklin and Bricklin (4) have made an important contribution to the understanding of the parents' role in dealing with the behavior of the child with severe learning disability.

Perceptual-motor training is also often employed with those children who appear to need this special kind of help. *The Frostig Program for the Development of Visual Perception* (9) attempts to develop proficiency in visual perceptual abilities. Remediation is based on each of the five areas measured by the *Frostig Developmental Test of Visual Perception* (8). Kephart (17) also has developed a training program for developing perceptual-motor abilities in children who have "suffered breakdowns in perceptual-motor development at one of the earlier stages."

## Conclusion

In the past ten years there has been a tremendous degree of interest in, and concern for, those youngsters suffering with learning disability. Perhaps as a reaction to the indiscriminate use of such labels as minimal cerebral dysfunction, dyslexia, perceptual handicap, etc., some professional disciplines have proposed the single unitary diagnosis of "learning disabilities." While the desire to move away from the often inaccurate "labeling" of children is praiseworthy, the conceptualization of a circumscribed area of learning disability is more than questionable.

We have emphasized throughout this paper the importance of establishing a conceptual framework upon which to base the diagnosis of the multifaceted aspects of learning disorders. A single unitary approach to the evaluation of learning problems is highly fallible. Rather, one must always begin with the axiom that there is no single cause for learning problems. These difficulties may be caused and sustained by any number of factors. Furthermore, in any comprehensive evaluation, one must view the youngster experiencing school problems as a physical organism functioning in a social environment in a psychological manner. The corollary to this is that in every child there exists a unique interaction of both functional and organic factors.

We must begin "to accept strawberries in January." We must stop looking at these issues through our own windows of specialization. We must let down our defenses and feel free to accept any help in solving the dilemma of bright, alert youngsters who experience severe learning disability and its concomitant pressures. There have been strides in medicine, psychology, neurology, psychiatry, etc., which have contributed greatly to the knowledge of learning, thinking, and behavior. We cannot ignore what has been assiduously acquired, but instead must develop the capacity and the wisdom to use this knowledge in a manner that is most beneficial to the child.

# 14

## *Audiological Disorders*

PHILIP E. ROSENBERG, PH.D.

---

### *Hearing Impairment: The Invisible Handicap*

Hearing impairment has often been called the invisible handicap. Many disorders of childhood and adolescence are directly observable. Blindness is certainly conspicuous; cerebral palsy draws dramatic attention to itself; many forms of mental retardation are recognizable to even the untrained observer; and numerous emotional disturbances exhibit bizarre and obvious behavioral manifestations. Each of these entities causes a reaction in the beholder. At best, this reaction is an understanding empathy; at worst, pity. Hearing loss, on the other hand, carries with it no such observable stigmata. The vast majority of hard of hearing or deaf children appear entirely normal to either the casual observer or the trained professional. Yet such children suffer from one of the most depriving of all disabilities. Due to their hearing deficit, they are deprived of that one touchstone of humanity: language.

Since hearing impairment is invisible and since its various manifestations can be quite subtle, the impairment is frequently misdiagnosed. It is not uncommon for children with a significant degree of auditory deficit to be labeled as mentally retarded, brain damaged, emotionally disturbed, or aphasic (10). Indeed, most deaf children have, at one time or another, had such appellations given them. Many have been entered into therapeutic or academic programs totally unsuited to their needs because of this misdiagnosis. Once the child has been in an improper environment for a length of time, he tends to become his diagnostic entity. In other words, if a deaf child is treated as if he were mentally retarded for several years, he will exhibit the typical behavioral symptomatology of the retarded person rather than that of the deaf. Once this has occurred, salvage becomes difficult indeed.

The causes of hearing loss are many (1, 5, 9). Some causes affect children alone, some only adults, and many affect both children and adults. Almost one half of all congenital hearing impairments are genetically determined. This is particularly tragic since almost all hereditary forms of deafness manifest themselves through a recessive gene. Unfortunately, in our society, the deaf tend to marry the deaf and the recessive genetic material is reinforced and becomes manifest. Slightly over half of the congenital deafness problems are the result of developmental factors. Primary among these is maternal rubella in the first trimester of pregnancy. Over the past several decades, this has been the major cause of congenital deafness. Interruption of the formation of the auditory nervous system caused by this relatively benign viral infection results in profound hearing impairment. Other maternal viral infections in the early months of pregnancy can also interfere with the development of the auditory apparatus and result in severe loss of hearing. Rh incompatability with the resultant erythroblastosis fetalis can affect the second or subsequent pregnancy so that, although the child is born with normal hearing, he loses it in the early hours of life.

Other forms of hearing impairment are acquired after birth. These tend to be not quite so profound as those associated with the congenital anomalies. They are no less serious, however, since their late arrival may catch the examiner unaware. Any viral infection in early childhood may cause a relatively severe sensori-neural hearing deficit. Mumps, measles, chicken pox, scarlet fever, meningitis, and other diseases are not infrequently accompanied by hearing loss. Less serious hearing handicaps are abundant in the youthful population. Serous otitis media as a result of eustachian tube blockage, upper respiratory infections, or allergy causes enough of a hearing loss to create a problem in social or academic situations. Otosclerosis, the fixation of the stapes in the oval window, is not unknown in children and can result in a moderate conductive hearing deficit that will certainly interfere with all communication. Even the normal accumulation of ear wax or cerumen can cause an auditory deficit of moderate degree that often remains undetected and results in behavior that is subsequently misinterpreted.

It is impossible to overemphasize the importance of early examination, detection, and diagnosis of hearing problems. Some of the pathologies such as serous otitis media or otosclerosis are immediately reversible through appropriate medical treatment or surgical intervention. Restoration of hearing in these cases is total and immediate. For those children whose hearing impairments are not amenable to medical or surgical treatment, other therapies are available. Amplification through a desk model amplifier or through a wearable hearing aid can be utilized even in the early months of life. Appropriate special training and educational techniques can be employed to assist the child to develop language and speech. Most important, however, is that an inappropriate and incorrect diagnosis be avoided. The early months and years of life are brief and if once lost are beyond recall. It is during these early months and years that the child is exquisitely receptive to specific therapies and to language acquisition (4, 7). If he is inappropriately diagnosed and inappropriately placed, irreparable damage has been done. No amount of later training can undo the damage that has occurred.

## Testing Hearing of Infants and Children

During the past several years many hospitals and medical centers have instituted a program of hearing screening of neonates (2). Although these programs are still in the experimental stage and have not yet been completely validated, they appear to show great promise in detecting those children who have severe auditory handicaps. The test is usually conducted on the day after birth and consists of exposing the newborn child to a high intensity, high frequency sound. The stimulus usually consists of a narrow band of noise centered about 3,000 Hz at approximately 100 dB sound pressure level. The responses range from a full Moro reflex to a clenching of the fists or a pulling up of one leg. It is not difficult to learn to recognize typical hearing responses in the newborn child. The particular stimulus is carefully chosen since children with severe hearing problems will not usually have any demonstrative hearing in the region of 3,000 Hz. It must be emphasized that the neonatal testing program is strictly a screening device and hardly represents a definitive diagnostic examination. Likewise, screening tests are available for children of any age through pediatricians, public health clinics, well baby clinics, school nurses, and public school speech and hearing therapists. These screening tests are all precursors to a detailed diagnostic audiologic examination. If the child fails any of the screening tests, such an examination should be mandatory.

The diagnostic audiologic evaluation must always be preceded by a thorough otolaryngologic examination. An otolaryngologist should inspect the ear canal and the tympanic membrane otoscopically. He should also examine the oral and nasal cavities, the naso-pharynx, and should perform a mirror examination of the larynx. Once these examinations have been performed, the audiologic evaluation should be done.

Techniques are now available for the detailed study of the hearing of any child at any age (3, 5). The basic stimulus for the audiologic examination should be the pure tone. This is a rigorously controlled and calibrated sound of a single frequency. More casual types of hearing tests such as those performed with noisemakers, keys, watches, hand claps, etc., should be assiduously avoided. Not only do they not provide a reliable and valid estimate of residual hearing, but they tend to yield dangerously misleading information. Pure tone audiometry, on the other hand, can be performed by a number of different techniques all of which result in a highly accurate representation of the child's auditory system. These tests are usually conducted in a very quiet sound-treated environment by skilled personnel utilizing well-calibrated equipment. Stimuli may be presented through headphones or through loudspeakers appropriately placed around the room. Frequencies tested range from 125 through 8,000 Hz since this range encompasses the entire important area for human hearing and communication. Older children are examined simply by having them indicate when they barely begin to hear the sound. Children between the ages of two and a half and four years can be tested by conditioned play techniques whereby they perform a meaningful task such as dropping a marble in a bottle when the sound is present. Children below the age of two and a half can be examined through a combination of behavioral and electrophysiologic techniques. Many infants will localize quite well toward that loudspeaker from which the sound emanates. Others will indicate by momentary cessation of activity that they hear the sound. For still other children and infants, more elaborate electrophysiologic methods must be used. These include the use of electrodermal audiometry (Galvanic Skin Resistance) employing a Pavlovian conditioning technique coupling tone and electric shock. This conditioning manifests itself in a change in the electrical resistance of the skin which is measured by means of a galvanometer. More modern techniques include the electroencephalographic response to auditory stimulation measured through a computer of average transients. This computer effectively eliminates all background noise and regular electroencephalic activity, yielding a graph containing only the time-locked auditory stimulus and the appropriate electrophysiologic response. It is also possible to measure directly from an electrode placed into the middle ear and record the cochlear microphonic and the VIIIth nerve action potential evoked by auditory stimulation. With modern techniques and equipment there is no longer any child who is truly untestable. Any youngster at any age can yield definitive auditory threshold information through one or more of the techniques described.

The diagnostic audiologic evaluation yields much more information than merely the existence and severity of an auditory handicap. The interpretation of the audiologic data may well include information indicative of a particular pathology. Most causes of hearing loss have their particular audiometric configurations. The experienced audiologist can often assist in the diagnosis of the hearing loss and suggest the possible etiologic factors involved. Hereditary deafness, rubella, otosclerosis, serous otitis media, meningitis—all yield peculiar audiometric configurations that are almost unique to the particular pathological entity.

In the examination of the very young child in particular, the audiologic examination should be accompanied by other specific evaluations. The psychological and neurological evaluations are of primary importance. The determination of the integrity of the central nervous system through behavioral or neurologic techniques should be mandatory in the total assessment of the child with a communication defect. Still other examinations are frequently of great help. The electronystagmographic examination can assess the function of the vestibular portion of the inner ear by the measurement of reflex eye movements in response to caloric or rotational stimuli. Since auditory function and vestibular function are intimately related, the examination of each portion of the inner ear system assists in the examination of the other portion (11). Certain radiologic studies have also proved to be invaluable. Plesio-sectional tomography of the temporal bones may reveal structural anomalies which would assist in establishing the total diagnostic pattern (6). Although all of these examination techniques are not yet widely available, they are obtainable in most large metropolitan areas and should be sought out when a diagnostic problem presents itself.

## The Deaf Child

The child who is deaf is different both qualitatively and quantitatively from the child who is hard of hearing. The deaf child is not merely one who has a greater hearing loss than the hard of hearing child but, rather, is one whose hearing impairment is so profound that the residual remnant of hearing is so small as to preclude the development of language and speech. Thus the deaf child and the hard of hearing child are two separate clinical entities and require different methods of habilitation and education (8).

Almost all deaf children have some residual hearing. Most often it consists of hearing only for low frequency sounds. The majority of deaf children have no testable hearing above 1,000 Hz. Frequently, deaf children exhibit audiograms showing normal or nearly normal hearing at 125 or even at 250 Hz. Some deaf children have residual hearing throughout the frequency range that may be measured on the pure tone audiometer. Unfortunately their threshold of hearing in the middle and high frequencies may be at levels of 90 or 100 dB relative to average normal threshold. Thus, although hearing exists, it is hardly usable without a great deal of amplification (12).

Since most language development and language formation are based upon early auditory experience, the deaf child is particularly deprived in these areas. All levels of language and communication are grossly deficient. He has neither receptive language, inner language, nor expressive language. Eventually he may develop a rudimentary receptive language based upon gesture, facial expression, and visual clues. He will never develop speech without intensive special training (7).

The young deaf child usually goes through a period of extreme disequilibrium between the age of two and three years. The frustrations of not understanding and not being able to communicate are overwhelming for him at this age. He will frequently have severe temper tantrums accompanied by loud screams which tend to unnerve the parent unless he has been prepared to expect this sort of behavior. The inability of the deaf child to determine what is expected of him and his inability to exert control upon his environment through communication must produce an intense frustration indeed. The child's reaction to this frustration is certainly understandable and can be alleviated through proper parent education.

Deaf children and deaf adolescents exhibit a remarkable consistency in their behavioral characteristics. They appear to be and, in fact, are very alert children. They must be since the normal method of scanning the background of life is missing and they must make up for it through particular attentiveness and the utilization of other sensory inputs. The deaf child tends to scan his environment visually utilizing a primary foreground sense to replace the missing background sense. He is particularly receptive to stimulation including auditory stimulation if it is within his hearing range. Loud sounds, vibrations, visual clues, and other environmental disturbances are readily noted by the deaf child and he responds to them immediately and appropriately.

Eventually, the deaf child develops a rich and broad gesture language which assists in his communication. This gesture language is not necessarily related to the language of signs which tends to be quite formalized and not at all realistic in many of its expressions.

The motor behavior of deaf children is frequently mildly impaired due to accompanying vestibular disorders. Many pathologies which affect the inner ear hearing structures likewise affect the inner ear balance mechanism. Therefore, a number of deaf children have poor balance and appear rather clumsy and awkward while walking or running.

The social perception of deaf children, predictably, is disturbed and their adjustment to social situations often presents problems. Since much social interaction is primarily communicative in nature, the deaf child will often withdraw to the fringe of a social situation and become a nonparticipant. He does not do this in a pathological manner but, rather, protectively since normal social intercourse is frequently beyond his ability. His sense of humor, too, tends to be undeveloped and many deaf children laugh but rarely.

Since the deaf child is in constant contact with his environment through visual and tactile means, his emotional development and eventual emotional integration, while retarded, approach normality. The young deaf child appears to be emotionally immature and he is. It is important that his immaturity not be taken for a sign of emotional disturbance or abnormal development.

Habilitation of the deaf child should begin well before he is one year of age. Training, guidance, and education should be under the supervision of a skilled professional. Once the condition of deafness has been diagnosed, there are many things the parents may do at home to establish communication with their child. All types of language stimulation are of utmost importance between the ages of one and two years. The child must be exposed to as many different experiences as possible. There are many nursery school programs for deaf children which accept pupils at approximately eighteen months of age. These are not play groups but rather true educational institutions where the children are taught language concepts, speech reading, and the use of their residual hearing. They also learn the concepts of discipline and limits which are so very important in structuring the life of the young deaf child. They learn to relate to the other children in the small group and to the teacher. Children from eighteen months to four years of age learn quite rapidly in these programs and frequently have well-developed language concepts by the time they are ready to begin school. Most deaf children go to schools for the deaf. Very few indeed are integrated into the normal educational programs of their community. Schools for the deaf usually begin at age four and continue to approximately age eighteen. Early emphasis is on language and speech development with increasing emphasis upon academic subject matter. Vocational training is increasingly important in the latter portion of the educational program.

The older deaf child and the deaf adolescent have particular problems partly as a result of their deafness and partly as a result of their isolation from the hearing world. Their friends are almost all deaf, as are their schoolmates. They have considerable difficulty in communicating with the hearing world. Even those deaf children who have developed speech have numerous articulatory defects and feel, quite properly, that their speech is conspicuous and unpleasant. They frequently avoid talking to people who are not deaf since they feel that they may be ridiculed. They often resort to the pad and pencil for necessary communication. The isolation that begins in school is maintained throughout life. Social interaction tends to be with other deaf people. They feel that hearing people simply do not understand their problems and, in this, they are usually correct. The concept "deaf and dumb" does not symbolize only muteness in the minds of many people. People who are deaf are often considered to be stupid by the majority of the population.

Most deaf children and adolescents can benefit greatly from the use of a wearable hearing aid. Although they are unable to make any speech discrimination through use of their residual hearing alone, amplification enables them to follow some of the rhythm of speech and hear some of the low frequency vowel sounds. Interestingly enough, the use of their residual hearing through a hearing aid will often result in a dramatic improvement in their lip reading ability.

Most deaf children learn the language of signs and finger spelling whether or not it is taught in school. This tends to become their primary avenue of communication among themselves and further isolates them from the surrounding community. Most communities have organizations for the deaf which will supply translators should the deaf person find it necessary to communicate in depth with the hearing world. These translators, who are often normal hearing children of deaf parents, can assist the deaf in court, in various therapies, and in other activities where communication in depth is needed.

The deaf adolescent frequently needs guidance in choosing further education or deciding about vocational aims. While some few deaf children manage to go through a regular college or university, this represents only a minuscule proportion of the total deaf population. There are several colleges specifically for the deaf in this country that provide good academic training. Vocational counseling, too, must be realistic. There are very few deaf doctors, lawyers, or professors. On the other hand, the relegation of the deaf to occupations such as printing, shoe repairing, and auto body work should not be final. Many newer occupations such as computer programming are ideally suited to the concrete-minded deaf. Most modern schools for the deaf provide detailed vocational counseling and such counseling is also available from local, state, and federal agencies.

## The Hard of Hearing Child

The hard of hearing child bears a much closer relationship to the normal child than he does to the deaf child. His hearing impairment, even if it exists from birth, is not severe enough to prevent the development of language and speech. Language concepts may be incomplete and speech may frequently be defective but neither are totally absent. Therefore the hard of hearing child does not exhibit the typical behavioral characteristics shown by the deaf (1, 5, 7, 13).

Many young hard of hearing children have conductive hearing losses. The pathology of these impairments affects the outer or middle ear and may be congenital or acquired early in life. Such losses can reach a level of 60 dB but not greater. These conductive losses may be due to chronic or serous otitis media, congenital ossicular malformations, congenital atresias of the ear canal, and numerous other pathologies. Fortunately for these children, once speech is made loud enough to hear easily, it is well understood. The vowel and consonant elements of speech are heard in their entirety and there is no particular difficulty in understanding verbal communication. As a rule, medical or surgical treatment will result in complete restoration of hearing for the child with the conductive loss. Occasionally surgery cannot be performed until full growth has been achieved. Most frequently, however, medical or surgical treatment can proceed immediately after the diagnosis has been made. For the hard of hearing child whose surgical correction must be postponed, amplification through a wearable hearing aid will usually yield essentially normal hearing and normal auditory discrimination.

The majority of children who are hard of hearing, however, have sensorineural hearing losses. There are many etiologic factors involved in this type of impairment. Among them are birth anoxia, viral infections, and hereditary factors. Paradoxically, most children with sensori-neural hearing losses do not have great difficulty with hearing acuity. Rather, the main problem is one of poor auditory discrimination. The hard of hearing child can frequently hear the words but is unable to interpret the vowel and consonant elements. Vowel sounds are often heard with ease while high frequency consonant sounds such as "s," "sh," "th," "f," "p," "t," and "k" may not be heard at all. In this manner, the intelligibility of speech is sacrificed while its volume may be perfectly adequate. Unfortunately, neither medical nor surgical treatment is available for this type of problem.

Amplification through a hearing aid may often restore hearing to nearly normal and improve discrimination. It is rare, however, for a hearing aid to provide absolutely normal hearing and understanding of speech. It is imperative that the proper instrument be selected with great care. It is often necessary to test the child with many different instruments before his potential for amplification can be realized. Even an experienced audiologist is often unable to predict the results of coupling a less-than-perfect amplifier with a defective auditory system. Children who are severely hard of hearing must wear the standard body type of hearing aid while those with less severe impairments can do quite well with a head-worn hearing aid. This latter type of instrument may be worn behind the ear, fitted into the temples of eyeglasses, or inserted into the ear canal itself.

Since the hard of hearing child has not suffered the profound sensory deprivation experienced by the deaf child, educational and rehabilitative techniques are quite different. The hard of hearing child should *not* be placed in a school for the deaf. This will only serve to make him "deaf" rather than enable him to take advantage of his residual hearing in a more normal environment. Some severely hard of hearing children require special classes which are often available within the public school system. The majority, however, should be integrated into the regular school program. With proper amplification and proper training, the hard of hearing child can function quite adequately in the average classroom. He will need some special attention, however, to achieve this goal. Auditory training and lip reading instruction should be provided as an adjunct to amplification by the school hearing therapist. Many school systems now employ hearing therapists for the express purpose of providing services to hard of hearing children in the regular classroom. The school speech therapist can also help the child to correct the defective articulation that frequently accompanies hearing impairment. In addition to the special therapies, academic tutoring may frequently be needed. The hard of hearing child, even with amplification and therapy, will not catch every word spoken by the teacher. In those areas where special vocabulary is common, some outside academic tutoring would be beneficial. With amplification, lip reading training, auditory training, speech correction, and academic tutoring, the hard of hearing child can almost always maintain grade level.

Once the child has been started in an adequate program, there is no limit to his attainment on the basis of his hearing loss. Unlike the deaf child, the hard of hearing child can select any career or educational avenue. He is not hampered by language limitations.

The hard of hearing child frequently has a rather stormy adolescence. It is then that he realizes that he is "different" and that his hearing aid is the thing that makes him "different." The child will often attempt to reject the use of amplification so that this conspicuous sign of his disability will not be able to reveal its secret. Needless to say, the hard of hearing child is much more conspicuous without his hearing aid than he is with it since he is then dramatically handicapped by the hearing loss itself. Wise and understanding counseling can usually get the adolescent hard of hearing child over this hurdle without any particular trauma. Once the child can be made to understand his problem and his dependence upon amplification, he will accept the necessity of the use of the hearing aid.

## Pitfalls and Misdiagnosis

The age at which hearing impairment is first suspected by the parent has dropped steadily over the years (5). Most parents are sufficiently aware of normal and abnormal development to be suspicious of any gross deviation from the normal pattern. This is particularly true where speech is concerned. Since the first indication of hearing loss is usually the lack of development of speech, most alert parents suspect a problem before their child is eighteen months of age. The child is then taken to the general physician or pediatrician for confirmation of these suspicions. It is most unfortunate that the physician frequently shrugs off the suspicions of the parent and states that if there is any problem the child will outgrow it. Whatever testing is performed in the doctor's office is usually less than adequate. The examining physician may use his voice, the sound of clapping hands, or noisemakers to elicit responses from the child. Should the child respond to this gross type of stimulation, he is diagnosed as having normal hearing. Most hard of hearing children and even many deaf children would respond positively to the low frequency elements inherent in these test signals. The only adequate examination of a young child with a suspected hearing loss is by pure tone audiometry in a well-controlled environment (10).

Further confounding the picture is the atypical behavior pattern of the deaf or hard of hearing child. Many of the behavioral characteristics of hearing impairment may well suggest other pathological conditions to some examiners. The psychiatrist or the clinical psychologist is apt to diagnose a hearing-impaired child as autistic or brain injured. The educational consultant, on the other hand, is apt to interpret his poor language and communication development as mental retardation.

Ideally, a team of examiners should evaluate each child who presents a communication deficit. This team should consist of a pediatrician, a neurologist, a psychologist, an otolaryngologist, and an audiologist. Still further consultative services should be available on an ancillary basis if more detailed studies are indicated. Only through a comprehensive diagnostic evaluation can a valid statement be made concerning the child's defect.

Habilitative and rehabilitative therapy are available for both the deaf and hard of hearing child. Educational institutions and programs are well established for the child with a hearing handicap. Amplification by means of a wearable hearing aid offers substantial help to the hearing-impaired youngster. Medical and surgical treatment also can assist a substantial number of hearing-impaired children. If all of these forces can be marshaled and brought to bear on an individual problem, the invisible handicap of hearing impairment becomes much less formidable.

# 15

# Speech Pathology

GEORGE W. GENS, PH.D.

Disorders of speech are found in individuals with physical handicaps, emotional conflicts, environmental deprivation, or with no evident abnormality. These people constitute one of the largest single groups of handicapped children and adolescents.

Many definitions of speech disorders have been proposed. These range from Van Riper's (18) widely accepted descriptive definition, "Speech is defective when it deviates so far from the speech of other people that it calls attention to itself, interferes with communication, or causes its possessor to be maladjusted," to the etiological concept that "A speech deviate is an individual who presents an underlying, abnormal condition, the symptoms of which manifest themselves in the speech process" (5). For the sake of prevention and correction, it is important, then, to consider that the particular speech defect in question may be symptomatic of a hearing loss, cerebral thrombosis, developmental difficulties, or any physiological or psychological dysfunction.

The fields of speech pathology, in the author's opinion (6), becomes one which recognizes that speech is an intelligible, communicative process which requires anatomical structures which function physiologically in a sociopsychological environment. This is a philosophy which should satisfy even the extremists, some of whom believe primarily in speech drills for the speech defective while others believe in pure psychotherapy. It may not lend support to those who believe that through a process of "osmosis" a child will learn to correct his own speech by listening carefully to the intelligible speech of others. Although speech pathologists may vary in their definitions of speech disorders, most will agree that a speech disorder is better described than defined.

The following discussion of speech disorders and their treatment should orient the reader to the complexities involved in understanding and managing the individual with a speech defect. Although there are many different types, degrees, and overlappings in speech disorders, they may be classified in four general types: disorders of articulation, voice, rhythm, and symbolization.

## Articulation

Articulatory disorders, known as dyslalias or dysarthrias, the latter being due to central nervous system involvement, comprise more than 70 percent of the speech problems found in schoolchildren. Generally, these articulatory defects are manifested by substitution errors in which the individual will substitute one sound for another. That is, he will use the "w" sound in place of the "r" sound so that "red" becomes "wed," "rabbit" becomes "wabbit." Similarly, other common substitutions are "w" for the "l"; "sh" for the "ch"; "ch" for the "sh"; "f," "s," or "t" for the voiceless "th"; "v," "z," or "d" for the voiced "th"; "t" for the "k"; and others. A very common type of substitution error is the lisp in which the individual substitutes the "th" for the "s" sound. Other errors in articulation include errors of omission. Some individuals distort their sounds to a degree in which the audible sound cannot be identified by any phonetic symbol. This distortion is a form of substitution error. Some examples might include a hissing, whistling, or a slushy "s" sound. Some children will add a sound such as the "t" before the "s."

In the author's experience, one of the most important considerations in speech therapy is the decision as to when a given speech pattern may be considered a speech defect. We are all aware of infantile speech known as baby talk which is characteristic of certain developmental phases in a child's speech. Using the principles learned in child growth and development, we realize that there are individual differences in the maturation of articulatory skill and that some children will have a later development of speech. Statistics indicate that 10 percent of the population has various types and degrees of speech disorders. Studies with the mentally retarded reveal that about 66 percent of this population has speech disorders (6). In some cases, the articulatory development of a mentally normal child may be so mutilated and unintelligible as to give teachers and laymen the impression that the child is mentally retarded. Psychological evaluation of a child which points out that the child is up to par in areas other than speech, considering at the same time the effect that unintelligible speech may have on the child, will disclose that a child of normal intelligence can have a severe articulatory defect. Nonverbal tests of intelligence and social rating scales can be of great help here. This type of evaluation is critical and can have long-lasting effects on the stability and adjustment of a child in our society. Psychologists, therefore, should be given courses in speech and hearing disorders as part of their clinical training. Cases are cited in which children with hearing impairments were not detected by psychologists, and were misdiagnosed as mentally retarded (7). It is encouraging to note that at the Vineland Training School routine speech and hearing examinations now precede the initial psychological evaluation.

Etiological factors to be considered in articulatory disorders may be organic or functional. Some of the more important organic factors include hearing impairments, cleft palate, paralysis of the soft palate, cleft lip, cerebral palsy, dental abnormalities and malocclusion, high narrow palates, tongue-tie, enlarged tongue, and injuries to the tongue. Poor chewing habits, especially the prolonged feeding of soft foods to children, prevent the tongue muscles from getting the proper exercise which is so necessary for speech and may result in a dyslalia.

There are no specific speech organs as such, as each so-called speech organ serves a primary purpose more basic for digestion than speech. Speech is commonly considered an overlaid function and, from an anatomical standpoint, it makes use of muscles which are used in sucking, chewing, and swallowing. It is logical to assume, then, that any interference with the development of, or injury to, these muscles may affect speech. We also have to look for functional causes of these defects insofar as speech is not an innate but a learned activity. Incorrect learning habits may be formed through poor speech models at home or through imitation of one of the parents who may have an articulatory defect. Some children do not have the opportunity to play with other children in the neighborhood and are unable to benefit from the advantages of socialization. Some mothers are oversolicitous in catering to a sickly child and may anticipate his wants or inadvertently encourage the use of gestures. Many children react to the attempts of anxious parents to correct too early and too often. Parents, too, must learn about individual differences and realize that the structures cannot function until they are ready. Constant premature nagging about a child's articulation, or any other speech problem, is poor psychology. The when and how of speech therapy, therefore, become very important.

Basic to the management of a child with a speech problem is the realization of the following principles. Speech defects are not outgrown. Results of ten years of orientation speech examinations of over 30,000 incoming students at the University of Michigan revealed that of this educationally select group, 3.8 percent had noticeable speech defects (13).

What may appear to be a speech defect to the laymen may be a manifestation of normal or slightly delayed development. Speech is muscle movement and is amenable to muscular training. Too many parents and teachers, unaware of basic physiopsychological principles, expect a child to imitate correct pronunciation. This is faulty pedagogy insofar as speech is a learned activity and the faulty articulation, whether due to organic or functional causes, is a well-established habit. Insisting that a speech-defective child imitate distinct speech is analogous to asking a crippled man in a wheel chair to get up and walk without the benefit of rehabilitation.

The actual treatment is not difficult. It is a matter of knowing the when and how. Many speech pathologists agree with the treatment advocated by Van Riper (18) and Johnson (9) who use the following procedures. After a phonetic analysis has been made through pictures, reading material, and spontaneous speech, and the articulatory errors have been analyzed, the findings should be correlated with any of the above-mentioned etiological factors. Before actual speech therapy is initiated, any of the factors causing or aggravating the defect should be minimized or eliminated. For this reason, an integrated team approach is a recommended one for some children with a speech problem.

When all factors have been considered and the diagnosis made, the following therapy with individual variations is followed. Although speech develops automatically, it must be brought to the level of consciousness for the purpose of therapy. The individual must be made aware of his errors. This will not present the psychological trauma that some people may anticipate. A person receives support when he knows that there is someone to help him with what is troubling him. Through an intensive program of ear training, he learns to recognize audibly the misarticulated sound and the correct sound, and to differentiate and discriminate between them. This differs quite markedly from previous parental attempts to correct his speech. He is now acquainted with the fact that he is not having trouble with words but with a sound. After he is able to identify the correct sound, he is then taught to produce the sound in isolation. This is usually carried out by having the child respond to a strong auditory stimulus and by having him told or shown kinesthetically, and with the use of mirrors, where to place his articulators for the sound in question. After reasonable success is experienced in producing the sound correctly, it may then be incorporated with vowels to produce nonsense syllables. This part of the therapy tends to break down the maladaptive habit patterns by isolating the sound from the word configurations. In essence, the misarticulated sound is not corrected but a new one is learned. After the sound is strengthened, it is then transferred into simple words which are within the experience of the individual. Again after sufficient success, it is then incorporated into normal speech. The speech therapist is acquainted with many techniques to get the individual to use a new sound consistently. Familiarity with the theory of learning, which stresses the importance of repetition and reward, serves as a basic tool for the clinician. As with any learned activity, there may be remissions but the trained therapist, exercising good judgment and patience, expects them and does not become discouraged.

Carryover into natural speech is a final step in the treatment of the speech manifestations of the child with an articulatory disorder. Concurrent with the speech treatment, the therapist counsels the parents in terms of building up the child's confidence by not expecting better speech than he is able to produce at any given time. Any program which emphasizes speech drills to the exclusion of parental counseling and education is doomed to failure. Prognosis in this type of speech disorder is generally good.

## Voice Disorders

Although dysphonias or voice disorders are not as prevalent as articula-
ory disorders, they call upon the resources of the speech therapist in
cooperation with allied specialists for proper management. Dysphonias may
be classified as disorders of (a) pitch, (b) loudness, (c) quality, or (d)
flexibility. To have a voice disorder, (a) one's pitch may be too high or
too low for the age and sex; (b) the voice may be too loud or too soft;
(c) it may lack resonance or be too nasal, aspirate, hoarse, harsh, strained,
etc.; or (d) it may be monotonous and lack expression.

Etiological factors in dysphonia may be considered as organic, functional, or psychogenic. Since phonation is produced by a stream of expired
breath which sets the vocal cords of the larynx in vibration, we can
assume that any organic pathology which affects the musculature of the
breathing apparatus or the larynx or the resonating chambers may result in
some disorder of voice production. Central injuries, such as cerebral
palsy, or peripheral trauma, such as direct injury to the larynx, or tumor-
ous growths are some of the causes of dysphonia. In some cases of cancer
of the larynx, the only symptom for some time may be chronic hoarseness.
Paralysis of the soft palate, cleft palate, or bulbar poliomyelitis may contribute to the hypernasal quality of the voice. Enlarged adenoids may
account for a denasalized voice which lacks resonance and sounds muffled.
A voice that is too loud or too soft may be symptomatic of a hearing
impairment. This variation in loudness in either direction may be a manifestation of the individual's attempt to adjust to the audible intensity
level of his own voice. In the conductive type of hearing loss, the individual's voice is amplified for him so that he tends to decrease the volume
of his voice until it sounds suitable to him. This loudness level, however,
is much too weak for the average listener. In the perceptive type of hearing loss the individual attempts to compensate for his voice which sounds
diminished to him, and he thereby speaks too loudly. Glandular dysfunc-
tions may account for some voices that are too high or too low.

Although these organic factors can account for some types of dysphonia
and even for a complete loss of voice, known as aphonia, psychotherapists
certainly have encountered individuals with dysphonias or aphonias that
are brought about by psychogenic factors as evidenced in cases of hysterical
aphonia. Many types of voice disorders are correlated with personality
characteristics and deviations: the shy, timid voice of a withdrawn or insecure individual; the bombastic voice of the high pressure salesman or
politician; or the shrieking voice of a hysterical patient. There are some
adolescent males who, being sensitive to pubertal voice changes, attempt
to keep their voices from breaking and retain the prepubertal voice. This
condition may be aggravated by society's reaction to the breaking voice.

Some of the functional causes of dysphonia are seen in imitation of poor models at home. An individual may use an unsuitable pitch level which results in a voice disorder. Some dysphonias may be of temporary or permanent nature owing to abuse of the voice, as in constant shouting at play or in witnessing sporting events. Vocal abuse is also in evidence in some occupations which produce laryngeal tension through speaking too loudly. Excessive smoking may also contribute to vocal abuse.

It has been common practice for elocutionists who work with voice disorders to strive for tonal projection and placement. Speech therapists use to advantage the technique of finding a suitable pitch level for the individual. This therapy may be helpful in many cases, but in view of the discussion above, it should be apparent that before any type of voice therapy is attempted by a speech therapist or prescribed for by a speech pathologist, medical clearance should always be obtained. In spite of the fact that the majority of the voice cases may be nonorganic in nature, it is always wiser to err in the direction of overreferring to the laryngologist than to prescribe voice therapy and aggravate a possible pathological condition. The same holds for potential etiological factors which may be psychogenic in nature.

Treatment by the speech therapist, once all organic and psychogenic factors have been taken care of, generally consists of making the patient aware through ear training that there is a difference in voice. This can be accomplished by recordings on wire, tape, or disc, after which specific retraining techniques are used.

In recent years new hope has been offered to thousands of laryngectomized patients who no longer have to use artificial or mechanical larynxes to talk. More natural methods of talking without the benefit of a larynx are learned by the technique known as esophageal or pharyngeal speech. Esophageal speech may be produced first by swallowing air into the stomach. Then by exerting pressure on the stomach muscles the air can be forced up through the throat and can be made to vibrate against the fold of the esophagus and other tissues to produce sound. In pharyngeal speech the air is trapped within the pharynx by manipulation of the tongue and then expelled to produce the sound. A new method of glossopharyngeal breathing for polio cases is described by Affeld and Hansen (1). In this type of breathing the patient draws a small amount of air into his mouth, abducts the vocal cords in the larynx by yawning, and then by a pumping action of the tongue forces air into the open glottis. A repetition of three respiratory strokes produces a large breath which is then allowed to escape. This process is repeated six or seven times a minute and provides adequate ventilation. Glossopharyngeal breathing thus acts as a substitute or supplement for regular breathing and provides a margin of safety for those parts dependent on mechanical equipment. The flexibility of the chest is increased, the patient gains confidence that he has some control of breath, and the volume of air can be built up in his lungs which enables him to cough and to talk.

## Disorders of Rhythm

Realizing that slight repetitions and hesitations may be common to most speakers and that there are individual variations in the rate of speech, we may consider these differences within the range of normal limits of rhythmic speech. Cluttering and stuttering or stammering, however, are considered as rhythmic disorders of speech.

Cluttering is characterized by an extreme rapidity in speech which tends to make the words unintelligible through slurring and partially articulated words. The clutterer may be clinically differentiated from the stutterer both from the standpoint of speech and accompanying manifestations. The person who clutters does not seem to be overly concerned about his speech nor does he show the hypertonic anxiety avoidance reactions of the stutterer. Treatment, therefore, is quite different and generally simpler for the clutterer.

The most extensive recent study of cluttering is offered by Weiss (22), who believes that it is a speech disorder manifested by the clutterer's unawareness of his disorder, by a short attention span, by disturbances in articulation, perception, and formulation in speech, and excessive speed of speech. He feels that there is a hereditary predisposition for cluttering and that it is a verbal manifestation of what he calls Central Language Imbalance (with no evidence of any neuropathology) which affects rhythm, reading, writing, musicality, and behavior in general. He finds clutterers disorderly, restless, hyperactive, and unable to concentrate. When the inability to concentrate becomes a cause of repeated failure they are likely to become explosive and difficult to manage.

Weiss points out that these characteristics are apt to be misdiagnosed as indications of an emotional disturbance. His treatment consists of making the individual aware of his cluttering, increasing his ability to concentrate, and focusing his attention on specific tasks such as reading or speaking. He presents specific exercises for each symptom. Whereas the clutterer improves when he pays attention to his speech, the stutterer becomes worse when attention to his speech is increased. Weiss feels that in some cases symptoms of stuttering result from the child's efforts to overcome his tendency to clutter. Speech pathologists are familiar with other individuals who are known to clutter and stutter.

Stuttering, from a speech standpoint, is manifested by repetitions of sounds, words, or phrases. Stammering is considered a blocking or hesitancy in speech. Speech pathologists consider these terms synonomously and generally refer to stuttering as a disturbance in the fluency of speech which is further differentiated into primary and secondary stages. Inasmuch as there still exists some disagreement as to when primary stuttering becomes secondary, some discussion of the developmental phases of stuttering is indicated.

Studies at the University of Iowa Speech Clinic (9) have indicated that most children between the ages of two and six years repeat words, sounds, and phrases with the average child showing 45 such repetitions per 100 words. This phase of speech development is known as the "nonfluency" period and is a normal developmental stage. When parents or relatives show concern about the situation and attempt to do something about it, they may create what Johnson (9) calls a "diagnosogenic disorder." They label the child a stutterer, from which point the stuttering becomes a learned form of hypertonic avoidance behavior. This is motivated by the child's anxiety concerning the anticipated occurrence of nonfluency and its social consequences. This theory by Johnson, which is widely accepted by many workers, is borne out by the writer's clinical experience. Once the adult layman interprets and diagnoses the nonfluency phase as stuttering, his attempt at therapy by telling the child to take his time, take a deep breath, think of what he wants to say, punishment or negative reward, tends to produce the tensions and speech blocks characteristic of primary stuttering. Van Riper (18) gives an excellent capsule presentation of "A Case Study of a Primary Stutterer" which should be read to advantage by anyone dealing with a stutterer. When the child reacts to these penalties and attempts to avoid his stuttering through facial grimaces, extraneous movements, tongue and lip protrusions, foot and hand tapping, blinking of the eyes, word substitutions or avoidances, withdrawal reactions, refusal to recite in school or to participate in activities, he passes into the secondary stage of stuttering.

Counseling parents when children are in the nonfluency phase seems to be of great help in the majority of the cases. A review of some of the landmarks in the development of speech, including the possibility of repetitions and hesitations as an expected phase of speech development, may give parents a clearer insight into speech as an emerging sensory motor process. This may help remove parental guilt feelings in those cases where the home environment is stable and non-tension producing. In those homes where parents are putting well-meaning but critical pressure on children, the relationship of these speech and nonspeech pressures on stuttering can be pointed out. Proper attitudes in handling these pressures can be discussed with the parents. They can be shown how to make speech a pleasurable and rewarding activity for the youngster and at the same time reduce the number of stuttering experiences for him through singing, rhythmic games, reciting in unison, and through many other activities known to the speech therapist. Parents must not only be told not to tell the child to slow down, to take his time, take a deep breath, etc., they must also be told why these attempts to help the child are contraindicated. In some cases parents must be referred to a psychotherapist for a more intensive parental counseling program.

Because stuttering is such a complex pattern of behavior dependent upon so many variables, a preventive program through counseling does not always bring improvement. Van Riper (18) points out that there are some children who do not improve or even become worse in spite of the removal of environmental pressures or because their parents and teachers cannot change their attitudes. He feels, therefore, that some provision must be made to "toughen the child against rejections and unhealthy attitudes of others." He describes his technique of building up the child's tolerance to stress and calls this "desensitization therapy."

There have been many other theories offering the following as etiological factors in stuttering: neuromuscular incoordination; change in handedness; lack of cerebral dominance; metabolic differences; anatomical differences; birth injuries; neurological complications; psychoneuroses; psychoanalytical considerations; and hereditary predispositions, among others.

The literature is rich in nonconclusive studies of the various aspects of stuttering. They point out the complexity of the syndrome and perhaps again remind us to respect the importance of individual differences. To follow a prescribed course of treatment for every stutterer should be apparent folly. To adopt a hit-and-miss approach is equally fallacious. In spite of the several proponents of different etiological theories, it is encouraging that the majority of speech pathologists are basically agreed on the need for an integrated etiological and symptomatic therapy. Differences in terminologies and points of emphasis play a secondary role to the agreement by the different proponents that the subgoals set up for the stutterer emphasize the need for reducing the patient's fears, forcings, and inadequate social behavior. Van Riper's books (18, 19, 20) give a much more comprehensive and detailed treatment of the nature of and therapies involved in stuttering, and it is strongly recommended that the reader become better acquainted with the complexity of stuttering through these books and their bibliographies.

In a candid appraisal of twenty years of personal experimentation in various types of stuttering therapy, Van Riper (20) concludes that there is no single cause of stuttering. It may evolve out of a background of emotional conflict, low frustration level, many fluency disruptions, or from poorly coordinated speech impulses. It may be diagnosogenic in origin, or may result from anxiety and strain felt by a child in attempting to please parents who are demanding a linguistic function higher than his capability. Van Riper stresses the point that whether one becomes a stutterer because of environmental or constitutional factors, or both, stuttering tends to maintain itself once it gets started. He feels that the determination of the original cause or causes of the stuttering may not be as important therapeutically as the determination of the factors which maintain it. It is his experience that psychotherapy by psychiatrists, analysts, and clinical psychologists has been disappointing. It is perhaps with tongue-in-cheek that he claims that psychotherapy may have made them happier people except when they stuttered. He emphasizes the point that psychotherapy actually may have hindered improvement in speech fluency by distracting and detaching the stutterer from his communicative problems. He points out that psychotherapy which is supportive rather than reconstructive can be more helpful. Van Riper feels that a stutterer needs a very good teacher rather than a psychotherapist.

As Weinstock (21) points out, some of the difficulty between psychiatry and speech pathology in the treatment of stuttering has been the lack of communication between these two disciplines. Generally, speech therapy focuses on the speech of the stutterer with an attempt to change the non-fluency pattern and his attitude in living with his speech problem. Psychoanalysts tend to oppose this speech-focused approach which concentrates on the symptom rather than on the etiology. They feel that the stuttering is a symptom of a more basic emotional conflict, generally between mother and child. They believe in a resolution of the symptom need rather than focusing on the symptom.

These opposing viewpoints have resulted in a dichotomy which need not exist since there is general agreement that the etiology of stuttering is multifaceted and highly individualized. This writer's personal experience has indicated that integrated efforts by speech pathologists and psychologists have been very effective. Speech pathologists should be aware that unless they have the clinical training in psychodynamics they had best refer some of their stutterers for a psychological evaluation. Psychotherapists should be aware that many of the psychological and social maladaptive behavioral characteristics of the stutterer may not be the cause of his speech problem but may result from his feelings about his stuttering. His stuttering behavior may be his reaction to the environment's reaction to his nonfluent speech.

## Disorders of Symbolization

If, as in the traditional point of view, we consider communication as an interchange of thought, we can appreciate that there are nonlinguistic as well as linguistic components of communication. Meanings can be conveyed by nonlinguistic devices such as pictures, gestures, facial expressions, or vocal intonations. A wink of the eye may express more than a hundred well-chosen words. The intonation of a female's "no" may mean no, yes, or maybe. The buzzing of bees may have more significance to them than the danger to us. Even one-celled animals have a communication system or language although it does not involve the spoken word. As we study the phylogenetic and ontogenetic development of language we can see the emergence of specificity from the lowest form of animal life to the more complicated form expressed by the human individual.

In the study of human language, different disciplines become involved in the various aspects of the question, "What is language?" Phoneticians study the sounds which are produced by the vocal organs. Linguists are interested in semantics. To the grammarian, syntax becomes the focal point. The lexicographer is interested in the derivation or history of words. All of these considerations are embodied in a study of language but, to the layman, language is what he uses to communicate with other people.

The biolinguistic (12) point of view interprets communication in its broadest sense as any process of interactions set up between parts of the organism or between the environment and the organism. Language is a specialized form of communication found in higher organisms. In its most highly developed forms, as in human speech, it involves the use of fully developed nervous, muscular, and glandular systems, which were not primarily developed for speech at all. According to biolinguistics, the primary function of language is not simply the expression of ideas but the mutual adjustment of the organism and environment. As organisms increase in complexity in the course of phylogenetic or evolutionary scale, and as tissue develops an even higher degree of specificity of function, the forms of communication become even more intricate until we reach the highest form known to us—human speech.

As we study the phylogenetic development of communication from the simple one-celled animal to the four-legged animal to the erect human being we are aware of the parallel phylogenetic development of the complexity of the brain. It is no mere coincidence that there is an emergence of specificity and refinement in the development of more intricate communication systems as the brain develops throughout the animal families. Likewise there is a similar ontogenetic development of communication and language in the human as his brain develops. Although there are many unsolved mysteries concerning the cytoarchitectural structure, physiological function, and electrical activities of the brain, there is no doubt that one aspect of human language development is especially dependent upon the structure and function of the brain. Human language, as expressed by speech, demands an integrative process involving the brain and other tissues of the body. Speech is a process so demanding that it sometime defies human comprehension.

Normal functioning structures do not operate in a vacuum. They need to be exposed to a home environment which stimulates them through language. Speech is learned by exposure to speech through recordings, picture naming, story reading, and just talking. Providing a sensory training program for the parents to carry out at home not only supplies the child with a rich stimulating language environment but it also satisfies the need for the parents to be doing something constructive in helping the child develop speech. Briefing parents as to how speech develops and advising them of the wide range of individual differences in speech development provide a healthier home environment for speech development. Parental education can make for a more accepting psychosocial environment and prevent other behavioral problems.

A repertoire of unlearned vocalizations is common to all infants. When the visual-auditory reflex is ready to function, the infant begins to associate sounds with the perception of objects. With neuromuscular and sensory maturation these prelinguistic vocalizations irradiate into the expressive and communicative aspects of speech. In the case of a common object, such as "cat," olfactory, tactile, and auditory images combine with the visual images in the perception of the object, and these become associated with the sounds heard by the child which constitute the name "cat." Nouns and common objects are learned first; other words such as verbs, adjectives, and prepositions involve the association of sounds with a greater degree of abstraction from the perceptual situation and are learned later. (In some types of language breakdown, as in aphasia, we see the nouns and verbs intact, with a loss of prepositions and adverbs.) As the child learns to speak, he tries to reproduce the sounds he hears and thus kinesthetic sensations from the muscles of articulation become associated with these auditory sounds. Later when learning to read, he associates visual signs (letters and words) with the sounds he has already learned. In writing, movements of the hand are employed to reproduce visual signs similar to those which form the basis of reading.

At the psychological level, then, the meaning of a written or spoken word is the result of an association of the given visual and auditory sensations with other forms of sensations in the past. A meaning is thus based on an integration of associations built up by experience. At the anatomical and physiological levels the basis of such meanings is supposedly a linkage of neurons.

Words, therefore, are symbols. As symbols they possess significance only in relationship with other words. The unit of meaning is, then, a phrase, a sentence, or a series of sentences. Speech may, therefore, be considered as the communication of meanings by means of symbols which take the form of written or spoken words.

An area of speech pathology in which differential diagnosis is especially critical is the one which deals with deficiencies in symbolization. The inability of the individual to handle oral, visual, or auditory symbols may be developmental or acquired. The Veterans Administration program has given a very necessary impetus to the study of language disorders which are recognized in acquired aphasia. As a result, not only have neurologists and psychologists become increasingly familiar with the etiology and nature of the symbolic losses which result from organic brain pathology, but they are becoming impressed with the rehabilitation potential of these patients.

Wepman (23) describes three concepts—stimulation, facilitation, and motivation—as forming the basis for recovery from aphasia. When these three concepts are operating at their maximum, aphasia therapy has its greatest opportunity for success. Aphasic patients must be stimulated to action through supportive and instructive therapy. Wepman points out that aphasia therapy becomes a process by which the therapist provides stimulus material in the area of the individual's greatest need at a time when his nervous system is capable of using it for the facilitation of cortical integration which leads to language performance. Facilitation is thus seen as the physiological strength of the drive to motivate action. Motivation is described in its simplest terms as the amount of goal-directed behavior which the patient possesses.

The author's earlier report (5) that Broca's area does not have to be involved either in the failure of speech development or in the loss of speech has gained support in Sugar's (16) findings that the motor speech area is not restricted to Broca's area. Perhaps too much emphasis has been placed by textbooks on Broca's area as *the* speech center.

Eisenson (4) in his manual treats the aphasic individual in terms of modifications of intellect and personality as well as linguistic disturbances. Here he discusses concisely but inclusively attention, memory, perseveration, rigidity and orderliness, concretism, catastrophic reaction, euphoria, and withdrawal tendencies which we recognize in aphasics in varying degrees.

Recently more attention has been centered around the child who may have symbolization difficulties. Of all of the speech disorders discussed in this chapter, with perhaps the exception of stuttering, the problem of the child with no speech or with unintelligible speech may be the one which is most often found in the office of the psychotherapist. Parents become concerned, and justifiably so, when at the age of three or four the child is either not speaking or cannot be understood. It is a known clinical fact that children have different rates of maturation and some of these problems may be maturational. However, if the child at the age of seven does not have speech or language as a communication tool, the speech pathologist usually looks for the cause in one of the following four areas:

*Congenital deafness.* If the child is born deaf or becomes deaf before the acquisition of speech, it is reasonable to expect that the child will not develop speech unless he learns through the specialized techniques used in teaching the deaf to speak. In spite of our present knowledge, however, we still come in clinical contact with deaf children who have been misdiagnosed as mentally retarded. In a study of 156 children suspected of having a hearing loss because of impaired or absent language or speech development who were referred to the Columbia-Presbyterian Medical Center in New York, Kastein and Fowler (11) reported that seventy-five had no peripheral loss and twenty-seven had hearing losses accompanied by brain injury, mental retardation, or emotional disturbance.

*Psychological maladjustments.* Kanner's description of the autistic child is well known. We see children who have been diagnosed as schizophrenic children who do not feel the need for speech. There are other children who do not feel the need for speech. There are other children who, as a result of overprotection by their parents, do not feel the need for speech. Any of the psychological aberrations with which the psychologist is familiar may account for the lack of desire on the part of the child with physical and mental abilities to communicate through speech.

Many writers have reported on selective mutism. A British study reveals fully developed speech exhibited toward some people and absolute silence in the presence of others. This problem is interpreted by Morris (14) as one of social maladjustment in that the child refuses to accept communal socialization due to extrinsic and intrinsic factors. Removal of the child from an undesirable environment served as a solution in some cases. Four of his reported cases were educationally subnormal. Therefore he believed the condition must be recognized in the defective as well as the dull and normal groups.

*Mental retardation.* In order for the mental retardation to be either a cause or a concomitant of the lack of speech development, it must be very severe in nature. A child may be so retarded in psychological and social maturity that we do not expect him to learn such a complex process as speech. It would be wise, therefore, to remember that once a valid psychological evaluation diagnoses one as a moron, the speech development may be delayed but this type of mental retardation should not preclude a later development of speech.

Although textbooks have given undocumented indication that there is a correlation between speech and intelligence or mental age, more intensive studies (7, 10) have shown that mentally retarded children have the same types and degrees of speech disorders but they are more frequent. Middle-grade imbeciles have been found who had very clear and intelligible articulation, whereas high-grade morons and non-mentally retarded individuals are found with unintelligible speech. No special type or pattern of speech was found to be pathognomonic of mental deficiency. Prognosis of speech therapy for retarded individuals depends on individual insight and motivation. Since delayed speech maturation must always be considered as a possible concomitant of mental retardation, it would be wise not to attempt direct speech therapy too soon. With these children, vocabulary building for communication would be a more realistic goal than therapy for clear articulation.

*Congenital aphasia.* Aphasia is a central linguistic symbolic disturbance which may be acquired as in the adult or developed as in the child (5). Congenital aphasia, then, implies that the brain is agenetic or has been damaged either before or during birth or shortly after birth before the acquisition of speech and language (7).

A significant number of these exogenous children do not present accompanying motor or paralyzing involvements (8). In many cases neurological examinations do not produce supportive evidence for neuropathologies. Without these positive findings there are those who would be reluctant to make a definite diagnosis of congenital aphasia. When these children respond to specialized aphasic training after the usual school teaching methods have failed, more support is gained for the tentative diagnosis of congenital aphasia.

In view of certain aspects of localization of function in the brain, Sugar (16) finds it difficult to accept the concept of congenital aphasia. Other workers (15, 17) are aware of the syndrome and report that they see it clinically. Eisenson (4) includes a discussion of testing the congenitally aphasic child in his revised manual.

The author agrees with Bangs (3) that two serious errors made in the diagnosis and consequent remedial work are: (a) the assumption that the maladaptive behavior observed with children is a reflection of a deep-seated emotional problem that is responsible for the deficiency in language or speech. Actually the paucity of language is organic in its origin, while the behavior may be a part of the child's adjustment to his environment (this may be true of any speech disorder); (b) the assumption, without adequate testing, that children who are delayed in speech or language are congenitally aphasic. We do not as yet have a standardized test or battery of tests or even a series of informal criteria that enable us to make this diagnosis with assurance.

It is extremely difficult to make a clear-cut positive diagnosis of congenital aphasia in children. Since by definition we are dealing with a language disturbance which is due to C.N.S. involvement we can expect a combination of central and peripheral dysfunction. We may have an aphasic child so handicapped by other cortical disorders that a diagnosis of congenital aphasia for educational placement and rehabilitation purposes would be unrealistic.

Differential diagnoses should not be made too early because our diagnostic tools are not sharp enough nor are they sufficiently refined. Differences in maturational levels may give one the impression that he is dealing with an aphasic child when in reality it is a child with a slower developing speech. Some children of normal intelligence are slower in speech development and the majority of mentally retarded children are delayed in their speech development. The inability to handle linguistic symbols at about age six along with speech retardation may be an important diagnostic cue. The type of inconsistent responses to therapy for language development that is noted in aphasic children may also serve as a cue. A differential diagnosis, then, between retarded speech development and congenital aphasia may not be too difficult unless attempted too early.

Congenital aphasia may be mistaken for deafness or severe hearing loss. Deafness should be obvious but auditory aphasia can be misleading. Clinical experience with the expressive aphasic child has not presented difficulties in audiometric testing. His responses have been consistent and reliable. The child with auditory aphasia, however, has presented an inconsistent and fluctuating pattern of responses to auditory stimuli in testing situations from day to day. Audiologists are becoming more sophisticated in their observations of children's responses in the testing situation. As we become less the tools of our testing equipment and more observers of behavior during the testing experiences, so we can rely more on clinical intuition. This may not be an objective approach but when we are lost in a network of uncertainties or when we are dealing with a relatively new area we cannot always wait for objectivity. Sometimes applied subjectivity leads to objectivity.

A differential diagnosis between aphasia and emotional disturbance may be beyond the scope of the speech pathologist alone. An aphasic child may be misdiagnosed as being basically a child with a severe emotional disturbance when actually his behavior may be the result of his reaction to his slower language development. It is important to determine whether for this "emotionally disturbed mute child" speech therapy is the answer, or whether psychotherapy is indicated, or both or neither. Although we know that in some cases speech therapy is the best form of psychotherapy, we must never reach the point where we think speech therapy is a panacea for everyone who does not speak. Autistic or schizophrenic children have been favored with the label "aphasic," which has led to unrealistic goals and hopes for anxious parents and to frustration for teachers and therapists. Poor speech stimulation experiences at home and other environmental factors may lead to emotional problems which may preclude the use of language.

Although speech development is expected to be slower, expressive speech is anticipated in trainable and educable mentally retarded children. These children do have language function of various degrees within certain limits usually commensurate with their mental development. Mentally retarded children have been misdiagnosed as aphasic and aphasic children have been misdiagnosed as mentally retarded. The latter have actually tested as mentally retarded on psychological tests involving language. Upon being retested using nonlanguage performance tests they were up to normal for their age or even higher. The mentally retarded child will have a more even, generally lowered level of functioning in all areas. Thus a significant discrepancy in the verbal and performance IQ in a child who has an impairment in speech and language development may be a critical clue in the diagnosis of congenital aphasia. This psychometric pattern has been found in children (8) tentatively diagnosed as congenitally aphasic who later made favorable progress with speech therapy.

A differential diagnosis, then, of aphasia may be made by eliminating other possible etiological considerations through careful integrative studies and diagnostic procedures by speech pathologists, audiologists, psychiatrists, psychologists, and pediatric neurologists. However, a diagnosis of congenital aphasia cannot be made simply by eliminating other possible known diagnoses. There may be other bases for language dysfunction of which we are not aware. We would prefer a more positive approach to the diagnosis rather than by elimination. In the light of our present knowledge, however, the positive approach is a difficult one and at times a near impossible one. The professional training, experience, and clinical integrity of the examiner may be more important than any technique or procedure.

This brief description of the four main categories of speech disorders is hardly to be considered as all-inclusive. It is obvious that there are certain disorders which overlap and result in any combination of the classifications. Cleft-palate speech may involve articulation and phonation. Extensive research findings have made the field of audiology extremely specialized. Any discussion of the psychological implications involved in the testing, diagnosis, and treatment of individuals with hearing impairments goes far beyond the space made available in this chapter. Cerebral palsy may include all four. Because of the multiphasic complexity of these disorders, the best management may be found in a team approach.

The speech pathologist, individually or as a member of a team, must be aware of the interrelation of the many professional disciplines. He must work integratively with plastic surgeons and prosthodontists in cases involving cleft palate; with neurologists, orthopedic surgeons, and psychiatrists in cerebral palsy, aphasia, or other neuropathologies; with orthodontists in cases involving malocclusions; with otologists in working with children with auditory impairments; and with other medical specialists depending on factors causing or contributing to the speech disorder.

He must also cooperate with clinical psychologists and psychiatrists in studying environmental factors related to the speech disturbance. Intelligent parent counseling requires knowledge of expected norms and of the parent-child, parent-parent, and child-parent relationships when these norms are not achieved. Proper parental attitudes present difficulties for parents of children who are apparently not handicapped. These attitudes may be thrown further out of line when a speech or any other handicap is present. Parental goals, expectations, and hopes for the child can be understandably out of balance through feelings of guilt, rejection, or through the unconsciously motivated need for overprotection. The reality of the existence of a handicap may be accepted by a parent intellectually but not necessarily emotionally.

Parents of those children who are either slow in developing speech or who have unintelligible articulation may benefit from counseling. Parents must be advised of the proper attitudes in handling such a child. Early evaluation by a speech pathologist may help discover an undetected problem or may remove many years of needless worry and anxiety on the part of the parents who are confronted with family and community pressures to do something about the speech. Conflicting advice from other people assuring them that the child will outgrow his speech problem just adds to the parents' confusion and leads them to "do-it-yourself" home speech therapy. This parental attempt at speech correction can only lead to an exacerbation of the problem. First, they don't know how to correct, and second, the child may not be ready for it. If speech therapy is carried out by either a parent or a speech therapist before a child is physically or mentally ready for it we can expect some psychological sequellae.

An understanding of the coined word "strunction" (structure and function) will set an operating basis and philosophy which should make one a better diagnostician. Strunction (12) implies that a structure will not function until it is ready. The determinants of readiness can be anatomical, physiological, or environmental. We can understand the rationale for premature or improper attitudes of parents in their management of their children with speech problems. Parents must, however, be counseled in the possible debilitating effects of their treatment. They must be told that when their expectations for achievement are greater than the child's capacity for accomplishment, a pressure is exerted on the youngster which is frustrating to him and may lead to further elements of asocial behavior. Since different children have different rates of speech maturation, meaningful developmental speech norms for speech handicapped children are difficult to establish. Because of the highly individualized nature of the speech problem these children should not be compared with other children in the family or community. Nor should these children be expected to be "chips off the old block." Overconcern based on lack of information can create pressures on the child with resulting secondary psychological problems that can be more severe than the primary speech problem. On the other hand, lack of concern with resulting lack of stimulation and exposure to language or overprotection which anticipates a child's needs may impede the development of speech. Early speech evaluation, then, with proper advisement and guidelines may prevent more serious behavioral pathologies.

The seriousness of speech disorders can be appreciated in the problems that they may produce. Children with speech defects appear to be scholastically retarded, and later fail to take advantage of college possibilities, out of proportion to expectations based on intelligence test data (2). Because speech and personality are so interrelated, the relationship between speech defective children and their parents and peers can be demoralized. Insecurity, resentment, withdrawal reactions, hostility, aggression, all of which may be reactions to frustration, can result from disorders of speech. Speech therapy, therefore, is not only concerned with development or improvement in speech, but also with the adjustment of the individual.

A competent speech therapist uses "psychotherapy" in all of his dealings with speech defectives, within the limits of his training. He should know when a problem is out of his scope and refer the patient to a psychotherapist. Considering all of these factors, the experienced diagnostician is aware that for some individuals the best type of "psychotherapy" is speech therapy.

# 16

## The Physically Handicapped Child

ROBERT C. PRALL, M.D.

### Introduction

It is of considerable importance to both professionals and parents and to the psychological development of the child to consider the ramifications of physical handicaps upon the child's budding personality. Many congenital and acquired physical disorders play a vital role in the psychic development of the infant and can extract a very heavy toll in terms of later personality adjustment, effectiveness of learning, social functioning, and productiveness throughout the individual's lifetime.

Literature is rapidly accumulating from careful studies of the incidence and causation of physical handicaps and their impact on emotional adjustment, personality, growth, and development. It is the task of this chapter to review briefly the present state of our knowledge of the etiology and incidence of physical handicaps and our understanding of their role in personality development and to present what is presently known concerning intervention and prevention which may be useful to those involved in work with physically handicapped children and their parents.

### Etiology

In recent years there has been a rapid acceleration in our knowledge of the relationship of congenital malformations to a wide variety of causes including infections, radiation, and toxic agents to which the pregnant mother may be exposed. Drugs, chemicals, environmental toxins, insecticides, the defoliants, and many other environmental poisons are being investigated to assess their teratogenic and toxic potential. The occurrence of prenatal injury in the fetus, which may result in myriad physical handicaps, may also be related to absent prenatal care, poor nutrition, and toxemia which have long been suspect in the occurrence of delayed development of the newborn, abnormal births, and congenital malformations.

Often, if not usually, multiple physical handicaps occur in characteristic groups based upon the age of the fetus at the time the toxic or infectious process had its effect during pregnancy. Our knowledge of prenatal insults is expanding so rapidly that it is impossible in this chapter to give a complete review of the literature. A brief overview must suffice to give the interested reader information as to sources for further reading on the subject.

## DRUGS

In recent years many drugs have been investigated for their possible toxic and deforming properties in respect to the fetus. Clinical observations and animal research have led to suspicion concerning a wide variety of drugs, some of which have been proven beyond any reasonable doubt to have profoundly toxic and/or teratogenic effects on the developing fetus, particularly at certain crucial points, e.g., the first trimester and just before birth. Since the damage may be done quite early, often before the mother may be fully aware of the presence of the pregnancy, it is of great concern for physicians to use extreme caution in prescribing certain medications to women of child-bearing age and to obtain a detailed menstrual history prior to and during drug therapy.

The worldwide publicity concerning the tragic results of the sedative and anti-emetic drug thalidomide as a teratogenic agent, following its detection in 1961, brought the attention of the entire world to the grave dangers inherent in the indiscriminate use of medications during pregnancy (23). As far back as 1959, Warkany and Takacs (78) pointed out that animal experimentation showed the possibilities of even such a ubiquitous drug as aspirin producing teratogenic effects in animals.

In a current pediatric editorial, Schwartz and Pearson (66) discussed the findings that aspirin has been shown to prolong bleeding time by its inhibition of endogenous adenosine diphosphate leading to failure of platelet aggregation and plug formation. The possibility that newborn infants showed altered platelet function due to maternal aspirin ingestion is being seriously considered and should be investigated thoroughly. Other pain-killing drugs, such as acetaminophen or Darvon (dextropropoxyphene), which do not alter platelet function should be used during pregnancy instead of aspirin. Platelet formation also is affected by glyceryl guiacolate, phenylbutazone, sulfinpyrazone, dipyridamole, and some antihistamines along with other substances.

With our population bombarded by hundreds of drug commercials on TV and radio, as well as through the other advertising media, self-medication by millions of people constitutes a potential hazard of tremendous proportions. Over-the-counter medications may contain drugs potentially harmful to the unborn child. For example, in Garb's (23) recent 1970 edition of *Pharmacology and Patient Care*, quinine is listed as absolutely contraindicated in pregnancy and yet it is available in certain drug store remedies (23a). Incidentally, it is also readily available in tonic mixer ("quinine water").

For a complete presentation of current pharmacological data on this subject see Garb (23) and Goodman and Gillman (25). Several categories of drugs are being investigated or have been proven to be related to fetal distress, retarded fetal growth, abnormal births, and/or teratogenicity.

Some have been demonstrated to lead directly to congenital malformations. Fraser (19) listed in 1967 potentially dangerous drugs suspected of teratogenic effects. A brief summary of the data presented by Fraser and other contributors follows:

*Alkylating agents.* These anticarcinogens are highly teratogenic in rats. Defects have been reported in humans when the mother has received the drug in pregnancy. Chlorambucil, cyclophosphamide, busulfan, and melphalan are included in this group.

*Antimetabolites.* Aminopterin, a folic acid antagonist, has been shown to be a potent teratogen in animals and has been incriminated in human infants as well. Its use as an abortive medication has resulted in widespread malformations. Milunsky *et al.* reported on cases where total dosages of 10 to 20 mg. of folic acid antagonists were given in the fourth to twelfth weeks of pregnancy. Of four live-born babies, all had congenital abnormalities, the most common being cranial ossification defects, cleft palates, and facial and ear deformities. Methotrexate, the methyl deriva tive of aminopterin, was the drug impugned in this report (47). Mercaptopurine, used in the treatment of leukemias, is also potentially teratogenic.

*Carbon monoxide.* Fraser (19) cited reports of malformation following maternal carbon monoxide poisoning during pregnancy.

*Antibiotics.* Fraser (19) stated in 1967 that there was no direct evidence of teratogenicity, but tetracycline was suspected in infant cataracts and discoloration and caries or enamel hypoplasia of infant teeth.

More recent literature reported the placental transfer of tetracycline and the incorporation of tetracycline into human fetal bones after maternal drug administration (76). Swift (75) has reported recently on the injury to human cells by tetracycline which can be demonstrated experimentally. The work of Cohlan *et al.* in 1963 described bone and body growth inhibition in infants due to tetracycline. Swift also reported the newborn infant's inadequate renal clearance of penicillin which is on the order of one fifth that of older children. The possibility must be considered that penicillin could be dangerous to the fetus.

The tetracyclines, including Aureomycin (chlortetracycline), Terramycin (oxytetracycline), Achromycin (tetracycline H Cl), etc., are potentially dangerous and should be avoided in later stages of pregnancy according to Mirkin (49). Albamycin (novobiocin) should be avoided especially near term, as should Ilosone (erythromycin).

NegGram (nalidixic acid) was reported by Anderson in 1971 to have caused intracranial hypertension with 6th nerve palsy and papilledema in a five-year-old child treated with nalidixic acid for urinary tract infection. The child's residual strabismus will probably require surgical correction. Borens and Sundström reported similar findings in a six-month-old child, according to Anderson (1). Buchheit's findings were similar and that report listed tetracycline, steroid therapy, steroid withdrawal, hypervitaminosis A, lead, and arsenic as toxins which can produce intracranial hypertension, papilledema with the possibility of secondary optic atrophy, and loss of vision (6). Garb (23) also lists nalidixic acid as not recommended in pregnancy and possibly dangerous.

Streptomycin was reported to be connected with impaired infant hearing following administration of the drug to the mother during pregnancy.

Macrodantin and Furadantin (nitrofurantoin), used in treatment of urinary infections, should be avoided in late pregnancy and early infancy up to one month of age because of the danger of infantile hemolytic anemia (49).

Ethionamide, used in tuberculosis, may be dangerous to the fetus and should be avoided (23).

The long-acting sulfonamides, including Gantrasin (sulfisoxazole), used in urinary infections, especially near term, seem to be implicated in hyperbilirubinemia and kernicterus (33, 49).

Chloromycetin (chloramphenicol), near term, has been related to cardiovascular collapse, the "Gray Syndrome," and fetal death (33, 49).

*Cortisone.* Fraser (19) stated that some evidence indicated that cortisone in early pregnancy may cause cleft palates as it does in mice and rabbits. In addition, steroids may suppress fetal adrenal activity. Aristocort, Kenacort (triamcinolone), Celestone (betamethasone), Hexandrol (dexamethasone), and Medrol (methylprednisolone) are not recommended (23).

*Quinine.* Fraser (19) cited some evidence of congenital deafness and malformation following quinine intake for abortive purposes but was not convinced of the causal connection. Garb (23) listed quinine as absolutely contraindicated in pregnancy. Mirkin (49) related quinine to thrombocytopenia in infants.

*Sulfonylureas.* Fraser (19) stated that Orinase (tolbutamide), an antidiabetic drug, was suspected of teratogenicity but that definite proof was lacking at that time. Since that time, Schiff *et al.* (65) indicated in a recent article that neonatal thrombocytopenia and congenital malformation are associated with administration of tolbutamide. Garb (23) also listed tolbutamide as absolutely contraindicated in pregnancy, as are acetohexamide and Diabinese (chlorpropamide).

*Anticoagulants.* The anticoagulants are dangerous to the fetus because of fetal bleeding and possible death (19, 33). Bloomfield (4) indicated that fetal death and malformation occurred with the use of coumarin derivatives in pregnancy. Pitkin (60) stated that heparin was preferable to coumarin because of the lack of placental transfer and its ready reversibility.

*Thiazides (Diuretics).* Fraser (19) indicated the danger of thrombocytopenia and bone marrow depression in the infant following administration of the diuretic thiazides. More recently, Gray (27) again implicated thiazide in fetal damage in pregnancy.

*Drugs in metabolic disorders and endocrine disorders.* Fraser (19) pointed out that insulin may interact with salicylates or chlorpromazine which raised the question of a possible connection with sacral aplasia noted in diabetic pregnancies. DBI (phenformin hydrochloride) should be avoided in pregnancy (23).

Thyroid and thiouracil derivatives, as well as potassium iodide, may depress fetal thyroid, increase thyrotropic hormone output, and result in fetal goiter (19). Prophylthiouracil has its effect later in pregnancy according to Mirkin (49). Radioactive iodine, from the fourteenth week on, appears to lead to congenital hypothyroidism (33).

Estrogens (stilbestrol) may well lead to masculinization of the female fetus and synthetic progestins, including Norlutin, etc., may be teratogenic more than progesterone. Oral contraceptives are contraindicated in pregnancy. Cafergot (ergotamine tartrate) is absolutely contraindicated (23).

The androgens are also contraindicated, including testosterone and methyltestosterone which may cause masculinization of some female babies and pseudohermaphroditism. Drugs not to be used among others include: Duraboline (nandrolone phenpropionate); Adroyd, Androl (oxymetholone); Anavar (oxandrolone); Maxibolin, Orgabolin (ethylestrenol); and stanozolal (23).

*Tranquilizers and sedatives (used as anti-emetics).* Meprobamate (Equanil, Deprol, Meprospan, Meprotabs, Miltown, Wyseals, etc.) according to Garb (23) is absolutely contraindicated in pregnancy, as is Thalidomide, a known teratogen. The phenothiazines (Compazine, Mellaril, Sparine, Stelazine, Thorazine, etc.) are possibly dangerous to the fetus. Serpasil (reserpine), which crosses the placenta, is more dangerous soon before delivery (23, 49). The safety of Librium (chlordiazepoxide) has not yet been established. Mirkin (49) indicated that phenobarbital may produce hemorrhage and an increased rate of neonatal drug metabolism.

*Antidepressants.* Tofranil (imipramine) and Triavil, Etrafon, Elavil (amitriptyline), etc., are contraindicated in pregnancy. Aventyl (nortriptyline H Cl) has not been ruled out as a possible hazard. Eutonyl (pargyline hydrochloride) is not recommended. The safety of Norpramin (desipramine hydrochloride) has not yet been established (23).

*Anti-emetics.* Torecan (thiethylperazine) is listed by Garb (23) as absolutely contraindicated and Bonine and Bonamine (meclizine), which is teratogenic in rats and suspected in man, should be avoided in pregnancy. Marezine (cyclizine), buclizine, and chlorcyclizine are listed as dangerous in animal studies (33).

*Antihistamines.* In addition to Bonine, listed above, other antihistamines have been suspected, but evidence is not yet conclusive. Vollman et al. (77) indicated in 1967 that no significant differences in the type and frequency of malformations were noted in the offspring of 34,240 mothers who reported intake of antihistaminic drugs in the Collaborative Project

Study on the outcome of pregnancy. (See Masland [44].) Garb (23) listed Marezine (cyclizine) as not recommended in pregnancy.

*Parasympathomimetic drugs.* Myocholine and Urecholine (bethanechol chloride) are, according to Garb (23), absolutely contraindicated in pregnancy.

*Antiparasitic drugs.* Aralen (chloroquine) was suspected by Fraser (19) and listed as definitely dangerous, according to Garb (23). Chloroquine has been used as an antimalarial drug as well as in the treatment of lupus erythematosus, rheumatoid arthritis, and scleroderma. Flagyl (metronidazole), used for trichomonas, is not recommended during pregnancy (23). Daraprim (pyrimethamine), an antimalarial, is teratogenic in animals.

*Anti-inflammatory agents.* In addition to the cortisones, pyrazole compounds, e.g., Butazolidine (phenylbutazone), used in arthritis, should be avoided (23). Salicylates have produced CNS, skeletal and eye defects in mice and rats, and large doses are suspected in possible damage to the human fetus (23, 33, 66).

*Analgetics.* Heroin and morphine near term are related to respiratory depression and neonatal death (23). Severe withdrawal symptoms have been encountered in the newborn infants of mothers who are addicts.

*Anesthetics.* Mepivacaine (carbocaine), near term, may possibly be related to fetal bradycardia and neonatal depression (33).

*Stimulants.* Some reports are beginning to appear on the occurrence of malformations connected with Dexedrine and Preludin, used in obesity in pregnancy (33, 74). Animal studies show a relationship between malformations and caffeine and Dexedrine (33). Serotonin has been shown to produce fetal death and deformity in rats and mice by constriction of uterine vessels and may have a role in toxemia of pregnancy (25).

*Depressants and anticonvulsants.* Meperidine, alphaprodine, pentobarbital, and promethazine were listed as dangerous by Sutherland and Light (74). Dilantin (diphenylhydantoin) may induce teratogenic effects, e.g., cleft lip/palate in rodents, and does pass across the placenta. Mirkin (48) stated recently that larger studies are needed to determine the true picture. He added that the concentrations of Dilantin in breast milk of mothers receiving the drug are very low and do not constitute a clinical hazard.

*Vitamins.* In large doses Vitamin A may produce congenital defects (cleft palate, eye damage, and syndactyly) while large doses of Vitamin D may cause excessive blood calcium and mental retardation. Vitamin K analogues in large doses near term may cause hyperbilirubinemia and kernicterus (33, 49).

Garb (23) listed large doses of Vitamin E as possibly suspect but definite evidence was not yet available.

Vitamin deficiencies are known to produce definable disease patterns such as congenital rickets, from insufficient Vitamin D.

*Miscellaneous.* Anisotropine, a parasympathetic blocking agent, is not recommended (23). The antihypertensive Aldomet (methyldopa) is not recommended (23). Hexamethonium bromide, a ganglionic blocking agent used in treatment of toxemia of pregnancy, has been connected with the occurrence of paralytic ileus and death in infants and should be avoided (23, 25, 33). Quinidine, used in auricular fibrillation, is probably dangerous to the fetus (23). The nitrites, e.g., nitroglycerine and vasodilators, may produce methemaglobin and reduced oxygen carrying capacity.

Heavy metal poisoning in the pregnant female from arsenic, lead, or mercury should be considered as a potential hazard to the fetus.

Fluid and electrolyte imbalance brought on by ammonium chloride, hypotonic solutions of glucose, or hypertonic solutions of mannital might influence fetal survival according to Sutherland and Light (74).

New evidence is constantly suggested adding still other drugs to the growing list of dangerous agents.

For other reviews of the effects of drugs see those by Nicholson (56), Karnofsky (38), Smithells (69), Stuart (73) and the bibliographies in (33) and (74).

This is by no means a complete list but represents some of the drugs to which the psychiatrist, psychologist, or social worker should direct attention in taking a pregnancy history of a child suspected of possible cerebral damage.

Physicians should avoid using these drugs with pregnant women and where pregnancy is likely. Public education as to the hazards could help to reduce the incidence of toxic effects and possible fetal damage and aid in prevention.

INFECTIONS

It has been quite well established that certain infections in the mother during pregnancy, particularly during the first trimester, are related to fetal abnormalities. A review of the literature reveals much evidence in this connection.

White and Sever in 1967 (79) indicated that there were then three known microorganisms proven to cause fetal malformations: (a) cytomegalic inclusion disease virus, (b) the rubella virus, and (c) the protozoan toxoplasma gondii. There also appeared to be other likely candidates to be added to this list in the future.

The defects associated with cytomegalovirus include microcephaly or hydrocephaly, microphthalmia, and microgyria. Signs and symptoms at birth include hepatosplenomegaly, jaundice, petechiae, and chorioretinitis. White and Sever (79) indicated a poor prognosis and the possibility of severe neurological sequelae including mental retardation, blindness, seizures, and spastic paralyses.

Rubella (German measles), first implicated in fetal damage more than twenty-five years ago, especially if contracted in the first trimester of pregnancy, may cause deafness, blindness, microphthalmia, congenital heart disease, microcephaly, and mental retardation with acute illness in the newborn often associated with prematurity by weight. When chronic infection remains in the infant after birth this constellation, with the malformations, is referred to as the "expanded congenital rubella syndrome" (79a). Many of the infants infected prenatally remain infected throughout the pregnancy and for long periods after birth.

Of those infants with the acute illness, many die in a few weeks. Of those who live, and while the virus shedding is gradually taking place, sometimes up to one year of age, cataracts may appear. Infection of the infant may occur even when the mother has had a subclinical infection without a rash.

Stern and Williams (72) isolated the rubella virus from an infected infant born with hepatitis and microcephaly both during life and after death from the liver which showed evidence of giant cell hepatitis.

Treatment includes repair of the structural defects and supportive treatment in the acute stage. Incidence varies with the epidemic nature of Rubella. In nonepidemic years, one case of Rubella was found in 1,000 pregnancies while in the 1964 epidemic 22 per 1,000 cases occurred. In 1964 20,000 to 30,000 damaged infants were born as a result of the epidemic. The chance of significant damage to the fetus from infections early in pregnancy is very high, with more than 50 percent of the pregnancies ending in abortion, stillbirth, or malformation.

Prevention by active immunization of all women *before puberty* and by short-term protection by a killed vaccine during child-bearing age would be desirable. Therapeutic abortion may be indicated with a carefully established diagnosis by antibody studies and virus isolation when infection occurs early in the pregnancy. Immunization during pregnancy should be avoided (79).

Toxoplasmosis, according to White and Sever (79), is a parasitic disease which produces malformations in approximately 20 percent of congenital cases, including microcephaly, microphthalmia, and hydrocephaly. Chorioretinitis (65 to 90 percent), anemia (55 to 77 percent), convulsions, jaundice, splenomegaly, and hepatomegaly are among the signs in infected infants. Neurological sequelae include mental retardation and seizures. Severe ophthalmic disorders may follow the chorioretinitis. Diagnosis is made by a Wright or Giemsa stained preparation of sedimented cells from cerebrospinal fluid. Incidence: Of 23,000 pregnancies studied, 6 per 1,000 pregnancies showed the disease. In addition, 17 per 1,000 showed antibody results suggestive of recent infection. In the pregnancies of mothers who showed a rising antibody titer 16.5 percent resulted in stillbirths, neonatal death, or definite congenital toxoplasmosis. Another 16.5 percent were suspected of having the disease. Transmission of the disease is poorly understood but it can be contracted from eating raw meat or contact with infected animals. The worst prognosis occurs with infection in the second and third trimester in contrast with Rubella.

Treatment by sulfa drugs may be helpful even though they may represent a potential hazard to the fetus.

Other infections which may cause fetal damage are not so common and include fetal meningitis, syphilis, diphtheroid bacterium, staphylococcus, and cryptococcus infection. Suspect infections also include influenza and mumps virus which may prove to be teratogenic according to White and Sever (79). The Coxsackie B-4 virus may also be involved in congenital heart defects and much work is needed to clarify other possible infections which may be teratogenic.

Since the White and Sever review in 1967, more recent work by Ermert has linked other virus diseases with fetal damage. Virus hepatitis during the first trimester may cause changes in the brain, blood vessels, spinal cord, lungs, and the crystalline lens in the embryo (15). Elizan and Fabiyi (12) stated that the placental barrier has been passed by Rubella, herpes simplex, and Coxsackie B viruses. South (70) related congenital malformations and higher abortion rates to herpes virus (type 2) genital type.

Other infections may be involved in causation of fetal damage. Recently mumps has been suspected in relationship to endocardial fibroelastosis (24). Laurence and Carter (39) indicated that virus influenza may play a role in fetal abnormalities. New work in progress will shed more light on this area of investigation.

MECHANICAL DAMAGE

Fetal damage has been associated with anoxia and hypoxia from a variety of mechanical causes. Cord constriction, cord wrapping around the neck of the fetus, prolonged and difficult labor, dry births, pelvic disproportion, breech and transverse presentations as well as placental separations and other placental abnormalities are but a few of the possible hazards.

Hypoxia may be connected with maternal anemia, high altitudes (19), and possibly with chronic air pollution, smog, and carbon monoxide toxicity.

Mulcahy (50) pointed to the increased risk of abnormal births and possibly of congenital deformities with increased maternal age, parity, and cigarette smoking.

Masland (44) also listed the following maternal factors as influencing the offspring: (a) nutrition, (b) emotional factors, (c) physical activity and occupation (occupational toxins?), (d) toxemia, bleeding, and infertility, (e) blood type, (f) endocrine dysfunction, diabetes, prediabetes, and thyroid dysfunction, (g) maternal immune reactions, and (h) maternal physique.

Baker and Rudolph (3) discuss exogenous factors operating in utero and review thirteen cases of congenital ring constrictions and intrauterine amputations. The etiology of these malformations appeared to be amniogenic due to fibrous bands of tissue which constricted parts of the fetus. The authors pointed out the relationship of the defects to early rupture of the amniotic membranes, maternal bleeding, and infection and reported on the evidence from animal experiments in which early amnionic sac puncture led to cleft palates in 100 percent of the offspring.

They indicated that the incidence of these abnormalities in humans is infrequent (1 in 10,000 births) but they raised the question about the possibility that amniocentesis might possibly lead to difficulties with amnionic tissues and called for careful study and caution in its use.

## ENVIRONMENTAL TOXINS

In recent years, much attention and controversy has centered around the effect on the developing fetus of a variety of readily available toxins. The U.S. Food and Drug Administration banned the use of cyclamates based on evidence from animal research which has been questioned as to its hazards in the human embryo (34). This chemical cannot be classed as an ordinary drug since it was in such widespread use as a sugar substitute.

A current controversy surrounds the use of the phenoxy herbicides (2,4–D and 2,4,5–T) used with picloram as defoliants in the war in Vietnam as well as for domestic uses. Newton and Norris (55) questioned the placing of restrictions on the use of these chemicals based on the lack of firm evidence of their human teratogenic properties in the dosage used. However, Galston (22) indicated that the spraying of twenty-seven pounds per acre of 2,4–D (2–4-dichlorophenoxyacetic acid) and 2,4,5–T (2,4,5-trichlorphenoxyacetic acid) could lead, after one inch of rain, to such concentrations in drinking water in the Vietnam area involved that a pregnant woman drinking one liter of water per day could have a dosage of 50 mg. per day, roughly 1 mg. per kilogram of body weight. This dosage is not far enough below the minimum comparative teratogenic dose in mice and rats to give any margin of safety. Galston urged caution and more careful study of the toxicity to the human fetus. Nelson (53) also called for further study and added to the list of possibly dangerous substances PCNB (pentachloronitrobenzene) and other pesticides which produce malformations in mice and rats.

Radiation in therapeutic doses (19) and atomic radiation as experienced at Hiroshima and Nagasaki (52) have been implicated in the occurrence of microcephaly and skeletal malformations. The high strontium–90 levels in milk and in human tissues as a result of fallout from atomic testing led to great concern as to the possibility of irreparable damage to fetal and infant development. The possibility of genetic mutations and defects in subsequent generations raises serious concern about the risk of atomic radiation (9).

Potentially dangerous heavy metals have recently been found in abnormal concentrations in widespread distribution in nature. Mercury, for example, is presently being detected in certain fish in dangerous amounts. Swordfish and tuna fish may prove dangerous to children and adults and the effect of such toxins on the unborn fetus must be carefully evaluated.

Lead from paint and other sources has long been identified as an environmental toxin of importance. The highly volatile organic lead compounds, such as tetraethyl lead in gasoline, are converted into toxic inorganic lead in the body and may constitute a hazard if inhaled in sufficient concentrations. Goodman and Gillman (25) indicated that substantial proof of the danger is not yet available, however.

Arsenic is judged harmful to the fetus.

Fishbein *et al.* (17) pointed out that only recently has there been a realization of the potential health hazards due to chemical mutagens. New methods of detecting and measuring their effects both in vivo and in vitro make it possible to explore these hazards more fully. We may hope for new information which will add to our understanding of other environmental dangers to the fetus which should then be eliminated.

Insecticides have been implicated in terms of potentially hazardous chemicals. The increasing concentration of DDT and Endrin, for example, in the food cycle chain, which has lead to massive deaths of fish in our rivers and to near extermination of certain fish-eating bird species, with failure of the chicks to survive due to excessive DDT concentrations in the body tissues, raises serious questions as to possible effects on human beings. Widespread occurrence of DDT concentration in human tissues poses possible hazards of this neurotropic poison to coming generations (9, 26). Reports abound of infant and child deaths from toxic doses of insecticides, particularly in farming areas, and questions must be raised as to the effect on the central nervous system of chronic sublethal doses of the wide variety of insecticides, pesticides, and herbicides in widespread use.

HEREDITARY DISORDERS

In addition to the various toxic and infectious processes enumerated above, it has been well documented that a vast array of hereditary disorders may cause birth defects. Apgar (2) in 1968 reported on 1,487 known hereditary conditions which caused birth defects. She added that the recent increase in our knowledge of pharmacogenetics and the role of errors in the construction of protein molecules has added greatly to our understanding and detection of birth defects. Specific metabolic deficiencies may have hereditary trends and familial studies are indicated whenever an abnormality is detected in a child. In 1960 Apgar mentioned thirty-five human conditions with chromosomal abnormalities; however, by 1968 she noted that there were well over 100 known. In addition, she noted that in cultures from spontaneous abortions, one fourth to one half of the cultures showed chromosomal abnormalities. She recommended an accurate history of spontaneous abortions and examination of the chromosomal structure which can be very useful in genetic counseling.

Newly developed electron microscopic techniques have enabled us to visualize the disordered chromosomes responsible for many of these anomalies and even to predict their occurrence in advance with fairly good accuracy (30).

Polani (61) in 1963 estimated the number of birth defects in the general population due to chromosome errors as 1 in 200. Lubs and Ruddle (41) in 1970 estimated the same rate (0.5 percent) or approximately 20,000 births per year in the U.S. with chromosomal abnormalities. They added that the rate rises with maternal age: mothers over age thirty-four (1.5 percent); age forty to forty-four (1.61 percent).

## Incidence of Physical Handicaps

Every organ system is subject to deformities or congenital malformations. Rubin (64) in 1967 in his comprehensive *Handbook of Congenital Malformations* listed all of the prevalent conditions by organ systems and gave the incidence, associated anomalies, hereditary factors, treatment, and outlook. The interested reader will find this a helpful reference book.

Another very useful textbook is Smith's *Recognizable Patterns of Human Malformation* (68).

Among the congenital malformations, many of these are genetically determined and may be due to chromosomal, metabolic, or enzymatic defects which may have hereditary tendencies. A detailed discussion of this is beyond the scope of this chapter. However, reference is made to the hereditary nature of many of these defects.

Malformations tend to occur in groups and therefore one should be on the alert for other abnormalities when any malformation is detected. Nelson and Forfar (54) gave a review of the occurrence of the association of congenital abnormalities with one another and gave tables on the percentage occurrence of association between various defects.

Smith (68) listed: (a) single malformations resulting in secondary defects (chapter one); (b) 135 syndromes of multiple primary defects (chapter two) with very helpful summary tables giving the diagnostic manifestations of each syndrome, the occurrence of mental deficiency, effect on stature, and the chromosomal or genetic patterns known to date (pp. 22–32); (c) an excellent section on morphogenesis with a table relating the malformations to developmental pathology and the age of the fetus by which the defects take place (pp. 314–315); (d) genetic counseling (chapter four); (e) the significance of minor malformations as indicators of altered morphogenesis (chapter five).

Smith's approach to a multiply defective individual is worthy of note and consists of: (a) information gathered by history and physical examination; (b) a developmental appraisal of the anomalies made to determine which one represents the earliest morphogenic defect. The developmental problem must have existed prior to that date and any environmental factor after that time could not be the cause. Next, determination is made of which defects are primary and have led to secondary defects as with a "single syndromic anomaly" as differentiated from "multiple primary defects;" and (c) overall diagnosis and counseling to include how the altered structures came about, their natural history, treatment, and etiology, and genetic risk of recurrence in subsequent siblings (68a).

A review of the literature on the incidence of congenital abnormalities reveals a great deal of variation based on the definitions used in the surveys. In some only major defects are considered, while in others, major and minor defects are combined. The number and scope of the conditions included vary to some extent from one study to another, making it difficult to make comparisons between studies in different geographical areas. However, in spite of these difficulties, it is possible to show that the incidence of congenital malformations does apparently vary with location, season, racial groups, age of the mother, and other variables.

Nelson and Forfar (54) in 1969 reported over a two-year period in Edinburgh an incidence of congenital abnormalities of 5.4 percent (major defects 2.1 percent and minor 3.3 percent). Since 17 percent of the babies with congenital defects were stillborn or died in the first week of life, the incidence of babies alive after one week was 4.9 percent.

McIntosh *et al.* (46) in 1954 in New York found an incidence of 7.5 percent. Nelson and Forfar (54) give a comparison table between different studies showing the range of percentages noted in various surveys.

In the collaborative study of the National Institute for Neurological Diseases and Blindness, as early as 1961, Masland (45) reported that, of the first 2,300 births followed for one year, a high percentage of infants, 11.8 percent, showed neurological signs at one year of age. He also reported the incidence in 9,300 pregnancies of (1) spontaneous abortion—3 percent; (2) stillbirths—2 percent; (3) neonatal deaths—2 percent; and (4) prematurity—8–10 percent.

From all of the many studies, it can be concluded that approximately 5 percent of births (200,000 births a year in the U.S.) have abnormalities, with about 2 percent having major defects and 3 percent minor defects while about 0.5 percent of infants show chromosomal defects.

This represents a major problem in our population since Jansen (36) stated that congenital defects are the principal cause of neonatal deaths at full term.

Apgar (2) pointed out that many cases (over 57 percent) are diagnosed long after birth, sometimes as late as in adolescence and even in adult life. Obviously much work must still be done to increase our knowledge and efforts toward prevention of these crippling disorders.

## Prevention

With the rapid increase in our knowledge regarding the etiology of congenital physical and mental handicaps, both endogenous and exogenous factors have been identified as important contributors to the incidence of these unfortunate defects. New steps are possible in terms of prevention of malformations, mental retardation, and cerebral damage which should eventually help to reduce their incidence and the severe emotional disorders which so often accompany them.

### PRENATAL PREVENTION

It is now possible with the aid of *careful genetic diagnosis and counseling* to prevent certain hereditary abnormalities which are connected with chromosomal defects, enzymatic and metabolic errors. Studies of the genetic, enzymatic, and metabolic patterns of the parents, grandparents, and siblings can uncover potential hazards which may lead to the birth of a malformed child. Of course, it is not the geneticist's role to determine whether a couple should take the risk of having a defective child. However, he can advise prospective parents as to the percentage risk of such a tragedy and then it is up to the individuals to make their own decision in view of the risk involved. Literature on genetic counseling is growing rapidly. An excellent text on the subject is that by Reed (62).

Genetic centers are now available in every state and many foreign countries, which represents a giant step forward compared with the facilities available a few years ago in 1964 when Gustafson and Coursin (30) listed twenty-eight genetic centers. Certain chromosomal defect diseases can be predicted with a high degree of accuracy. For example, adult carriers of Tay-Sachs Disease, a recessive genetic disorder that kills its victims in the second to fourth years of life, can now be identified by a simple blood test based on a decrease of the enzyme hexosaminidase A in their blood. This disease affects predominantly those with an ancestry of Ashkenazi Jews of Eastern Europe, which includes about 90 percent of the Jews in this country. Approximately one in thirty people from this ancestry carries the Tay-Sachs gene. Mass surveys are being undertaken to identify the carriers and it is theoretically possible to eliminate the disease with our present knowledge (37). Should a couple have a pregnancy after the discovery of the likelihood of an affected fetus, prenatal intrauterine diagnosis is possible and a tragedy can be avoided (see below, O'Brien *et al.* [58]).

Cystic fibrosis, a nonsex-linked recessive condition in which the carrier excretes ten times the normal amount of salt, is also a predictable disease. A sweat test for concentrations of sodium and chloride reveals the presence of the latent abnormality in the carrier (30).

The sickle cell anemia trait in a carrier can be readily detected by examining a drop of blood under low oxygen tension. Hemophilia, in the clinically normal female carrier, can be detected by chromosomal studies, as can numerous other disorders.

The complexities of diagnosis and prediction of recurrence after the birth of one abnormal child are illustrated by Down's syndrome (mongolism) which is associated with extra chromosomal material. However, three different subtypes occur with varying rates of recurrence, as described by Gustafson and Coursin (30).

The Trisomy 21 "standard" type, the most common, is related to advanced age of the mother and is usually not familial. The 15, 15/21 or "translocation" type can occur in women of any age. Risk of recurrence is high and it is transmissible through families.

Counseling can provide very helpful data when previous pregnancies have led to infants with congenital malformations, retardation, or to spontaneous abortions or stillbirths. Chromosomal studies of the parents, siblings, and grandparents can shed light on the likelihood of recurrence of the conditions in subsequent children and percentages of likelihood can be given to the parents (29, 62).

Rubin (64) gives the likelihood of recurrence in subsequent offspring for many of the congenital handicaps listed in his handbook.

It is particularly important for prevention of subsequent deformed children to accomplish chromosomal studies on stillbirths, spontaneous abortions, and handicapped children so that attempts may be made to detect parental genetic defects which may affect the siblings.

In view of the unquestioned increase in the incidence of fetal abnormalities, serious deformities, and mental retardation with increasing age of the mother as well as with higher numbers of pregnancies, it is obvious that counseling of parents should include increased caution with advancing age of the mother. At present there does not seem to be any definitive evidence relating the age of the father to fetal abnormalities with the exception of exposure to radiation which may effect the male germ plasm.

In regard to psychological factors, one of the most important aspects is the parents' readiness for a child and *planning of pregnancies*. Unplanned and unwanted pregnancies very frequently result in parental, particularly maternal, feelings of guilt, remorse, rage, and rejection of the unborn child, sometimes, after birth, amounting to serious neglect and even child abuse and infanticide.

Every infant has tremendous emotional needs and demands which, along with the physical demands he makes on the mother, can only be met adequately when the mother feels comfortable and reasonably warm and accepting toward the baby.

Sensible planning and spacing of the pregnancies can help the parents to be better prepared emotionally and physically to provide for the child's physical and emotional needs. Studies of mothers of twins and those who have children quite close together reveal how burdensome these circumstances can be for an average mother. Case studies of such children confirm the impact on the offspring of the heavy demands upon the mother.

Thus careful family planning, spacing of children, and readily available birth control are essential to the prevention of emotional disorders in children.

Apgar (2) stated that it has been shown that the age of both the sperm and the ovum at the time of fertilization has an effect on the viability and prognosis for a normal fetus. The older the oöcytes (i.e., the longer between ovulation and fertilization for the ovum, and between spermatogenesis and contact with the ovum), the higher the chance of abnormalities in the fetus.

Thus, for the best chance of fertilization between a healthy ovum and sperm, when planning a pregnancy, ideally, the prospective parents should have intercourse every twenty-four hours from the tenth to the twenty-fifth day after the beginning of the last menstrual period to insure early fertilization of the ovum by young, viable sperm, thereby *planning conception*.

In addition, Apgar stated that breaks in oral contraceptive pill routine may be related to abnormal pregnancies due to the effects of the progestins on the fetus. Therefore she advised when planning pregnancy one should stay off the pill and also avoid pregnancy tests with ingested or injected steroids which may be teratogenic.

Prevention of maternal malnutrition, vitamin deficiencies, physical disease, anemia, and other debilitating conditions in advance of pregnancy can aid in the prevention of fetal defects. Pregnancy in women with endocrine and metabolic disorders calls for particularly careful medical attention when considering pregnancy.

Detection of blood type incompatibilities should be accomplished routinely by blood type studies of both parents in order to avoid serious consequences in the newborn. Apgar (2) indicated in 1968 that it would soon be possible to prevent 5,000 deaths per year and thousands of stillbirths by eradication of erythroblastosis due to Rh incompatibility through the development of a new vaccine for Rh-negative women and Rh-positive husbands.

Combating of cigarette smoking during pregnancy as well as the more serious drug addictions can help to save fetal insults. Infants of mothers who smoke weigh less than those of nonsmokers. In known heroin addicts, Methadone maintenance programs can spare the severe signs of fetal withdrawal and possible deaths seen in the newborn babies of addicts (13).

Prevention of the infectious processes known to involve fetal damage can be accomplished to some extent by early and comprehensive programs for immunization against such diseases as rubella. Unfortunately, even though much is now known about prevention, 100 percent protection is not being taken advantage of in this country. Evidence for our inefficiency and ineffectiveness in immunization programs can be seen from the fact that the incidence of measles, which dropped dramatically after 1963, when the measles vaccine became available, to a low in 1968, increased in 1969 and 1970, and figures available to date indicate that the rate for 1971 will be still higher. In some "backward" countries such as Gambia in West Africa, where universal immunization programs have been carried out, measles has been virtually wiped out (16). The lessons to be learned from this data are quite clear. We must develop a far more comprehensive public health program if we are to reduce the potential hazard to unborn children from such preventable diseases.

Vaccination against Rubella should be done early (prepuberty) and should be avoided in women of child-bearing age because of possible harm to a fetus.

Public education regarding the risks of exposure to the known deforming diseases particularly in the first trimester of pregnancy could help to avoid damage.

PREVENTION DURING PREGNANCY

With the knowledge we have gained about the teratogenic and toxic effects of certain drugs, education as to the dangers of self-medication and indiscriminate use of drugs is urgently needed. Further drug research and controls on the distribution and release of new drugs are essential in the prevention of such tragedies as occurred with the use of thalidomide. Particularly in the first twelve weeks during the rapid proliferation of the nervous system and the limbs, great care is required in the use of medications.

Environmental toxins such as Strontium–90, the heavy metals, pesticides, and carbon monoxide, which have become suspect, will pose a major problem since there is no simple answer to the problem of environmental pollution. However, public education and efforts to obtain stronger legislation on environmental sanitation may be able to reduce the ever-increasing burden on the future infants which our pollution and waste disposal problems have inflicted. It is possible with enough determination to interrupt the downward spiral of environmental degradation which has gained so much momentum. Exposure to radiation can be reduced by restricting the use of unnecessary X-rays in pregnancy and by cessation of atmospheric nuclear explosions in the world.

Much of the *mechanical damage* to the fetus can be prevented by careful prenatal care and good obstetrical care during labor and delivery. New diagnostic techniques for placental displacements and abnormalities can prevent fetal damage by planning caesarian section before labor begins, thus avoiding such hazards as ruptured placenta, bleeding, and placental separation.

Fetal monitoring by electrical recording of the baby's ECG can detect distress in time to use obstetrical intervention to avoid damage to the fetus. Phonocardiography and ultrasonic cardiography are extremely sensitive new methods of detecting fetal distress and have proven 100 percent reliable in determining the presence of a live fetus.

New techniques of *early prenatal intrauterine diagnosis* are now available which make it possible to diagnose with a high degree of certainty the presence of certain abnormalities of the fetus early enough to permit therapeutic abortion where there is a certainty of deformity. For example, in a recent study by O'Brien *et al.* (58) using amniocentesis, a simple procedure for removing amniotic fluid by needle through the abdominal wall, the presence or absence of Tay-Sachs Disease was determined in fifteen cases. In pregnancies with a history of previous siblings with the disease, amniotic fluid and cells were assayed for the enzyme hexosaminidase A. Of the six fetuses diagnosed as affected by the disease, the diagnosis was confirmed in all cases after therapeutic interruption of the pregnancy. Of the nine cases diagnosed as not having Tay-Sachs Disease, the six born so far were all free from the disease. Three were not yet born.

The diagnosis of Down's syndrome can be made readily by amniocentesis in time to permit termination of the pregnancy and thus prevent the birth of a mongoloid baby. This method can be extremely helpful in the diagnosis and prevention of seriously handicapped infants.

Brady (5) recently added two hereditary genetic disorders, Niemann-Pick disease and Fabry's disease, to the list of conditions which can be diagnosed in utero in time for intervention.

Fortunately, liberalization of abortion laws and public acceptance make this method even more useful.

However, caution is indicated until further studies can answer the question raised by Baker and Rudolph (3) of whether amniocentesis may result in premature rupture of the amnionic sac with the possibility of fibrous bands and constriction of the fetal limbs.

Intrauterine photography has been introduced recently by means of introducing a flexible glass fiber hysteroscope into the amnionic sac which permits visualization of fetal defects.

Needless to say, prevention of maternal infections is as important throughout the duration of pregnancy as it is earlier.

To prevent fetal damage in later pregnancy maintenance of adequate nutrition, vitamin, iron, and other mineral intake throughout pregnancy is essential and the avoidance of excessive weight gain and the accumulation of fluid in the body tissues are also important. Toward the end of pregnancy, particularly, adequate prenatal care can help to avoid such dangerous conditions as eclampsia and hypertension which may jeopardize the newborn infant's condition.

Assessment of fetal viability is possible by means of analysis of the maternal urinary excretion of steroids according to Reynolds (63). Heys (32) indicated that a sudden drop in urinary estriol excretion below normal levels reflects deterioration of the condition of the fetus. When the estriol level falls below 6 mg/24 hrs., the risk of intrauterine death within forty-eight hours is 30 percent. Lowered levels of excretion are also found in cases of retarded fetal growth, premature delivery, toxemia, and placental insufficiency. Heys recommended weekly determination of urine estriol level after thirty-two weeks of pregnancy in patients with suspected retarded fetal growth, previous unexplained stillbirths, and hypertensive toxemias with albuminuria.

When danger to the fetus is expected, as with toxemia, prolonged gestation, pregnancies in women over thirty-five years of age, maternal diabetes or Rh sensitization, and after treatment for sterility, special care should be taken throughout pregnancy. In these cases amnioscopy may be done to determine the fetal condition and amniography may be used for the detection of congenital malformations (28).

### PREVENTION IN INFANCY AND EARLY CHILDHOOD

If the infant survives all of the hazards of intrauterine life and the possible trauma of delivery, there is still the possibility of damage to the central nervous system after birth. Careful pediatric infant management in the immediate postnatal period can help to avoid these dangers. Thorough pediatric evaluations immediately after birth and at regular intervals may uncover treatable abnormalities in their early stages.

Prevention of infections which may lead to encephalitis and cortical damage in the child should be accomplished. Many of the childhood infectious diseases which can result in brain damage or other serious consequences, including rubella, measles, diphtheria, pertussis and mumps, may be prevented by prompt immunization. Controversy still exists about the timing and use of certain of these immunizations on a universal scale because of the possibility of infection spreading from a child in the process of immunization to a young woman of child-bearing age, and some authorities question the use of mumps vaccine other than with puberty-age boys since it may be preferable for the young child to develop a permanent immunity from the disease rather than a temporary one from the immunization.

Many chronic parasitic, bacterial, and viral infections can adversely affect the growth and development of the young child. Continued pediatric care through the use of well-baby clinics or private medical care is of great importance to the child's future health and development, both mental and physical.

Adequate nutrition, vitamin, iron, and other mineral intake are essential in the avoidance of a wide variety of deforming and debilitating diseases of infancy including such deficiency disease as rickets (Vitamin D), scurvy (Vitamin C), and anemia (iron). Regular pediatric care should help to prevent these disorders.

Prevention of drug toxicity in infancy: as can be seen from the above section on toxic drugs which can affect the fetus before birth, it is apparent that certain drugs may also affect the newborn or young child adversely. As was pointed out, certain antibiotic drugs are not well tolerated by the young infant and should be used with great care. These include, among others, the tetracyclines, penicillin, nalidixic acid, nitrofurantoin (1, 49, 75), and chloramphenical (74).

Great care should be used in prescribing any medication to infants in order to avoid those that are potentially harmful and one should watch for possible toxic side effects. The avoidance of self-medication of infants by their parents is essential.

Drugs which affect growth and metabolism should be used only with great care. Such drugs as the estrogens may be inadvertently introduced indirectly through the use of oral contraception with nursing mothers since the estrogens are secreted in the maternal milk. Oral contraception should be avoided by nursing mothers.

Accidental poisoning of infants and young toddlers is extremely common and constitutes one of the preventable damaging events in early childhood which requires the attention of all those working with parents and children. A massive educational program is needed if we are to avoid much needless damage to children.

Aspirin poisoning is one of the commonest causes of death in childhood. Each year between one and two million cases of poisoning occur in the United States with over 3,000 deaths. One third of these occur in children under five years of age who are attracted to bottles and containers easily within reach. The actual figures are undoubtedly much higher. Deeths and Breeden (11) reported recently that, of 1,057 cases of poisoning in children, the incidence of the etiologic agent was: aspirin—35.3 percent, barbiturates—4.2 percent, tranquilizers—4.2 percent, amphetamines—3.7 percent, and miscellaneous drugs—10.7 percent (total 58.1 percent). The remaining poisonings (41.9 percent) were from substances other than drugs.

Environmental toxins are also of great importance in the occurrence of poisoning in childhood, and knowledge of the dangers is important in the prevention of damage to children from such poisonings. In addition to drugs which are so readily accessible to children, a wide variety of toxic substances is easily available in the average household kitchen, laundry, and bathroom. Lye, bleaches, cleaning compounds, insecticides, moth-proofing compounds, cooking substances, and a vast array of caustic and poisonous chemicals are within easy reach of nearly all little children who love to imitate their parents by "cooking" or preparing "food" and by eating what they have mixed.

In the study by Deeths and Breeden (11) referred to above, the remaining 41.9 percent of child poisonings were due to the following chemicals: hydrocarbons (e.g., charcoal lighting fluid, kerosene, gasoline)—18.4 percent, mothballs—2.9 percent, lead—7.0 percent, arsenic—1.9 percent, miscellaneous nondrugs—12.6 percent.

Many of these toxic drug and chemical reactions, if death does not occur, may result in brain damage, convulsions, and/or impairment of various bodily functions which may interfere with the child's future growth, psychological development, and educational progress.

Efforts to combat this tremendous problem are being made by local and national medical groups coordinated by the National Clearinghouse for Poison Control Centers. The control centers offer information on toxicity and emergency treatment twenty-four hours a day and collect information useful in research and prevention.

The impact on children of television advertising of drugs, various sprays, and cosmetics cannot be overemphasized. Efforts should be made to curtail the exposure of such advertising when children are watching.

Among other environmental toxins, lead plays an important role. Parents should avoid the use of lead paint on furniture and toys used by small children where chewing on the painted surface can result in ingestion of toxic amounts of lead.

Another group, the toxic hydrocarbons, should be kept out of reach of children, as should detergents, cleaning fluids such as benzene and naphthalene, and the various bottled and spray-can products around the home such as antiseptics, astringents, and deodorants which contain toxic aluminum and zinc compounds.

Another attractive hazard lies in a variety of plants and shrubs whose toxic bright-colored berries or leaves and roots are poisonous. Children should be taught to avoid ingestion of all such potentially dangerous plants.

Head injuries frequently result in brain damage affecting various functions including speech, learning, and motor performance. Automobile accidents account for a sizable number of head injuries in young children where the unrestrained child is catapulted against sharp protrusions or the windshield. Crash research has shown conclusively that a properly designed child's restraint harness can prevent many head injuries. Children should always be made to sit down and to use restraints and never be allowed to ride standing up in an auto since sudden stops or turns can cause serious blows to a child's head.

Accidents in the home are also very common and can be avoided to some degree by such preventive measures as removing sharp and dangerous objects (e.g., razors and knives) to a safe place, and using nonslip rugs and bath mats and child-proof electric plugs for light sockets. It is impossible to remove every danger, but adult supervision of small children can help to avert much harm.

The importance of head injury to the child can be seen from a study of 624 cases of cerebral palsy acquired after birth: 18 percent resulted from skull trauma, 57 percent from encephalopathy, and 12 percent from meningitis; 65 percent of the cases were acquired before age two years and 92 percent before eight years (59). Thus avoidance of head trauma as well as infections would help to reduce the number of injuries to the brain.

An important concept in prevention is the identification of high risk infants, i.e., those children who merit special attention because of the possibility of developmental difficulties and/or the occurrence of physical handicaps which may develop after birth. The high risk group includes: (a) premature and postmature infants, those born with a prolonged, complicated, or precipitous delivery, and those newborns who showed a low Apgar score; (b) presence of a family history of mutant genes, central nervous system disorders, and allergies, as well as low socio-economic status; (c) certain conditions in the mother: diabetes, hypertension, thyroid disease, cardiovascular renal disease, radiation or chemotherapy, and short stature; (d) previous obstetrical history of stillbirths, abortions, toxemia, and abnormal birth weight infants; (e) in the present pregnancy: maternal age under sixteen or over thirty-five years, multiple births, polyhydramnios, pyelonephritis, medications, radiation, anesthesia, toxemia, and fetal-maternal blood-group incompatibility; (f) placental infarction, separation, placentitis, and amnion nodosum; and (g) neonatal conditions: single umbilical artery, jaundice, abnormal head size, infections, convulsions, failure of weight gain, congenital defects, and disproportion between weight or length and gestational age (10).

Since proper and timely medical management can correct many potential defects if they are detected early, it is important for those working with parents to bear in mind these danger signs and to help parents get adequate and prompt care for their child. Particularly in the low socio-economic disadvantaged group, many treatable conditions go undetected for too long a period of time, often until severe or irreversible pathology sets in.

In spite of every effort at prevention, many children will unavoidably show congenital or acquired physical handicaps. With these children we should be on the alert for the development of psychological difficulties which all too frequently come to overlie the physical handicap.

## Psychodynamic Considerations

Many of the congenital malformations and acquired handicaps discussed above may have serious effects on the psychological development and emotional adjustment of the unfortunate victim.

NORMAL CHILD DEVELOPMENT

In order to understand the impact of the handicap on the emotional life of the child it would be helpful to review briefly the theoretical constructs of child development from which the psychodynamics will be discussed.

At the outset, it may be stated that the normal child's development results from an interplay between his hereditary, constitutional endowment and the forces of his environment with which these inborn tendencies interact. If a child survives the prenatal and neonatal period intact, given an average endowment of physical and ego apparatuses and an "average expectable environment" (Hartmann [31]), and, in the sense of Winnicott, "good enough mothering" (80), his psychic development may be expected to proceed along reasonably steady lines keeping pace with the biological maturation and physical growth which unfold according to genetically predetermined schedules.

Satisfactory psychological development is largely dependent upon a close, meaningful relationship with the mother or mother substitute, as pointed out by Jacobson (35). Since it promotes the establishment of stable, enduring libidinal cathexes, parental love is the best guarantee for normal ego and superego formation.

Winnicott (80) spoke of maternal devotion as a necessary quality in child rearing, required by the infant. He stated that success in infant care depends on the fact of devotion by the mother, not on cleverness or intellectual enlightenment.

Mahler (42, 43), in her studies of normal child development, indicated that it is the mother's "libidinal availability" to the child which is the principal effector of the child's emotional development. In her construction of early normal development, the child is said to pass through the following developmental phases: (a) "normal autism" where, during the first three months of life, the major site of libidinal investment is in the infant's own body, particularly the gastrointestinal organization; (b) as the child's development progresses, a close mutually need-fulfilling relationship gradually develops which Mahler refers to as "normal symbiosis" from approximately three to six months of age, reaching its height at four to five months; (c) during this period of close mothering and meeting of the infant's physical and emotional needs by the external ego of the mother, the infant begins to emerge from the symbiotic web into the phase of "separation-individuation." The libido is gradually withdrawn from the mother and becomes attached to the infant's own bodily parts and functions. During this rather complex stage of development, which Mahler and her coworkers have carefully delineated into four subphases, the infant begins to develop its own sense of identity, self-image, and body-image and begins to function as a separate individual.

It is of importance to the consideration of the various physical handicaps which follows to briefly adumbrate these subphases.

First, in the "differentation" subphase, which lasts from approximately age five or six months to about ten or twelve months, the infant begins to differentiate between the self and the external object. Stranger anxiety is commonly noted at about six to eight months as the child develops a firmer awareness of the mother and begins to differentiate non-mother more clearly.

Second, in the "practicing" subphase, from about ten to twelve months to sixteen to eighteen months, as the younger toddler develops independent locomotion, he begins actively to move away from and separate himself physically from the mother in contrast to the earlier separations which were experienced passively. As the ego functions of perception, motor control, and cognition, recognition, and recall develop, the toddler experiments with the process of separation and return to the mother. At certain times, after a period of time away from the mother, he will look for her as though to check on her presence or may return to her side briefly for "emotional refueling" (Furer's term).

One can see that these activities would be severely disrupted by a wide variety of physical handicaps such as blindness or congenital defects which interfere with locomotion. I will return to this later in regard to specific handicaps.

As the toddler develops increased motor skills, he appears to experience a "love affair with the world" (Jacobson) during which he explores his environment and increases in his mastery of upright locomotion as well as the development of language, control of his aggression, mastery of self-feeding, and other bodily functions.

Third, in the "rapprochement" phase which lasts from approximately sixteen to eighteen months to twenty-two to twenty-four months, there is somewhat of a return to the closer ties with the mother as ego development increases.

Further individuation occurs during this period. Differentiation of the self and object representations increases and consolidation of the sense of identity and self-image takes place.

The object relationships with the mother, father, siblings, and others take on increasing significance during this phase. The specific fear during the separation-individuation phase is the fear of object loss.

Fourth, as the child's inner mental representation of the mother becomes firmly established, the phase of "object constancy" gradually evolves between about twenty-five and thirty-six months of age. At this point the maternal image has become intrapsychically available to the child as the actual mother had been libidinally available. Now the specific danger becomes the loss of the love of the libidinal object, although some fear of object loss may remain.

The child's ambivalence and aggressive impulses in the oral-sadistic and anal-sadistic phases aggravate the danger of loss of love and of object loss. According to Mahler,

By the end of the second and the beginning of the third year, the fear of loss of love is compounded by castration anxiety.

It is the mother's love of the toddler and her acceptance of his ambivalence that enable the toddler to cathect his self representation with neutralized energy. Where there is a great actual or fantasied lack of acceptance by the mother, there is a deficit in self-esteem and a consequent narcissistic vulnerability . . . (43).

## THE PSYCHOLOGICAL DEVELOPMENT OF THE
## HANDICAPPED CHILD

*Development of object relationships.* Many of the physical handicaps may interfere with the smooth progression of these developmental phases described above. It may readily be presumed that any defect which intrudes itself into the child's developmental path may impinge in two ways upon his progression.

First, from the child's point of view, a physical defect such as blindness, for example, would markedly affect the course and vicissitudes of the development of his object relationships. Also such motor handicaps as congenital hip dislocations or other deformities of the lower extremities would detract from the smooth passage through the early separation-individuation subphases, particularly the practicing and rapprochement subphases.

Second, from the point of view of the mother, it is apparent from our clinical observations that any physical defect in the child may lead to interferences in the mother's capacity to cathect her infant and in her capacity for libidinal availability to the child. Feelings of anguish, guilt, shame, self-degradation, self-blame, and depressive attitudes are extremely common among mothers of infants with any kind of physical defect whether congenital or acquired sometime after birth.

Commonly the parents search for "the cause" in themselves, blaming themselves, each other, their heredity, and an array of possible etiological factors. Family tensions often ensue.

The anxiety on the mother's part often interferes with the smooth development of a close symbiotic need-fulfilling relationship with her baby. Guilt feelings and the unconscious wish to get rid of the child often become disguised in efforts to make up for inflicting the defect on the child with subsequent compensatory efforts. The tendency to prolong the child's infantile dependent position is quite frequent. Thus maternal feelings of guilt and the wish to compensate for the deformity often lead to prolongation of the symbiotic phase and disturbances in the subsequent separation-individuation process.

Oversolicitousness and overprotection tend to delay separation-individuation by keeping the child closer to the mother and more dependent upon her than is advisable. The defects in the early mother-child symbiotic need-fulfillment phase also contribute to the failures in progressing smoothly into separation-individuation, which process requires a relatively satisfactory prior symbiotic phase for adequate resolution of the symbiosis.

Failure to develop a comfortable, satisfying symbiotic phase is noted very frequently, particularly where there is maternal depression and withdrawal of the mother's libidinal cathexis from the infant. Consequently, regression to and/or fixation at the autistic phase of development occurs with some handicapped children and accounts for the large number of physically handicapped children we encounter in our work who are also noted to function on an autistic level.

Stranger anxiety may be greatly exaggerated at six to eight months in the handicapped child where there has been a partial failure of the close symbiotic relationship. The basic "sense of trust" (Erikson [14]), which has its foundation in the early mother-child interaction, is often lacking. Fixation at a quasi-symbiotic stage may result from such inadequate need fulfillment with the possibility of subsequent borderline personality adjustment.

In the practicing subphase the handicapped child's delight in mastery and in experimenting with independent locomotion may be impeded by many of the physical handicaps.

Medical and surgical manipulations, repeated examinations, painful experiences, and necessary separations from the mother, before the child's ego is sufficiently developed to cope with such trauma, add to the already overburdened ego's capacity to cope with its situation. Regression may occur at any point in the child's development and is frequently encountered at key points, particularly in the separation-individuation phase where even the most normal child needs help in mastering untimely separations from his mother.

Repeated or prolonged hospitalizations for reconstructive surgery, as with the cleft-palate child, for example, extract a very heavy toll from the child's beginning object relations (see also Anna Freud [21]).

Spitz (71), in his studies on "Hospitalism" many years ago, showed the striking effects of separation from the mother on the child's psychological development.

Prevention of undue trauma is possible to some extent with necessary surgical and medical interventions for handicapped children by careful psychological preparation, timing, and by assuring the child of the mother's presence throughout a necessary medical procedure or hospitalization. Treating the handicapped child as an individual and as one who deserves consideration, extra kindness, and tact in handling can help in prevention of some of the trauma which may occur when handled in an unfeeling, insensitive manner, as happens all too frequently in a busy hospital.

As the child begins to develop his sense of identity, his body image, self-image, and sense of self-esteem, many of the more obvious physical handicaps as well as the more hidden ones begin to interfere with these processes.

From the child's point of view, the defect may interfere with his achieving the gratification of ego-building experiences which independent functioning, mastery of locomotion, hand-eye coordination, and bodily processes provide. Defects in the body image, self-image, and self-esteem result and the child develops a concept of himself as different, inadequate, clumsy, stupid, deformed, inferior, or unwanted and unloved.

Mahler's (43) statement that "where there is a great actual or fantasied lack of acceptance by the mother, there is a deficit in self-esteem and a consequent narcissistic vulnerability" in the child is of great importance here. Since the child's sense of self-esteem emanates from the mother's acceptance of him as a person, much work is often necessary with the parents of handicapped children to help them overcome their guilt and to be able to accept their child and to offer the basic necessary early relationship which can assist the child in developing some sense of trust and self-esteem in spite of his handicap.

Later on, during the third to fourth years, when the child should be progressing well into the phase of object constancy, the earlier defects in object relationships show their mark in the inevitable delays in acquisition of object constancy which show clinically in prolonged separation anxiety and other symptoms.

*Libidinal development.* Considering the child's progress from the point of view of stages of libidinal development, one can readily see how a variety of congenital handicaps would interfere with the processes involved in each of the early stages: oral, anal, and phallic.

For example, cleft lip and cleft palate and other oral or esophageal defects, as well as pyloric stenosis, pose grave threats to the feeding process particularly in the oral phase, roughly during the first year of life. Danger of aspiration of liquid is present as it is in conditions such as cerebral palsy and other diseases which affect the pharyngeal and esophageal musculature. Surgical intervention is often necessary along with such traumatic procedures as tube feeding, anesthesia, and restraints.

Feeding difficulties in the early oral stage due to such defects leave an indelible mark on the development with subsequent oral fixation points.

If a handicapped child survives the first year of life, there often ensues a period of intense struggles in the anal phase of development.

We know that normal children are prone to anal struggles particularly if the quality of the oral gratification or the symbiotic relationship with the mother has been less than optimum. Thus, with the defects in the object relationship sphere in the symbiotic phase and early separation-individuation subphases which tend to occur with handicapped children, severe mother-child struggles frequently occur during the anal stage along with heightened ambivalence on the child's part and a failure of neutralization of aggression, in the sense of Hartmann (31).

In the phallic stage, the physical defects and the defects in body image and self-image heighten the normal tendency to castration anxiety.

Bodily defects assume tremendously important roles in the establishment and undermining of the self-esteem and frequently leave a residue of greatly exaggerated narcissistic vulnerability.

Niederland (57a) has described the narcissistic ego impairment in patients with early physical malformation and their "compensatory narcissistic self-inflation, fantasies of grandiosity and uniqueness, aggressive strivings for narcissistic supplies from the outside world, [along with their] impairment of object relations and reality testing [and their] excessive vulnerability." He pointed out that "an early body defect tends to remain an area of unresolved conflict through its concreteness, permanency, cathectic significance, and its relationship to conflictual anxiety (primitive body disintegration anxiety, castration fear)." Niederland added that patients with congenital or early acquired malformations suffer from permanent disturbance of the self-image which if severe may reach delusional proportions. In all of his patients the defenses of denial and undoing were present, which has also been observed frequently by the author.

Niederland (57b) observed that, when a physical defect is found early in infancy, there often ensues a marked disequilibrium in the relations between mother and child which hardly ever fully subsides. The overstimulation of the body which results from medical and orthopedic procedures such as immobilization, braces, etc., and the resultant inadequate discharge of aggressive and libidinal energy and the threats to bodily intactness accentuate the traumatic influence of the defect upon psychic development.

## PSYCHODYNAMIC CONSIDERATIONS OF SOME
## SPECIFIC PHYSICAL HANDICAPS

*Blindness.* One of the handicaps which has a potential for severe impact on psychic development and especially on the formation of object relations is blindness. In her careful studies of blind children, Fraiberg (18a) indicated that "the early development of blind babies is perilous." She added that " . . . not blindness alone but tactile-auditory insufficiency in the early months will prevent the blind baby from making the vital attachments to his mother, and to the human world." She also pointed out that the blind baby's hands must be trained in special ways since adaptive hand behavior follows a very different pattern in the blind infant. Delayed creeping and walking were noted with all of the blind children in her study.

Since the visual image of the mother's face is missing, the development of the specific symbiotic mother-child tie may be disturbed. Auditory and tactile-motor cues must replace the visual ones. Delays are often noted in the separation-individuation process since locomotion is frequently delayed and also the child cannot visualize the mother from a distance to check on her presence. Fraiberg stressed the role of vision in forming stable mental representations. The blind child is delayed in this process and is reduced to helplessness and panic when he cannot verify the existence of the mother.

However, she added that under favorable circumstances with adequate mothering, "blindness need not be an impediment to the establishment of libidinal object ties in the first year of life. But the stability of these ties, and hence the stability of the early ego organization, can be imperiled through the prolongation of infantile dependency and helplessness and the limited adaptive solutions open to a blind child" (18b). Fraiberg (18b) stated that the sequence of visual recognitory experiences which contribute to the establishment of the identity of the mother in the sighted child "is a progressive synthesis of visual-auditory-tactile experience in which the picture unites all sensory data. The term 'synesthesia' is exact here. . . . "

It is my impression, from clinical work with blind children as well as sighted autistic and retarded children, and from normal child developmental observations, that the role of the olfactory sense in the process of establishing the identity of the mother is of great importance. Fraiberg and other observers seem to have overlooked the olfactory sense in their observations.

Sighted babies may be seen to react to olfactory stimuli emanating from the mother, for instance, if she is dressed up and wears perfume. With blind children I have frequently noted that they explore human and inanimate objects by carefully smelling them and they appeared to rely quite heavily on the sense of smell.

I assume that in the blind infant the olfactory sensations blend with those from the auditory-tactile-motor spheres in establishing the identity of the mother in the young infant's mind.

From the point of view of defensive operations, Fraiberg found that the blind child in the second year, when experiencing danger, cannot "fight back" and shows primitive motor discharges, e.g., tantrums and tic-like symptoms, without the motor patterns for aggression used by the sighted child, e.g., hitting back. She added that " . . . *regression remains the chief defense of the blind young child in . . . the second year*" (18c).

Blindness can produce striking effects in the development of the ego. Fraiberg has developed an educational program for blind babies and their parents which can help to overcome the deficiencies which she has noted to be very common.

Other authors who have made important contributions to the understanding of the psychodynamics of blind children include Burlingham (7, 8), and Nagera and Colonna (51).

*Strabismus.* Another physical handicap which has an impact on personality development is strabismus. Lipton (40) indicated that strabismus is quite common, occurring in about 2 percent of the population and in half of institutionalized brain-damaged and retarded patients.

Strabismus may occur at any age, with most cases beginning between two and a half and three and a half years. Feelings of confusion occur with the double visual images with subjective discomfort along with disturbances in balance and orientation in space. In addition to the subjective symptoms, the reactions of the environment are of considerable importance, as with all handicaps. Lipton pointed out that the mother-child relation may become distorted because of the child's defect and that the mother's anxiety about the condition may conjoin with other maternal conflicts. The mother may also become concerned about what other people will think of her child and of herself. Parental anxiety may be communicated to the child and make the child anxious. The mother's anxiety may be "experienced as aggressive overprotection by the child" (40a). Inhibition of aggression resulted in several of Lipton's patients.

As with various other physical defects, repulsion is often felt by the observer of the child with the handicap, which adds to the child's discomfort.

Treatment programs such as glasses, eye patches, or exercises may become battlegrounds for parent-child struggles, particularly during and soon after the anal phase. Lipton added, regarding the extreme anxiety of a castration or annihilation type, that "when these struggles occur during the anal-urethral and phallic-oedipal phases, they are not only intensified but may very easily become part of sadomasochistic and activity-passivity conflicts" (40b).

"An important factor in the child's ability to cope with trauma is his use of the mother as an auxiliary ego, his capacity to borrow her ego strength" (40c). As with other defective children, the strabismic child requires greater borrowing of ego strength to compensate for the defect, and thus he is more vulnerable to poor mothering.

In terms of superego development, Lipton pointed out that lying and self-deception are common in these children. These traits are connected with the defensive operations involved in trying to hide the defect. The low self-esteem is related to the outside world's reactions of repulsion, rejection, and taunting with which the child has identified and, in so doing, he has adopted a rejecting attitude toward himself. In addition, character traits, including passivity and dependency, may result from a continuation into later life of the early defensive operations used by the ego.

Eye operations can result in psychic trauma since separation from the mother and the temporary blindness from having the eyes covered, along with anesthesia and restraint, can result in considerable anxiety unless conscious efforts are made to forewarn the child and to offer constant external ego support, preferably from the mother. Even with the utmost care in preparation for surgery, many children show anxiety following such operative procedures. It is possible to help the young child to work through and master the anxiety connected with medical and surgical procedures by offering him the opportunity to re-enact and talk about or play out the experiences. Young toddlers may be observed spontaneously playing out traumatic procedures with their dolls or teddy bears—for example, taking out the doll's tonsils with a spoon. This kind of self-expression should be encouraged in order to avoid the repression of the feeling of fear, helplessness, and rage which can contribute to later symptom formation.

*Motor defects.* A variety of motor handicaps can interfere with the personality development of the growing child. Congenital dislocations and deformities, which require casts, splints, and operations with subsequent immobilization, interfere with the child's mastery of locomotion as well as with the separation-individuation process. Here, again, psychological preparation for operative procedures and assuring the mother's presence during hospitalizations can help to avoid some of the traumatic aspects of the necessary procedures.

In later childhood obvious motor defects frequently lead to taunting and ostracism by peers with consequent withdrawal and feelings of inferiority and self-negation.

The adults can help a deformed child to compensate for his physical handicap by accepting him in spite of his defects and by helping him to develop alternative and compensatory skills. Many noteworthy examples of healthy compensation might be cited, for example, blind musicians, artists, poets, and authors with physical handicaps and similar successful adjustments in spite of lifelong handicaps. The child with a defect need not grow up to lead a miserable and lonely life if efforts to help him deal with and accept his handicap are made by the parents and other adults in his environment.

These few examples can serve to highlight the kinds of reactions experienced by the handicapped child and his parents. Each specific defect tends to have certain characteristic personality implications but, in general, the reactions of children and their parents to a wide array of defects tend to be somewhat similar.

## Work with Parents

From the foregoing considerations of the psychodynamic aspects of physical handicaps, it is apparent that the impact of the child's defect upon the parents may be quite severe. It is of greatest importance to both the newborn child and his parents, siblings, and larger family circle to offer prompt and effective advice and counseling to the parents of a child with any type of physical malformation.

As pointed out by Freeman (20), skillful and ongoing diagnoses are essential, since misdiagnosis and poor handling of the presentation of the diagnosis by the professional worker contribute to the parents' anxiety, distress, and confusion and may threaten possibilities of initiating an adequate treatment plan when a correct diagnosis is established. Diagnosis may be helped by seeing the child in his home or school setting as well as in the clinical setting. Freeman pointed out the need for tolerance of the parents' anxiety, hostility, and frustration, which is understandable. Parents must be helped to overcome their tendencies either to reject the "helpless" child or to overprotect him and to prevent his optimum development by allowing excessive regressive and passive behavior. They also need assistance with what to expect at the time of surgical intervention to which children often react by showing anxiety, regressive behavior, hostility to the parents, or clinging, demanding behavior and sleep disturbances. Parents should be forewarned to expect such behavior, since, if they do not react adversely, it will often be transient. If such behavior persists unduly, referral for professional help for the child and parents may be necessary. Freeman listed the indications for referral as well as the factors conducive to good adjustment which the interested reader may find valuable.

The author has found that parents often require considerable emotional support and help with accepting the diagnosis of their child's disability. Rather than giving them the information and allowing them to "shop around" for other professional opinions, it is usually most helpful to arrange for immediate follow-up work with the parents to help them to accept, to understand, and to work through the feelings which they have about the diagnosis. Often groups composed of parents with similar or closely related problems find considerable support in a brief group therapy situation. Often parents can see each other's blind spots and help each other to accept the diagnosis, and it is especially helpful to realize that they are not alone in their grief and mourning for their child.

Group therapy and/or individual supportive therapy or casework may be necessary for long periods with some parents who find it more difficult to accept their problems and to work with their child. Occasionally, individual psychiatric treatment may be necessary for certain parents, particularly those with severe depressive reactions.

The study by Fraiberg (18) referred to above points to a specific kind of educational work that is necessary for the parents of blind children and which can help the blind child to overcome many of the developmental handicaps that would otherwise occur.

Each developmental defect tends to have specific pitfalls with which the parents need guidance. For example, a study of mother-child interaction in severe cases of nonverbal, nonambulatory cerebral palsied children, by Shere and Kastenbaum (67), found that the mothers fostered passivity and failed to provide adequate stimulation for cognitive development.

For the child with motor handicaps, parents must be encouraged to allow their child to take his knocks and bruises in order to learn to cope with the world of reality, since overprotection deprives him of his chance to develop autonomy and individuality. These efforts must, however, be titrated with a reasonable degree of protective watchfulness to minimize the child's feelings of being neglected and abandoned.

In general, one might say that each individual child requires a special individual kind of handling based on the type of difficulties and the stage of development. Some parents can do an exceptionally fine job intuitively, and others can be helped to be sensitive and alert to their handicapped child's needs. The professional worker must offer emotional support and intelligent, appropriate advice and guidance in order to assist parents to bring out their child's maximum potential.

# 17

## Milieu Therapy

JOHN R. KLEISER, PH.D.

---

### Introduction

The term "milieu therapy" is an understandable but highly generic term, acting as an umbrella for a wide range of elements presumed to contribute toward the treatment of disturbed individuals. The term seemed to grow out of psychiatric hospital settings as professional workers in them considered their own process. In earlier, less sophisticated days the idea seemed to be that mentally ill persons were placed in a mental hospital in which they were treated with the medicine of psychotherapy. The hospital itself provided containment and care of the physical needs, but the therapeutic process was presumed to originate from the psychiatric treatment itself. The fact that improvement sometimes occurred in the absence of psychotherapy and also that forces within the hospital, other than psychotherapy, clearly seemed to bring about positive changes led to the idea that the hospital itself could operate as a therapeutic device. This further led to the idea that the "environment" or the "milieu," if properly designed and organized, could bring about improvement. The thinking then seemed to become that everything in a hospital setting, other than psychotherapy, was considered to be milieu therapy.

This is not to say that psychotherapy and milieu therapy are in any sense antithetical or that milieu therapy can make individual psychotherapy unnecessary. There are children who can improve or even get well with milieu therapy alone but others, especially with some degree of neurosis, will not. In the latter case, psychotherapy is necessary to increase the likelihood of a good prognosis. Most frequently the ideal treatment for most rapid and favorable progress includes both psychotherapy and milieu therapy operating in harmony together.

Just as there can be an infinite variety in an environment, so there can be a very wide variation in what can be subsumed under therapeutic milieu. In his discussion of this particular term, Redl (5) discusses seven facets of the term "therapeutic" and twelve facets of the word "milieu," including consideration of the physical setup, flexibility of treatment, interpersonal relations, social structure, etc.

In a brief review of the development of the concept, Cumming and Cumming (1) reported that "the use of the word 'milieu' to mean a scientifically planned environment appears to have come into the literature during the late thirties and early forties." They then gave due regard to Harry Stack Sullivan's (7) observation about the behavior of schizophrenics on the ward, the development of Menninger's (4) idea of prescribed attitudes, and the work at Chestnut Lodge (6) involving the therapeutic use of ward personnel. For the purpose of Cumming and Cumming's work, which included an exposition of the theory and practice of milieu therapy in a hospital setting, they came up with the definition "a scientific manipulation of the environment aimed at producing changes in the personality of the patient." While this is a clear, straightforward definition, as the term is actually used in the literature it almost always refers to residential treatment rather than, say, manipulations in the home situation.

The recent popularity of the term itself can perhaps be best illustrated by the following table indicating the number of references subsumed under "milieu therapy" in *Psychological Abstracts*:

$$
\begin{array}{ll}
1965\text{--}1967 & 31 \\
1962\text{--}1964 & 7 \\
1959\text{--}1961 & 0 \\
1956\text{--}1958 & 1 \\
1953\text{--}1955 & 2 \\
1950\text{--}1952 & 0 \\
1947\text{--}1949 & 1 \\
\end{array}
$$

The current discussion is addressed to the question of milieu therapy in the area of behavior pathology in children. For this purpose the term will be used interchangeably with residential treatment in accord with customary usage.

## Advantages of Residential Placement

In recent years there has been a philosophical withdrawal from the idea of residential treatment, with its possibilities for milieu therapy, by many of the people engaged in mental health treatment of various sorts. The trend has been away from large state-supported custodial institutions placed in rural areas, with long-term, if not permanent, placement of patients. Instead, the thrust has been toward community-based mental health facilities, with the idea of maintaining the disturbed individual within the family constellation at all costs. The idea has been that the entire situation should be corrected by means of community clinics, special classes, therapy for parents, family therapy, etc. No one can quarrel with the concept of the healthy child in the healthy family, but attaining this ideal is fraught with many difficulties and, in many instances, impossibilities. Unfortunately the controversy has taken on the aspect of an all-or-nothing issue as though the choice of treatment models was limited to custodial institutional care on the one hand and multifaceted home treatment on the other. In truth, the selection of a homebound or residential treatment (both of which have many varieties) depends in the final analysis upon the particular situation. There are many instances in which good residential treatment (which need not be large, rural, or custodial) is the treatment of choice and improvements can be obtained in no other way.

The kinds of problems that may profit from milieu therapy encompass nearly the whole range of childhood behavior pathology but perhaps particular mention might be made of the psychoses, the intellectually retarded including delinquency, and, to a lesser degree, the neurotics. However, the determining factor should be the gestalt of the child and his situation and not the diagnostic label.

It is the purpose, then, of this discussion to point out some of the indications for, and advantages of, milieu treatment in the residential setting.

## SEPARATION FROM NOXIOUS MILIEU

Individuals engaged in residential treatment are familiar with the many cases in which the referral problem often seems to be at least half solved as soon as the child is placed. Often the disturbed behavior described in pre-enrollment materials does not occur after placement, and very often the child seems different from the one described on paper. This seems to be the result of separation of the child from a noxious and insidious environment.

Often the child and his parents are caught in a circular pathological interaction from which they cannot escape so long as they are confined within the bounds of the home. For example, take the instance of a child who steals because of deep-seated feelings of parental rejection. Each stealing incident induces expressions of rejection from the parents because of the unacceptability of this behavior, which in turn increases the child's unconscious need to steal. It is often difficult to know which came first, the adversive mechanism in the child or the parent, but it is clear that they are locked in a mutually destructive interplay. Often there is a dramatic improvement in the child's behavior as a result of the relief from pressure which occurs to both the parent and the child following placement away from home. This phenomenon, of course, is not universal but occurs frequently enough to make clear the advantage of milieu changes. At times too there occurs a therapeutic circular interaction to replace a previous pathological one between parent and child. In the example cited above, the child's stealing behavior may improve as a result of the reduced pressure after placement which induces some support and acceptance from the parent, in turn reducing the child's need to behave poorly and so on.

The variations in the pathology of the disturbed family situation are of course legion, including such things as divorced and remarried parents, psychotic and neurotic parent or parents, economic deprivation, community rejection, and so on. In residential treatment an effort is made to surround the child with a healthy milieu in substitution for the noxious one from which he was withdrawn. An attempt is made to substitute healthy models in the way of trained and knowledgeable staff for the pathological parental models from which the child, for the time being, is separated.

It is well recognized that emotional maturity is attained through interactions with prime figures in the environment beginning with the nurturing mother as suggested by French and Scott (2), so that it is necessary to supply, carefully, individuals to substitute for those who would usually be available to the "normal" child living at home. Since the child is removed from his real parents, the new environment must provide substantial parent surrogates as well as other significant figures.

By means of providing relationships and avenues for positive identification, the hope is to reverse the adverse processes thus far in operation. In many cases the poor environment from which the child is taken is noncorrectable or at least noncorrectable in time to have a positive effect on the child. For instance, the child could grow to maturity before therapeutic inroads might be made upon a psychotic or neurotic mother. Even if such a parent were treated successfully it would be too late to provide the beneficial influence that the child needs during the period of his life when he is more amenable to change than he is at maturity.

It should be made clear that separation from a noxious milieu is only one indication for residential placement and this is not to infer that parents are universally responsible for the pathology in their children. Their effect upon the child is often beyond their own control (as clearly illustrated by the psychotic mother) or it may be due to circumstances (such as the death of one or both parents) or it may result from nonfamily pressure (for example, the neighborhood abuse of a retarded child).

It might also be pointed out that the effect of the noxious environment on the child is partially the result of the way in which the child's ego reacts toward that environment. Some succumb very easily, others do not, and still others in some way capitalize upon the circumstances. Some of our most eminent people have arisen from wretched circumstances as illustrated by Goertzel and Goertzel (3). The explanations for these contradictions and paradoxes are yet to be derived.

## CONSISTENCY OF PROGRAM

One of the problems in treating a disturbed child in the home situation is the fact that in general he operates under dual or multiple jurisdictions there. Typically his home life is supervised by parents and his school life by teachers and school administrators. There may be other jurisdictions as well, such as therapist, church, and recreational organizations. Each of these jurisdictions usually operates with a measure of autonomy so that, in fact, the child often has to operate under two or more distinct frames of reference. For instance, the home may be permissive and the school structured and direct, or vice versa. Normal children make the transition and adjustment with relative ease but in the case of children with behavior pathology, particularly in cases of organic involvement, such a shift may not be possible and disturbed behavior results or is aggravated from this conflict of jurisdiction. In the case of residential treatment, there is the possibility of greater consistency of program so that the milieu can be more or less controlled over a twenty-four-hour period. To a greater degree than at home there is an overriding administration and therefore hopefully greater persistence of therapeutic effect.

For example, suppose that a child has a specific reading disability (dyslexia) and is therefore in need of specialized techniques to learn reading (usually at a painfully slow rate). In order for treatment to be successful he needs, in addition, understanding of his problem and an absence of criticism and pressure in relation to his reading. In a normal situation he may be traumatized and alienated from reading by an uninformed teacher, parent, peer, etc., quite unintentionally and unwittingly. Of course, the same thing can occur in a residential setting but there are opportunities for greater controls, communication, and training so that the chances for destructive influence are reduced. The dyslexic child is thus surrounded by praise and support for his slow progress (an achievement for him) rather than condemnation and ridicule.

This is not to say that a uniform, consistent therapeutic program is easily or automatically obtained in even the best settings devoted to milieu therapy but relative success is more feasible.

HOMOGENEITY OF PEERS

There seems to be the possibility that a therapeutic effect may result from the grouping together of children with behavior pathology. If the usual classroom teacher is approached about members of her class, she will usually report that one or two of them are problems for her. If these problem children are taken out of the teacher's class and grouped together in a special class with a special teacher, after a short time the special teacher will usually report that one or two of them are her problem students. The point here is that to a certain degree behavior pathology is relative to the group in which the child is a member. In a group composed of children with behavioral problems it is almost inevitable that a wider range of abnormal behavior will be tolerated and regressive acts less severely punished than in a group of more or less normal children. This toleration for pathology and reduced punishment may, in itself, produce positive effects, at least with some children. Perhaps best illustrative of this point is the retarded child, who in the normal classroom is faced with constant failure, ridicule, and punishment. When placed in a special class with children at his own level of intellectual ability, he is no longer subjected to these kinds of pressure, a situation which may result in his making greater use of the limited resources which he does have.

Another therapeutic effect results from the fact that problems can sometimes be attacked more easily when there are others "in the same boat." It sometimes helps a disturbed individual to realize that others are struggling with the same kinds of problems and there is sometimes a certain amount of positive interaction in such instances. This, of course, is a familiar phenomenon in the area of group therapy and it is certainly illustrated in the effectiveness of such organizations as Alcoholics Anonymous with its principle of mutual support. Although this peer support may be used with design and intent, the effect also often occurs spontaneously and should be fostered when it does.

It goes without saying that the homogeneity of the group allows for a treatment process appropriate to that group whereas a deviant individual in a normal group may not be afforded such a therapeutic process. For example, one hyperactive child in a normal class must follow the routine established and his being unable to do so causes endless problems for the teacher and the class, but when he is placed with others like himself, a program of action-oriented projects, shorter class periods, personnel to take him when the pressure mounts, etc., can be designed.

### SPREAD OF RESPONSIBILITY

Working with disturbed and problem children is almost, by definition, a trying and nerve-racking experience. Most people find it is difficult to understand and handle the unusual, and often unexplainable, behavior that is so often encountered. It is thus rather obvious that children of this sort require more people to deal with them and opportunities for such people to have relief from the emotional pressure involved in dealing with them.

The parent in the home has to deal with not only his deep emotional involvement with his own child, but also overlong periods of time in trying to cope with behavior that is difficult and poorly understood.

In school classes for normal children and very often also in special classes in public schools the number of children assigned to one teacher may preclude her devoting the time to the child necessary for effective teaching and influence. In a properly constituted residential placement there is a spread of responsibility among staff with opportunities for relief. The point is that a staff member is able to put in his hours of duty and then, ordinarily, to leave the responsibilities in the hands of someone else and to turn to other aspects of his life, thus maintaining a balance and equilibrium not available to the unrelieved parent or overburdened teacher.

There is, of course, the disadvantage that the child has to deal with a variety of personalities, but experience would suggest that dealing with several individuals who have opportunities for proper relief is better than dealing with a smaller number of people who are near the end of their tether.

One individual pushed beyond the limits of his toleration for disturbed behavior may in one outburst of anger destroy weeks of therapeutic movement in the child. Even the best intentioned parent, teacher, therapist, or whoever needs relief and opportunity to develop facets of his own life independent of the disturbed child.

## EVALUATION AND DIAGNOSIS

It is obvious that evaluation and diagnosis of behavior pathology are not dependent upon residential placement and complete milieu manipulation. Such problems can, and are, studied effectively in out-patient clinics. However, in a milieu treatment center there are greater opportunities for twenty-four-hour observation of the individual under study. There are greater possibilities for integration of observations in school and in the home, as well as in the testing situation. Such observations can be systematized and organized in the way of behavioral ratings and observations, with more objective reporters than are to be found among family members at home. Also in a residential situation, possibilities for integrating diagnosis with treatment may be a little more positive because of a more unified administrative setup. Possibilities for communication among professionals are enhanced by physical proximity and also, hopefully, administrative unity.

Mention might also be made of the maintenance of more unified, consistent records of diagnostic and treatment processes. Not only do such records have value in terms of research potential but also in the practical world of funding. There has developed a complex patchwork of support for the residential study and treatment of children including state programs (all different in extent, requirements, and supervision), federal programs, insurance support, and private agency funding. All of these sources of money require reports (all different) to justify the expenditure of their funds.

Residential centers also have the opportunity for maintaining staffs schooled in multiple disciplines, sometimes to a greater degree than small out-patient clinics. In any event, evaluation and diagnosis is an important part of the process of milieu therapy.

## BREADTH OF PROGRAM RESOURCES

In a residential center which brings together many children with similar problems, there is an opportunity to develop program resources appropriate to those problems. These specialized resources, of course, carry over into afternoon and evening activities, which is not always possible in an out-patient treatment center. For instance, it is feasible to organize athletic activities with other children of equal abilities and interests. The poorly coordinated child who is an outcast on the baseball field being used by normal children is an integrated member of the team when he is in a similar situation with other equally handicapped children. In like manner, scouting activities can be made available to problem children in such a setting, when they would be excluded by their peers in a conventional scouting organization. Appropriate physical facilities can be developed and also the specialized staff needed to handle such children in such activities can be trained.

## Problems in Milieu Therapy

Once it is agreed that milieu therapy is indicated for the treatment of at least some cases, it becomes logical to turn attention to the problems met in trying to implement this treatment.

### TREATMENT COST

One of the major problems involved in milieu therapy is the very basic one of cost. There is practically no limit to the variety, complexity, and, of course, cost that can be utilized in the treatment of exceptional children. Professional services, in the way of psychotherapy, psychodiagnostics, medical studies and treatment, and program specialties are all expensive and becoming more so as the demand increases more rapidly than available personnel resources. What is badly needed is a measure of emotional improvement per dollar spent. Of course, in the present state of our knowledge, this is impossible, so that a great deal of unconfirmed judgment enters into attempts at solving this problem.

It is further complicated by the fact that each of the specialists working with these children operates under the natural bias of his own importance. If a child improves, is it due to his therapy, the kindness of his housemother, his victories on the athletic field, his improvement in reading, or social work with his parents. Of course each of the specialists is struggling for improvement so that when it occurs it is only natural that he should feel that it is the result of his efforts and that he should push for a greater influence in the treatment of future children.

Even though it is agreed that improvement in many cases is due to a combination of factors, the relative importance of various aspects of treatment continues to be a nagging problem. As a result, public facilities are likely to squander money on ineffective treatment and private resources are constantly operating under the temptation to cut corners in order not to put themselves out of business by skyrocketing costs.

In social terms, the problem resolves itself into the question of how much money should, and can, be spent on one child in relation to antici-pated improvement. There is, of course, a point of diminishing returns, but since the commodity being purchased is so ephemeral and unmeasur-able, how is one to know when it is acquired? And when the amount of available money is established, how is it to be distributed? Should there be more recreation and less psychotherapy or vice versa? Should there be higher paid housemothers and less comfortable furnishings or vice versa? The choices and balances are endless and many of the problems incapable of ideal solution.

The answer, of course, lies in some kind of a balance of all of the factors involved, employing the best possible judgment available. It is the attain-ment of this balance that is the difficult, but crucial, task of administrative leadership.

In any event, milieu therapy is bound to be expensive and there is the question as to where the funds are to come from. Two notable trends might be mentioned here. First of all is the tremendous increase in public monies being channeled into this area both in the development of public institutions and agencies and in the application of public funds to the support of children in nonprofit private facilities. The other notable trend is the increase in insurance funds, notably major medical policies, which are being made applicable in this sort of treatment.

In spite of increasing sources of funds, the vast number of untreated children continues to be a vexing and pathetic problem.

## HETEROGENEITY VS. HOMOGENEITY OF GROUPING

One of the decisions to be made in milieu arrangements involves the grouping of children together, with such basic questions as the size of the groups and the kind of problems under which the individuals are operating.

One of the controlling factors is, of course, the nature of the referrals to the particular institution and this would vary not only with the agency but with time in a particular agency. Changes in sources of funds will in-fluence the nature of referrals and there seem to be changes on a purely chance basis. The very complexion of an institution, or groups within an institution, can change with the flow of cases that are enrolled and discharged.

Of course, to a certain degree a treatment center needs to define for itself the kind of children it can handle in terms of its own available services but its nature is also dependent upon the clients who actually come to it.

As far as the size of groups is concerned, it has been generally recognized that in dealing with problem children, the size of the group should be small and the staff-to-student ratio high. In academic areas, for instance, six to eight children is regarded as optimal with individual work in some areas. As far as rooming arrangements are concerned, there has been no general agreement. In many cases single rooms would probably be ideal but beyond the practical reach of most organizations. Double rooms pose problems in the way of supervision of behavior, particularly sexual behavior. In general, next to single rooms, probably three or four to a large room is advisable.

The problem as to how homogeneous groups should be is a very subtle and really unsolved one. Certainly some degree of homogeneity is necessary for treatment and the factors that are probably most relevant are those of age, intellectual level, and severity and nature of the problem. At first blush one might feel that the more homogeneous the group, the better, but in terms of practical experience this does not always seem to be the case. Sometimes progress has been noted in quite heterogeneous groups and sometimes diverse problems complement each other in positive fashion. One term used for this interactive force is "group balance," which is a meaningful if not clearly defined term. Particularly in the case of delinquent problems, groups can sometimes absorb a certain number of such children, but then a point is reached at which the group balance is threatened and there may be an outbreak of undesirable behavior.

One of the frequent fears of parents in the placement of children is that the undesirable symptoms of other children will be picked up by their own child. While this is a very natural kind of fear, once again in actual practice it seems to occur with surprising infrequency. This is probably because the expressed symptoms are based on such deep motivations that such a superficial influence as the behavior of adjacent children is not as influential as might be thought, and in the event that the symptom of another child is acquired, it is probably based on a readiness that would bring out the acquisition in almost any case.

One danger of heterogeneity does lie in too great a variation in intellectual level. In this event, it may occur that more able children will take advantage of those less able to protect themselves.

In any event, the answer at our current level of inadequate information seems to be that a certain amount of homogeneity is beneficial in terms of age, intellectual level, and severity of problem, but that such a principle should not be made a fetish or carried to extreme degrees.

### DISTRIBUTION OF AUTHORITY

Almost by definition, milieu therapy involves a multidisciplinary approach to the problems of the children being treated. While certainly the idea that a wide range of knowledge should be applied in the treatment of the children is a worthy one, this approach also raises the problem of the integration of disciplinary influences in the treatment program. The fact that each discipline views the child from a different vantage point leads to conflict of opinion and the need for some attainment of consistency. There are some decisions about a child that clearly belong to one discipline in which there is not likely to be conflict of opinion. For example, the treatment of measles would belong clearly to the medical doctor, hospitalization for a psychotic episode to the psychiatrist, the selection of an intelligence test to the psychologist, the construction of a classroom examination to the educator, and the collection of background historical information to the social worker. However, there are also a great many decisions about the child that cut across disciplinary lines and should, in fact, involve most or all of them. Such decisions include admission to the institution, termination of treatment, major transfers within the institution, disciplinary measures, major program policies, etc. It is the process by which such decisions are made that is crucial to the particular treatment effectiveness and program. In the traditional out-patient clinic, the triumvirate of psychiatrist, social worker, and psychologist has frequently been dominated by the psychiatrist. In residential settings, the necessary inclusion of education and medicine has further complicated the scene.

This problem area has led to the widespread espousal of the multidisciplinary team approach, the idea being that representatives of the various disciplines get together, thrash out their differences, and arrive at some consistent decision and program. This can, however, lead to a great many expensive professional workers spending long hours in endless routine meetings rather than in treatment and contact with the children under study. For this reason, great care needs to be taken in the administrative setup under which the multidisciplinary function operates. In order for such interaction to be effective, the meetings need to be well chaired, efficiently run, and limited in time. Experience has suggested that the effectiveness of such teams is dependent in large part upon the positive interaction and good will of the team members, rather than only upon the training, skill, or formal qualifications of the individual members. In other words, there is a gestalt to such a team which is not the same as the sum of its individual parts. Personality clashes can destroy the effectiveness of the best intentioned teams and, on the other hand, good will between members can overcome major obstacles. Anyone who has worked in a residential treatment center is familiar with the subtle covert power struggles between individuals and between disciplines.

As in the operation of all groups, there are possibilities for the extremes of authoritarian and democratic operation. Does the individual directly responsible for the program of the child operate with the advice of other disciplines or is he responsible and subservient to them? At one extreme is the danger of unilateral decisions and on the other endless debate and inefficiency. Actually, many of the enigmas in this area are really unresolved, although some middle ground seems to be the most likely desirable administrative setup.

## HOME CONTACTS

A child placed away from home for purposes of milieu therapy continues to need some sort of relation and contact with his family. It is very rare that an institution can, or should, completely substitute for "family" and "home." Once again the degree and frequency of such contacts depend upon the individual circumstances of the case, but certain general guidelines can perhaps be suggested.

Immediately after placement, experience suggests that a period of separation of perhaps six weeks to allow for working through of separation anxieties on both sides seems advisable. Of course, contact by mail at all times, including this period, is generally supported and encouraged, but even this may need some judicious counsel and control. The anxious mother who writes two or three letters a day and sends a package every other day needs guidance to space her communications more judiciously, as does the family who does not write for weeks on end. Similarly, telephone calls will need to come under scrutiny and control.

There is more or less general agreement that milieu treatment should be on a twelve-month rather than a nine- or ten-month basis. Interruption of two or three months during the summer, in many cases, would have a disruptive effect. The general compromise has been a twelve-month program with two or three vacation periods at home of two or three weeks. Experience has further suggested that in many cases even a three-week vacation is too long and that a maximum of two weeks is probably more advisable. Of course, while the individual is in treatment, it is also advisable that steps be taken, if possible, to modify the noxious home situation, including counseling or therapy for members in the home where indicated.

It is essential that efforts be made toward establishing the situation in which both the home and the institution are working toward the same goals. Parents who, for one reason or another, do not support the efforts of the institution can have a devastating effect upon the treatment program. Parents who bypass rules, make unwarranted promises to children about termination of treatment, who complain about minor lapses on the part of the institution, are all well known. It is necessary to take steps of all kinds to see that the family understands and supports the treatment program. These steps include correspondence, individual conferences, parent institutes, the help of professionals at home, etc.

All of these efforts are directed toward physically separating the child from the home, and at the same time maintaining as healthy a psychological contact with it as is possible.

## CONFLICTS BETWEEN INTERESTS OF GROUP
## AND INDIVIDUAL

One of the persistent and knotty problems in residential milieu treatment arises from the conflict of the needs of the individual in relation to the needs of the group of which the individual is a part. It is easy to speak of a high degree of individualization of program in order to surround the person with forces necessary to his positive growth, but such an individual can not, and should not, live in isolation.

In practice the point of confrontation comes between the staff member who works on an individual basis, such as psychotherapist, tutor, speech therapist, etc., and staff members who are charged with working with the group, such as teachers, recreation workers, etc. For instance, it might be indicated that one student, because of his particular constellation of problems, should be allowed to walk out of classes at any time he wanted to, and this would be quite therapeutic for him, but the teachers would contend that if all students were permitted to do this, the classrooms would be empty most of the time. They would contend that if other students are not allowed this same privilege, they will feel unfairly treated. And, of course, it is recognized that the interaction in any one-to-one situation is frequently different than in a one-to-group relation.

In practice, there must be some kind of a compromise; certainly a treatment institution needs to be much more flexible than a normal situation, but some limitations are necessary to avoid chaos. It is possible to develop a certain level of understanding in the group so that the members come to realize that each individual has different problems with different requirements, so that there can be a reduction in the expectation of exactly equal treatment. However, this takes a great deal of skill and experience, as well as a certain amount of good will between group and individual workers.

The importance of leadership in the residential setting is particularly highlighted in relation to these competitive struggles of disciplines and individuals. It is necessary that the leadership project a definite and equal respect for all disciplines involved, meet with those involved equally, and expect and instill as much as possible a working rapport among the disciplines. Such a rapport can not be entirely legislated but a tone can be expressed and a way of operating set which can reduce to a minimum the adversive friction.

## PRECEDENCE OF ACTIVITIES

As the treatment techniques are expanded and compounded, it is inevitable that the problem of the relative importance of these elements should come into question, in relation to which takes precedence. Does an appointment for psychological testing warrant canceling a therapy session? Is participation in a soccer game more important than a dental appointment? Should speech therapy or a remedial reading session be canceled if one must go? It is clear that the meshing of schedules becomes both difficult and crucial as services to the children are improved. Flexibility, a certain amount of frustration, and infinite patience are required on the part of all staff members. A therapist learns early that a rigid schedule is not only difficult to maintain but leads to ineffective therapy. The child who is deprived of a trip to the zoo, a visit from a parent, or participation in an important athletic event by a therapy session is not likely to profit from it and may indeed react negatively in a generalized fashion toward therapy.

Any institution needs to develop its written and unwritten rules of precedence, and the more that they can be communicated among staff, the less will be the sources of conflict. For instance, it may develop that a one-shot psychological diagnostic evaluation would take precedence over ongoing therapy sessions and therapy sessions, where necessary, may have to cut into some academic classes. Special events and trips, having great meaning to a child, take precedence over nearly all other activities. Problems come, of course, where the ground rules are not universally understood and where a lack of preplanning leads to last-minute changes. Minimization of problems in regard to these details seems to rest upon good communication and good will between staff, so that all are informed, and, in instances in which there are inevitable conflicts, there is a certain amount of give and take to overcome them.

CONTROL OF ACTING-OUT BEHAVIOR

In a residential treatment center, one of the major problems in management is the control and handling of acting-out behavior, particularly physical aggression against other students and staff, sexual acting out, and elopements, because of the danger to the individual and to other individuals. Theoretically, an effective program of milieu therapy should keep these kinds of behavior at a minimum, but in practice, since techniques fall short of perfection and also because progress is based on a process taking a period of time, these kinds of behavior can be expected to occur. It might be noted in passing that these behaviors, while posing problems, are not always adversive or regressive. For instance, an aggressive act on the part of a passive, withdrawn child may represent a step forward. Similarly, an elopement may represent a crisis in a student's life, which can be used therapeutically to make further strides forward.

In general, control in this respect rests very clearly upon adequate supervision. Nearly always these outbursts occur under circumstances in which the students are, to some degree, left on their own. Of course, the exact amount and the nature of supervision depend on the type and severity of the problem being dealt with. In some cases it amounts to the literal presence of a staff member with a small group of students at all times; in less severe instances it means an adult in the general area of activity. Of course severely disturbed children may need to be supervised in closed facilities in which it is physically impossible for them to express such needs as the elopement.

In cases of significant incidents, it is advisable to have available facilities for the rapid removal and placement of the individual involved, until a decision can be made as to disposition. It is usually best if this is a closed and psychiatrically supervised facility of some kind. The reason for this is that it solves the immediate aspects of the problem, assures the safety of the individual and other individuals, and allows time for the process of rational decision-making and the involvement of key figures. For instance, supposing a child elopes and is picked up by the police (a relatively infrequent but dramatic example of acting out). To return him to his group might lead to subsequent elopement and also contagion and disturbance to others of the group. Therefore, in this instance, the child would be placed temporarily in an available closed facility while the circumstances of the elopement were investigated, the therapist notified, the family involved, etc. Then a decision can be made as to placement back in the group, transfer to another facility, return home, or whatever. It is, of course, advisable to consider the precipitating events leading up to such incidents in the hope that future recurrences can be reduced by modification of the treatment program.

While proper supervision and restraint are necessary to control acting-out behavior, they are only the first steps in the amelioration of the problems involved. It is necessary to encourage the sublimation of the underlying impulses into acceptable channels. In many respects the major goal of residential treatment is to strengthen the ego through the development of socially useful skills of all kinds. This provides the child with the means of discharging his tensions, aggressions, and impulses in ways which will be useful and acceptable both to himself and those around him. Take for example a slow-learning adolescent boy who has been faced all his life by demands from his home and school for academic achievement beyond his capability. His frustration leads to a fury which explodes in destructive acts such as destroying school property. When he is placed in a well-structured vocational training program followed by a sheltered workshop and then employment in the community, his skills are increased, his aggression sublimated, and his acting out eliminated.

## TERMINATION OF TREATMENT

Depending upon the effectiveness of milieu therapy, a point is reached at which the problem of termination of treatment becomes crucial. In some cases, of course, treatment continues into adulthood and may be necessary for a lifetime. In this latter instance, the specialized milieu becomes a way of life and a permanent need. However, in most cases the problem is one of returning the child or young adult to the normal community.

For some children this means a return to the homes from which they came. Hopefully, any pathological forces existing there have been ameliorated during the period of treatment. In order to make this transition it becomes advisable for the child to have more frequent contacts with home in the latter part of his residential placement. This may be effected by more frequent weekend visits, where feasible, and possibly spending summers at home rather than at the institution. Professional agencies in the home situation need to be given information to help them in the program designed for the child at home.

In instances in which there is considerable improvement in the child, but the home situation continues to be noxious, the transition needed may be into a more normal situation but not with the family. This may take the form of placement in a normal boarding school which provides the child with a more normal milieu but with continued limitation in contacts with his family. It may, in other words, be necessary to bypass return to the noxious family by schooling away from home followed by further college or vocational training with the attainment of adult life relatively independent of the family.

The transition into the community may be difficult for some students who have found a protected life in the residential treatment center. For these children, an intermediate step may be necessary in the way of half-way houses which combine some of the aspects of institutional protection with some of the aspects of normal community life. In these settings the students are gradually given more responsibility for their own management and can gradually engage themselves in community life by means of training or jobs outside of the institution, with participation in community organizations. Finally, the point may be reached at which complete separation from institutional ties can be effected.

## Conclusions and Outlook

It seems clear that in spite of the many problems encountered in milieu therapy in a residential setting, it is the treatment of choice in many instances. Certainly the concept will continue to be developed with its elements subjected to ever greater scrutiny and development. Undoubtedly current knowledge in the field and its application will be considered primitive and unscientific in the near future as more rigorous research and development of techniques are effected.

# 18

## Child Psychiatry in the School

WILLIAM STENNIS, M.D.

### Historical and Theoretical Perspective

Education had its beginnings in preliterate societies through the association of children with their elders. The elders did not really see themselves as teachers; the children did not really feel like pupils. This primitive beginning eventually became formalized, first through initiation rites at puberty as the child was passing from childhood to adulthood. This transition—the passing from childhood to adulthood—continues to be one of the major purposes of education: to help the child pass through childhood and become a successful adult. At these early initiation rites, the child was taught the origin of the earth and his tribe. From this he gained a tribal and self identity. The myths that were told him about the origins of the earth and of his tribe were often quite characteristic of the character traits of his people (13).

For example, in the creation myth of the Ute Indians of southwestern Colorado, it is said that God was sitting around His heaven one day and became quite bored. To relieve his boredom, he decided to make something. Accordingly, he began to gather together a large amorphous mass of material that surrounded him, shaped it into a round ball, and pushed it through a round opening in the heavens, thus creating the earth. The Utes' culture is extremely aggressive and has other rather direct anal characteristics. The word "Ute" is derived from the Indian word "Nuwinta," which in effect means "person" as distinguished from bear, lion, or deer. The word "Navaho" also means "person" in the same sense (12).

In addition to learning his tribal and self identity, the child learned that certain restrictions were placed on his impulses, such as the tribal taboos toward food, behavior, and sex. Eventually the control of these initiation rites was assumed by a sort of priest-medicine man-teacher. Thus the past reveals that the professions of teaching and medicine have a common origin.

When man developed written language, he used it for two purposes: first, to carry on the religious tradition of the people, and later, in keeping records of business transactions. In the beginning only the priests, still really a combination priest-medicine man-teacher, were allowed to have the skills of written language. This gradually became the province of businessmen as well, and the school took on the added task of education for mastery of the world. While medicine eventually split itself off from the priesthood, religion and education continued to be closely associated. In the early days of our own country, the church saw education as its responsibility. Although the Supreme Court has separated the public schools from the church, the school still holds itself responsible for the proper behavior of the child. Social institutions have the task of finishing what the family has left undone, that is, mastery of pregenital impulses and resolution of the oedipal conflict.

The specialty of child psychiatry is in actuality little more than fifty years old. The official subspecialty became a reality in 1958. I prefer to trace its origins to France in the early 1800s when Jean-Marc-Gaspard Itard, a young physician at the Paris School for the Deaf, set about trying to help a severely deprived child. In the *Wild Boy of Aveyron*, Itard tells the story of a ten-year-old boy captured in the woods of southern France who had been living for some years wild as an animal. The most eminent psychiatrist of the day, Pinel, saw this child and pronounced him an idiot, but Itard took it upon himself to educate this boy, who had no speech and who literally behaved like an animal. In 1825, Itard longed for a science that would:

Bring to bear all the resources of their present knowledge in order to develop him physically and morally, or, at least, if this proved impossible or fruitless, there would be found in this age of observation someone who, carefully collecting the history of so surprising a creature, would determine what he is and deduce from what he lacked the hitherto uncalculated sum of knowledge and ideas which man owes to his education (10).

The boy was captured in September of 1799 by three sportsmen. Itard writes of Pinel's report:

Proceeding first with an account of the sensory functions of the young savage, Pinel showed that his senses were reduced to such a state of inertia that the unfortunate creature was, according to his report, quite inferior to some of our domestic animals. His eyes were unsteady, expressionless, wandering vaguely from one object to another without resting on anybody; they were so little experienced in other ways and so little trained by the sense of touch that they never distinguished an object in relief from one in a picture. His organ of hearing was equally insensitive to the loudest noises and to the most touching music. His voice was reduced to a state of complete muteness and only a uniform guttural sound escaped him. His sense of smell was so uncultivated that he was equally indifferent to the odor of perfume and the fetid exhalation of dirt with which his bed was filled. Finally, the organ of touch was restricted to the mechanical function of the grasping of objects. Proceeding then to the state of the intellectual functions of this child, the author of the report presented him to us as being quite incapable of attention (except for the objects of his needs) and consequently of all those operations of the mind which attention involves. He was destitute of memory, of judgment, of aptitude for imitation and was so limited in his ideas, even those relative to his immediate needs, that he had never yet succeeded in opening a door or climbing up on a chair to get the food that had been raised out of reach of his hands. In short, he was destitute of all means of communication and attached neither expression nor intention to his gestures or to the movements of his body. He passed rapidly and without any apparent motive from apathetic melancholy to the most immoderate peals of laughter. He was insensible to every kind of moral influence. His perception was nothing but a computation taught by gluttony, his pleasure an agreeable sensation of the organ of taste, and his intelligence the ability to produce a few incoherent ideas relative to his wants. In a word, his whole life was a completely animal existence (10).

Itard set for himself five goals:

1. To interest him in the social life by rendering it more pleasant to him than the one he was just leaving, and above all more like the life which he had just left.
2. To awaken his nervous sensibility by the most energetic stimulation, and occasionally by intense emotion.
3. To extend the range of his ideas by giving him new needs and by increasing his social contacts.
4. To lead him to the use of speech by inducing the exercise of imitation through the imperious law of necessity.
5. To make him exercise the simplest mental operations upon the objects of his physical needs over a period of time, afterwards inducing the application of these mental processes through the objects of instruction (10).

Among other things, Itard had the boy match shapes of triangles, circles, and squares.

Although his success was limited, he began an important trend. His pupil was Seguin, whose form board is a part of our present-day Stanford-Binet Intelligence Test. Seguin's pupil was another physician, Marie Montessori, who worked so diligently with the retarded children of Rome and contributed so much to kindergarten education.

The early part of this century saw the development of psychoanalysis in Vienna, and through association with her father, a young schoolteacher, Miss Anna Freud, began applying psychoanalytic principles to education. Her fellow teachers, Mrs. Berta Bornstein, Mrs. L. Peller, and Mrs. Emma Plank, eventually became well-known child analysts. Dr. Fritz Redl, one of our country's foremost authorities on delinquency, also began as a teacher in that Viennese group. Even in modern times child psychiatry and education have common origins and interests (1, 13).

In spite of our common origins and the fact that psychiatry and education have tended to mutually fertilize one another, there remains considerable disagreement over just what the school should be doing and whether or not we, as physicians and child psychiatrists, have any business there. This is not a new controversy.

Consideration must be given to the question, what constitutes education and what is the proper way to be educated. At present, there are differences of opinion as to the proper task to be set; for all people do not agree as to the things the young ought to learn, even with a view to virtue or with a view to the best life, nor is it clear whether the study should be regulated more with regard to intellect or with regard to character. And confusing questions arise out of the education that actually prevails, and it is not at all clear whether the pupil should practice pursuits that are practically useful or morally edifying, or higher accomplishments—for all of the views have won the support of some judges (8).

This is an opinion first propounded only twenty-three centuries ago by Aristotle.

It was from Plato's *Republic* that Rousseau built his thoughts about education. Plato saw education as the central concern of any well-ordered government and the preoccupation of man throughout his life. He felt that education should free the mind of the prejudices of those around him and motivate him to accept responsibility for helping others achieve the same goal. For Plato, one of the effects of true education was to make a man profoundly dissatisfied with what he had been previously taught, and he felt that formal schooling culminated not in a finished body of knowledge but in the mastery of a method for the lifelong pursuit of wisdom. With Plato's philosophy behind him, Rousseau emphasized the development of the child's natural latent abilities through education. Pestalozzi emphasized developing powers of observation and perception. The man who founded kindergarten, Froebel, emphasized the process of learning through activity. Piaget has awakened us to how much we need to know about the evolution of cognitive processes in children and, with Froebel, believed education should be an active exploring experience.

Dr. Robert Waelder said, "It is the task of education to tame the instincts without damaging them." The child is born with drives, both sexual and aggressive. These drives cannot be allowed completely free expression lest the individual have no control over his behavior and end up a psychopath. Although we must help a child to bridle his instincts, we must never forget that these same instincts are the driving force behind all great human accomplishments. If controls are too loose, the resulting product cannot live in harmony with society. If controls are excessive, the very strength of the drive is weakened. If overcontrol persists, we have a crippled and restricted personality, no different from a withered arm or leg (17).

In the treatment room it is our goal to understand the individual child. We want to know what things are blocking his move toward maturity.

We communicate our understanding of this block to him in such a fashion that his easily damaged narcissism is not injured. Once we have managed through understanding to release whatever is blocking his maturation, we try to educate him toward successful and acceptable sublimations. In a broad sense, our treatment task is similar to that of the teacher. There are marked differences, however, in how we go about this. These, I think, have given rise to some unfortunate misconceptions. In the treatment room we deal with one child. The atmosphere we attempt to create is one of unique permissiveness. The child is permitted to say anything, anything he wishes, and we place as few restrictions as possible on what he does, short of saving our bodies and offices from total destruction. This permissive air is designed to help the child relax his defenses so that he can talk about his worries and fears and, through verbalized understanding, overcome them.

The same air of permissiveness is not desirable in most classrooms. Unfortunately, some have suggested that this atmosphere be encouraged in the classroom. The technique has great value in the consulting room; it has little place in the classroom.

What kind of atmosphere should be created in the classroom?

The tools of education are: (a) a loving relationship with the teacher, (b) punishment and reward, and (c) stimulation of curiosity.

For a successful educational experience, any child must begin with a comfortable, kind, mutually respectful, loving relationship with his teacher. He must receive before he can give. In order for a child to have this with a teacher, he must first have it with his parents and his peers. These love relationships with parents and teachers are the preservers of the instincts. A child who comes to a teacher without having received this love at home is a challenge for the best teacher, but many teachers do succeed even with them. As our school system expands, including younger children from culturally and emotionally deprived homes, we will succeed even more. To establish this kind of relationship with her pupils, the teacher must be available to them. Large classes dehumanize this relationship and give it a mechanistic flavor. The teacher must not overidentify with the emotionally disturbed child nor blame his parents too quickly for all of his distresses. Neither must she be intimidated by his parents or constantly strive to make the child do what his parents want him to do rather than what he can do. Her relationship with him must always be that of a reasonable adult. If she can establish this loving relationship, the teacher who is sure of her own feelings, who is not ambivalent about establishing controls, generally finds it easy to instill discipline. The child who is disciplined is one who has received reasonable external controls from a loving adult and who has made these external controls part of himself. The teacher will find it necessary to exert a constant pressure on her pupils to perform, but this pressure must be accompanied by a tolerant respect for the child's wish not to perform. The impulse itself is not condemned. One must show a tolerance for the impulse while at the same time asking that it be controlled.

In this setting the greatest of rewards is approval, and the greatest of punishments is disapproval of a loved human being. When the impulses are controlled, the drives behind the impulses likewise become easily directed into curiosity and the desire to learn.

It has been said so often that it has become a virtual cliché that "children want to learn." The cliché is correct but it does not go far enough. Children want to learn because their all-consuming passion is to be grown up. They play at almost nothing else and they want to be in school for the simple reason that that is where you learn to be grown up.

It is the task of the teacher and the child psychiatric consultant of the school system to help each child to grow up to meet his maximum potential; and in order to do this we, as consultants, must be experts on every aspect of the child—anthropologically, psychologically, neurologically, and educationally. We must not be afraid to use all of the knowledge gained from all of the behavioral sciences to help every child achieve his maximum potential. But in using this knowledge, we must bear in mind that our major task is translating it into usable classroom procedures.

The generalizations just presented are fairly definite. In the educational field, theoretical foundation is not nearly so well structured. Many professional educators are often confused about what is health and what is illness. The vast majority of times health simply means conformity. This is conformity particularly from a behavioral standpoint, and becomes especially important when classes are very large, as they frequently are in new growing communities and in certain other schools. Many educators are intolerant of the usual turmoils of adolescence. Often overconforming, basically disturbed adolescents without evidence of behavioral difficulty may be overlooked. Even experienced teachers have difficulty differentiating when a child is disturbed and when he is passing through a maturational phase. Because of many divergent theories of educational practice, teachers are torn between whether to create a permissive class atmosphere or a highly structured one. "If a teacher demands too much docility, the pupil may some day have trouble thinking independently and imaginatively; if too much time is spent in 'free expression,' mastery of basic skills may suffer" (2). This is the conflict often facing the teacher, and in this context it is well for us to bear in mind that the training of teachers, like the training of psychiatrists, has different theoretical orientations.

Consider briefly the three main theoretical orientations of teacher training. They are subject-centered teaching, child-centered teaching, and teacher-centered teaching.

In subject-centered teaching the approach places an emphasis on the teacher's knowledge of his subject. Those who support this view hold that education courses are basically of little value and tend to interfere with the teacher's mastery of his own field. They also hold that good teaching is something that cannot be taught. They maintain that if a teacher knows his subject well, his personal characteristics are not important. A more moderate view holds that the teacher's personality does influence his pupils and that mere knowledge of subject matter is not sufficient. This is counterbalanced, they feel, by the teacher who knows what he stands for and has enthusiasm for his subject. Through this he may stimulate thinking and aid the integration of the pupils' personalities (2).

The second type of teacher education, child-centered teaching, has perhaps been strongly influenced in the twentieth century by the impact of psychoanalytic theory, which recognizes the importance of the early years of life—years which offer opportunities not only for growth, but for personality damage. The backers of this child-centered theory of teaching hold that the teacher should perhaps be the most expert individual in our culture, and that the mental health of the child should be her specific preoccupation. Emphasis is on helping the teachers gain a thorough understanding and knowledge of the child not only in the classroom, but also in relation to his parents and the community at large. This philosophy has had such a significant impact on our culture that legislative acts have been passed requiring specific courses in educational or developmental psychology as a prerequisite for teacher certification. But this approach has created many problems, in that frequently teachers are unable to absorb the insights they have gained through this training. It has also created confusion about the role of the teacher. There are teachers who become more concerned with "helping" individual children than educating them. The aim, of course, in the ideal situation would be for the teacher trained in this philosophy to create a classroom atmosphere that makes learning, reasoning, exploring, and mastering possible for all of her pupils (2).

The most recent trend in teacher training seems to suggest a new emphasis on teacher-centered training; the teacher rather than the child is seen at the center of the educational process. Backers of this approach insist that the teacher candidate must have an ability to relate to children, to relate to authority, and to show evidence of emotional strength. Their philosophy is summed up in two fundamental principles. They hold that, first, the teacher needs perspective about himself and some insight into his own dynamics. Second, the teacher should have a knowledge of his role as a teacher distinguished from other roles that may be a part of the educational setting. It is held that teachers with this orientation will foster a consistent classroom atmosphere that encourages the development of healthy personalities.

The majority of teachers, however, feel that their own educational experiences in teacher training have been inadequate. There is a need for a re-evaluation of the entire system of teacher training.

This consideration of the theoretical aspects of consultation in the schools would be incomplete without a discussion of the elementary and secondary guidance counselors. Secondary guidance evolved from the need to aid adolescents in their struggles through what Dr. Erik Erikson called "the identity crisis" (5).

"Now that I am through with high school, where do I really go from here?" I am told that there was a time in Europe when a late adolescent who was struggling with this crisis could take a year or so after high school to work and give his personality time to settle. In America, we are less tolerant of the late adolescent's need for time. To help us with our wish that the adolescent get on with his education, the secondary guidance counselor was established. He was to help answer practical questions like "What college should I attend?" or "What course should I take?" or "What am I really suited for?" Since his approach was a practical, logical, sensible one, he was soon given the task of preparing rosters, sending out transcripts, pleading with colleges to take a certain child, placating anxious parents. In the midst of all of this he was saddled with myriad time-consuming clerical details that could often be handled by fairly bright high school sophomores. With the current increasing awareness of mental health, he has now been given the additional task of handling all of the emotional and adjustment problems of the most complex and difficult of ages. And certainly he is a logical choice, for in the process of helping late adolescents, he soon discovered that it was more complex than just finding the right college or best roster for them. He found that this strange group of unpredictable human beings, whom he would so much like to help, did not always respond in a reasonable, logical fashion and that his persuasive skills were far less than he could have hoped for. Being a diligent man, he turned to psychology and intelligence tests and aptitude tests and interest tests, ad nauseam, which sometimes left him more perplexed than ever. He frequently discovered that when adolescents and parents are presented with the results of these tests, they choose to ignore them or accuse the counselor of invasion of privacy or favoritism or other things that parents do when they are distressed. Such a situation is enough to make anyone retreat to the security of preparing rosters or transcripts.

There are, however, a few brave secondary counselors who have begun to suspect that the answer may lie in the unconscious struggles of the adolescent and that through careful study of his personality, both conscious and unconscious, his anxiety diminishes and more answers are available. This is a truly courageous step for it means changing one's entire orientation from conscious thought processes that are logical and reasonable to an additional consideration of unconscious thought processes that often seem illogical and unreasonable.

The secondary counselor's student has some very important differences from those seen by his elementary counterpart. Some of the adolescents come to him of their own accord and ask for help. They complain of anxiety, of depression, of confusion, often directly, more often indirectly in the form of concern over their curriculum or worry over whether or not they will get into college. The counselor, sensitive to the unconscious, will easily see the internal struggle. He can obtain a description of the pupil's behavior not only from his teacher but from the pupil himself. He can glimpse the internal dynamics through the adolescent's telling him what is wrong. Though often tied and responsible to his parents, especially in our culture, he is in the process of breaking his childish tie with them and establishing himself separately from them both physically and psychologically, and he is receptive to outside help in the struggle.

Such is not the case with the younger child. He is deeply dependent on his parents, and most of the time he is brought to see the elementary counselor rather than coming on his own. It is extremely unlikely that he will be able, without special interview techniques, to verbalize his real concerns. The child between six and ten and a half years who replies, "I don't know," when he is asked why he behaved in a particular fashion may well be telling the truth, especially if one translates what it means—"I don't know why consciously! The reason is not available to me for verbalization." This does not mean that a child of this age does not know all of the time. He may know, but to put things into words is a more difficult task for him. He is still too close to action. He may fear, for example, that if he says that he is restless and disrupts the class because of anxiety, when he returns to class the mere fact that he has said this to you will increase the chance of it happening again. Or if he tells you that he has nightmares of monsters eating him up, this telling the fear might cause them to be worse that night. In addition, his own self-esteem is so low and insecure that he has tremendous shame over what you will think of him as a person and sometimes actual fear of what you as an adult will do to him for thoughts he feels are bad—because for him thoughts are still so close to deeds. The child in pre-adolescence is in an even more difficult situation. These children can say very little about anything because of their internal anxieties. These result chiefly from the hormonal changes of puberty. The girls wonder when menstruation will come, who will be first or last in class, and as their bodies change, whether they will be pretty or ugly, and whether they really want to have menstruation begin at all. The boys are repeatedly pulling their shirttails and sweaters down to hide their involuntary erections evoked by all sorts of nonspecific stimuli. A thirteen-year-old male patient of mine said to me, "Boy, that principal of ours is a rat fink—he won't let us wear our shirttails out or long baggy sweaters. Doesn't he know why we need them?"

The elementary guidance counselor finds herself too often trained along the same lines as her secondary counterpart and often with a descriptive rather than a dynamic model of childhood. She knows that a seven-year-old should behave in this fashion and an eight-year-old in that, but she has difficulty recalling all of the norms, and often if she can, she does not know how they will help the third-grade teacher with Bobby. The role of the guidance counselor needs to be more clearly defined on both secondary and elementary levels.

## The Technique of Consultation

### INTRODUCTION

In my capacity as consultant to the school system in Bucks County, Pennsylvania, for many years, I functioned in a number of practical roles that I will describe in some detail.

1. The service role of diagnostician.
2. The administrative role of developing a program of elementary guidance.
3. The preventive role of teacher education.
4. The research role of developing more individualized instruction.

Before I begin a consideration of each of these areas, let me set the stage for the atmosphere you find in most schools.

Many educators feel that child psychiatry and psychoanalysis have something to offer, but they fear us as well. They fear we will turn some kind of mystical power on them and discover their innermost secrets. They fear that we will see their mistakes and tell the school board and the community. They fear our knowledge will supplant theirs and that cherished pedagogical theories and techniques will be overthrown wholesale. They fear we will "take over," but what they really fear is that we will discover their sadistic or sexual impulses toward the child. Like the English schoolboys in William Golding's *Lord of the Flies* (7), like each of us in our own personal analyses, like all human beings throughout the ages, they fear mostly the depths of their own unconscious. Their unconscious will fight against being understood and will show its resistant head in countless unique, surprising, and frustrating ways. But if they find us helpful, they will ask us back.

### DELIVERING DIAGNOSTIC SERVICES

On one of my first days as a school consultant I was met in one of the schools by a conscientious guidance counselor who told me that he had eight cases for me to see that day. At one time in my training career, I was the only psychiatrist for some 350 very ill patients and I had considerable empathy for his pressure and distress. At the same time, I also had a realistic view of my own capacity to adequately evaluate this many children in one day. I knew that I could make a few educated guesses about some of them and I knew that some of these guesses might be helpful, but I also knew that I owed it to each child to give him or her very careful consideration. The decisions I made could conceivably influence the rest of his life. I was aware that should I make a mistake in judgment it is unlikely that any of these children would die a physical death of that mistake, but I was keenly aware that a mistake could leave them crippled psychologically, which is certainly no less tragic than a physical death or a muscular paralysis.

I also considered that if I listened to the thoughts and observations this counselor presented and then gave omnipotent sounding advice, I was likely to create the impression that I could actually evaluate eight children in one day. Also, if I made judgments on minimum data, he would have no chance to follow the steps of my reasoning, no chance to see the data on which I based my recommendations, no chance to acquire some of my knowledge and skills. I decided that it was not only my task to adequately evaluate children but to enhance the skills of this counselor so that he could see more children and possibly prevent the necessity for psychiatric intervention. I am convinced that one of the best ways of teaching preventive psychiatry is through careful and intensive study of one child. We are a rapidly growing nation. According to a conservative estimate made in 1962, there are approximately sixty million children below the age of fourteen, comprising some 30 percent of our population (3). This need to increase the understanding of children is made even more urgent by the fact that we, as a nation, are realizing that children and their education are our most precious investment for the future, and we are increasingly sensitive to the need to bring more of them to their maximum potential. The current two thousand certified child psychiatrists cannot accomplish this task alone.

My first practical suggestion to anyone doing school consultations is to limit the number of children you see and help as many people as you can to understand those you see to the fullest.

## WHAT DOES THE SCHOOL WANT FROM YOU?

In most schools, the teacher tries to handle the child she has concern about through her classroom contact with him or through consultation with his parents. The problems she cannot handle she refers to the principal. Those he cannot or does not wish to handle either with the child directly or with his parents are referred to me or to the guidance counselor if he has one. When I enter a school (I think it is infinitely preferable to go to the school rather than having the child brought to you) I meet first with the principal and teacher, find out what questions they want answered, and try to get some idea of what they think I can do for them. This is often not easy to do. Their wishes may range all the way from "get this kid out of my hair" and "please help this over-anxious teacher" to "help me get back at this kid's parents who gave me a hard time at the last PTA meeting." Most often, however, their concerns are about a child who is a behavior problem or who has a learning disturbance. As the chief complaint is discussed with you, make sure that the school records are available. Usually when a child is being referred for psychiatric reasons, you have some kind of IQ on him, and if you are lucky enough to have a psychologist with you, he can begin doing testing while you see the parents.

### HOW DO THE PARENTS FEEL ABOUT THE EVALUATION?

If the school is willing to spend time, money, and effort on a child in a psychiatric referral, it is reasonable to expect that both parents come to the school for a meeting with you. It is my own practice to refuse to see a child whose parents refuse to come to the school. In a period of some twenty minutes, I make an effort to explore the parents' concerns with the typical questions of: "When did it begin?"—"What seemingly related or unrelated factors were associated with its beginning?"—"What makes it worse?"—"What makes it better?"

Be prepared to hear the parents state that the child has no problems and that it's all the school's fault. It is better to allow this defense and try to understand why it is necessary. After the chief complaint has been delineated, I then explore as rapidly as possible the development of the child—a history of pregnancy and birth, searching carefully for organic factors, the developmental milestones in the first year of life, weaning, toilet training, phobias in the oedipal period, school adjustment in latency, and sexual disturbances or anxieties in adolescence. I ask a few brief questions about the parental backgrounds, such as the size of their families, the personalities of their parents, brief memories of their early childhood, their aspirations during adolescence, and the current family anxieties. You may wonder whether or not this can all be done in twenty minutes. Recall how long it took you to take a history the first few days of your internship and compare that with how long it took you by the ninth or tenth month. It can be done if you know what you're looking for and you try to get it done in the time you have. This interview with the parents serves not only to get historical data but to establish a relationship on which your later recommendations can be based.

### PSYCHIATRIC, PSYCHOLOGICAL, AND NEUROLOGICAL SURVEY OF THE CHILD

I next spend anywhere from ten to twenty minutes with the child, gathering as much data as possible in a short period of time. I invariably ask him why he thinks I am seeing him, his problems, worries, or fears related and unrelated to school, his dreams, and what his ideas are about why he is having problems in school. I explore with him who is at home and what kind of relationship he has with them. I ask about what he wants to be in the future. My approach is easygoing, free, and very active. If I don't have a psychologist along, I'm not at all averse to asking him to copy circles, triangles, diamonds, or Bender cards. I frequently ask a child to draw a house, tree, and person, and from time to time I present Rorschach cards and ask him to respond to them. If I strongly suspect the presence of significant organic factors, I do a brief neurological examination with particular emphasis on the so-called subtle neurological signs. Bucks County Schools has produced a film and television tape demonstrating the technique of neurological examination of children (14). I am especially interested in the child's coordination, his ability to balance, his ability to touch his nose with his finger, walking heel to toe, the simultaneous touch test, the ability to oppose finger and thumb, pronation and supination, his extra-ocular eye movements, undetected strabismus, the activity of his upper and lower deep tendon and abdominal reflexes, the presence of ankle clonus or Babinski. Why do I go to these lengths? Because I have found an inordinately high incidence of children with significant organic dysfunctioning of the central nervous system and because I want to know the total functioning of the child. I am, in these consultations, neurologist, psychiatrist, physician, psychologist, and friend, making as many observations as I possibly can. In some of my work in Bucks County I have had an opportunity to have a psychologist along with me. This is an invaluable aid because the psychologist can administer reading tests and has more skill with projective tests.

After I have examined the child, we get together and discuss our findings. Generally, I try to classify a child from the standpoint of the three D's, that is, descriptively, dynamically, and developmentally. Descriptively, I will fit him into one of the broad diagnostic categories— ego disturbances, developmental arrests, oedipal conflict. Dynamically, I look at his defensive structure and classify his major fears: (a) fear of loss of the primary love object, (b) fear of loss of love, (c) fear of castration, (d) fear of punishment by his conscience. Developmentally, I ask myself where does the child fit with respect to the appropriateness of his behavior? That is, does he behave predominantly like a three-year-old, a four-year-old, or a ten-year-old, and of course, I keep in mind Anna Freud's developmental lines. I make an effort to pull together material from the history, from classroom observations, from the psychiatric-psychological-neurological examination, to form a theoretical picture of why the child is behaving as he does at this point in time. I have no concern about whether or not the psychologist or teacher or principal is right and I am wrong. I assume that all of us are searching for data in good faith. It is my responsibility to explain the majority of this data with one major hypothesis.

PLANNING CORRECTIVE MEASURES

Now I have to plan what can be done for the child within the school system. Children who are mentally defective need a diagnosis. Many of these children have never been diagnosed etiologically. This often requires specialized tests, such as electroencephalograms, chromosomal studies, amino acid studies, dermatoglyphics, etc. A child who is mentally defective can be placed in special classes within the school, and it is sometimes possible to help prepare the parents for the eventual hospitalization of a severely deficient child. Children with organic brain syndromes respond remarkably well to specialized teaching techniques as described by Cruikshank (4) and Kephart (11), emphasizing the environment of the child in the classroom, structure, consistency, specialized teacher material, and especially athletics. For the younger child with an organic brain syndrome, the techniques of Marianne Frostig (6) and the materials developed to complement the *Illinois Test of Psycholinguistic Abilities* (9) are often of inestimable value. Children who border on severe ego disturbances or psychosis can often be helped with medication administered through the family physician. The neurotic child, of course, most often responds best to psychotherapy, but even he can be helped if the teacher understands he is struggling with an internal anxiety and not being outwardly delinquent. The developmental arrests very often reflect an attitude on the part of the parents which indicates a large investment in the child's maintenance of the immature behavior pattern. The school must always encourage and support growth, and if the responsibility rests with the parents it should be placed there.

Teachers and principals alike often have difficulty distinguishing behavior which outwardly is antisocial but reflects a defense against internal anxieties and behavior which is the result of the direct expression of unacceptable impulses. In the latter instance, the child often has simply not had sufficient controls from the parents and they are giving him permission to act out in a school setting. It is remarkable what definite limits can do for these children and it is equally remarkable how often educators restrain themselves from setting these limits when they are needed for fear of hurting a "neurotic" child. Generally, of course, the neurotic children respond much better to a permissive attitude than they do to structure. In making recommendations, remember the principle of priority. It may be easy to make many suggestions about what to do with a child. Frequently, however, some suggestions have to follow others. For example, before you can begin teaching a child, he must have some control over motility. With another child, who is acting out unconscious parental rebellions, first parental limits must be set, and if they are not, you are likely fighting a losing battle.

When the decision has been made about what should be done with the child, I meet again briefly with the principal and teacher to discuss the practicality of my recommendations. When a consensus has been arrived at, I meet again with the parents to discuss my findings and recommendations.

The last fifteen to twenty minutes of this two- to two-and-a-half-hour marathon is taken up in the dictation of a report, which contains the following headings:

1. The identifying information on the child.
2. Reason for referral.
3. Significant background information.
4. Psychological examination.
5. Psychiatric-neurological examination.
6. Conclusions.
7. Recommendations.

A copy of this does go to the school and is filed in the school's locked vault under my own personal name, thus making the report confidential medical information and not usually subject to subpoena in the community.

## IMPLEMENTATION OF RECOMMENDATIONS

The guidance counselor is an invaluable ally in the implementation of recommendations, but standards of training and definition of his role are far from complete or adequate. The guidance counselor should be the school's resident expert on children with a versatile knowledge of all behavioral sciences. The guidance counselor should know how to take a good psychoanalytic, chronological, developmental history. He should know how to administer psychological testing. He should know how to interview and observe the child in the classroom and individually. He should be able to do brief follow-up counseling of a child, and most important, he should be able to translate the study of an individual child into practical classroom application. In Bucks County, we have established a group of guidelines for training in elementary guidance. We believe that these people should have training in both education and psychology, that they should be able to do psychological testing, and we have strongly recommended that they have a clear understanding of normal development utilizing psychoanalytic theory. Responsibility for teaching them history-taking, interviewing techniques, and brief counseling should be that of the child psychiatrist. With this type of training they should be able to help many children without the necessity of formal psychiatric evaluation.

TEACHER EDUCATION

The third major function within the school system is the education of the teacher toward a better understanding of the child. I have already mentioned how the teacher is involved as much as possible in the evaluation.

Teacher education is a most rewarding experience, for teachers are eager to learn. Informal seminars for teachers of a specific grade are the best kind of structure since they afford an opportunity to compare behavior that is expected of a particular age group with deviations that are significant. I would advise the new consultant to begin in kindergarten and work his way slowly upward. The child psychiatrist will learn a great deal from teachers as well.

For a year I met once monthly with the kindergarten teachers in one school district. A practical suggestion we considered was what to do with the child who is immature emotionally and maturationally. It is the feeling of most of these teachers that to promote a child who is emotionally immature to the first grade is a gross error, that his emotional and maturational level is far more important than his academic progress. It was also their feeling that there are a number of children who come to kindergarten in a state of immaturity and simply need more close attachment to a maternal figure. They suggested that when these children are identified early, they should be placed in a class of fewer children so that they can have an emotionally corrective experience in the form of more attention from a maternal figure. We did not strive to make these teachers therapists but to help them make the educational experiences more therapeutic or more growth promoting for more children.

Another role that the child psychiatrist may have in the school system is that of a consultant to special classes. Many school systems have established classes for emotionally disturbed and "brain damaged" children. Often in the establishment of these classes the child psychiatrist will be involved in the diagnostic study or selection of the children and perhaps in the construction of the therapeutic milieu. At times, he may be involved in educational groups with parents of the children involved, but his most useful function is consultation with and support of the teacher who bears the enormous responsibility of caring for these children on the firing line of the classroom every day. Frustrations, anxieties, and angers that develop in these teachers are enormous. In addition, they frequently bear the brunt of the age-old wish to isolate those who are different. They need enormous support. The psychiatrist is the most logical and best equipped person to do this. While recognizing the importance of the specially constituted class for children with specific kinds of difficulties, we should strive against isolating the child who has difficulties.

Wherever possible it is preferable to keep a child in the normal classroom with tutoring from special instructors or his teacher given training on how to meet his particular needs than to place him in a class that is isolated from other children. Without question, children borrow ego strengths from their normal peers and in isolating them we deprive them of this valuable maturational aid.

## RESEARCH IN LEARNING

The Elementary and Secondary Education Act of 1965 made available to local districts funds for innovative programs in the field of education. This provided an excellent opportunity for us to learn more about learning. Many of these programs are making strides toward more rapid application of modern technology and learning theory to the schools, and the benefits that will evolve from these studies will continue to be evident for many years to come. What we desperately need, however, are more ecological studies of individual children in an average classroom. In our pursuit of rigidly controlled studies we appear to forget how much Freud and the child analysts have learned about children from studying intensively a relatively small number of subjects. Piaget has used essentially the same techniques with remarkable skill.

In one of the Title III projects of the Bucks County Schools we made an attempt to apply our understanding of children of a first-grade class to a large group of elementary schoolchildren. Two classes of "normal" first-grade children in two consecutive years were examined by a clinical diagnostic team (child psychiatrist, psychologist, social worker, master teacher) with developmental histories, psychiatric and neurological examinations, traditional intelligence and projective tests, and specialized testing (speech-hearing-vision). The diagnostic team reviewed its findings on each child, including a developmental, dynamic, and descriptive formulation, with an educational team of curriculum specialists in language arts, science, mathematics, and social studies. An "educational prescription" was written for each child to serve him throughout the second-grade year. The classroom teacher received frequent consultations from the diagnostic and educational team members within the classroom during this school year.

In order to bring the results of this study to more children, the children in these two classes were organized into three broad diagnostic categories (those manifesting evidence of oedipal conflict, developmental arrest, or ego disturbance) which were matched with teaching strategies that had been effective during the school year. The diagnostic scheme is one that both educators and clinicians can hopefully use effectively. This scheme was based on a grouping of factors derived from (a) consistently recognizable behavior patterns, (b) specific historical anlagen, (c) intrapsychic conflicts uncovered in interviews or in testing, and (d) workable teaching strategies.

A gross screening instrument was also devised that correlated the teacher's most reliable observations with clinical data. The twelve-statement questionnaire was used first in screening twenty-six additional children referred for school difficulties that were subsequently checked with more intensive investigation. It was then applied to an entire elementary school (grades kindergarten through six) of 600 children. All children in the school were thus classified into three diagnostic groups. Each teacher was supplied with a manual of teaching strategies for each group. After a three-month trial in this single school, the method of grouping was tested in three additional schools totaling 2,500 students, with most favorable results. Since the initial study the work has been expanded to include over twenty-five thousand children throughout the United States.

The complete findings of these studies are published by the Bucks County Schools, including a manual of teaching strategies (16). Perhaps a brief statement of some more specific findings might be of value.

We discovered that approximately 20 to 25 percent of the children in a normal classroom have impairments in the functioning efficiency of their central nervous system that significantly influence their learning. The use of carpets on the floor significantly reduces the noise level in the classroom, enabling these children to learn more efficiently. Is this not as important as good lighting?

For many years in educational circles a number of seemingly diametrically opposed concepts have flourished, such as active versus passive learning, a structured versus an unstructured classroom approach, phonics versus whole-word teaching of reading. We have learned that active learning in which the teacher poses questions and then provides tools to discover answers is infinitely preferable. But we have also learned that some children must passively receive or be led along discovery steps before they can take a more active part in learning. Some children need a structured classroom approach, others need to be unhampered. Phonics confuses some children who just don't learn other than with a whole-word approach.

When teachers become overburdened with the responsibility for growth of their children they occasionally react like the surgeon who must inflict much pain. They shield themselves from the anxiety and fears of children, forcing the child to retreat to fantasy for some degree of relief. Only support and education and practical suggestions can relieve their anxiety. All of us in the behavioral sciences must get into the classrooms. We have much to learn and much to teach.

A child who has reached the third or fourth grade with limited educational success has had almost half of his life marred by failure in the most significant areas of his life and is highly susceptible to more serious emotional disturbances. If we can enhance and individualize the learning process, have we not taken a significant step toward preventing mental illness? Where should the responsibility for preventing mental illness lie? Should it rest in the hands of the understaffed community mental health centers? Or should it be in the schools? I believe that it should be in the schools simply because that is where the children are.

# 19

## Child Psychiatry and the Law

JONAS ROBITSCHER, J.D., M.D.

All of the problems that arise in adult legal psychiatry—the questions of degree of competency and degree of responsibility, the maintenance of confidentiality, the fairness of procedures by which we label a person as mentally disabled, and the question of what rights we then accord this patient—arise in the field of child legal psychiatry. In fact, they arise with greater complexity caused by the presence in the child-therapist situation of third parties, by the problems caused in consensual situations by the consenter's lack of majority (which may be superimposed on a lack of mental ability), and by the lack of a clear concept regarding the civil rights of minors.

Down through legal and psychiatric history, the child has been seen as possessed of few rights and he has often been granted scant respect. In therapy there has been little concern for confidentiality. In delinquency proceedings, where the fiction prevails that a child is in the custody of the courts for therapeutic rather than criminal disposition, little respect has been shown for due process. In the disposition of the retarded and those labeled as defective delinquents, few legal safeguards have been available.

Recent years have witnessed a great increase of emphasis on the rights of minority groups and the rights of those accused of crimes. There has been some increased emphasis on the rights of the mentally disabled and some slight increased emphasis on the rights of children, the rights of child-therapy patients, and on the obligations that the physician, the therapeutic facility, and the community owe to minors. This "trickle-down" of social concern to the condition of children has been evidenced in at least the following four ways.

1. The child has received greater attention in such complex therapy modalities as crisis-oriented therapy, family therapy, and as the subject of community psychiatry practice. This emphasis has raised questions about the consent of the child to his treatment and the maintenance of confidentiality in treatment situations where families interact with teams of therapist/administrators, and with schools, clergy, courts, and social agencies, all of which may have a legitimate interest in the progress of the child.

2. The courts have evidenced greater concern for children when they are caught up in the criminal process but because of a special status—

juvenile, retarded, or defective delinquent—the children are not accorded the protection of adult criminal procedure but instead are considered to be subjects for therapy.

3. The courts have made some strides in more clearly defining the rights of the retarded and the defective delinquent so that determinations made during childhood will not continue to determine the individual's status when majority is attained.

4. There has been greater legislative concern for the well-being of children, evidenced in legislation ranging from "battered child" laws, and obscenity statutes, to compulsory testing for phenylketonuria.

Some of these concerns of child legal psychiatry affect only a small fraction of children, but two topics—also of prime importance in adult legal psychiatry—the topics of confidentiality and of informed consent, are of crucial importance in child legal psychiatry and cut across all categories of patients and all evaluation and therapy situations.

## Confidentiality and Privilege

Most psychiatrists fail to distinguish between privilege—which affects only a minority of child patients, since it is invoked only when a patient is the subject of his therapist's testimony in court—and the broader and less legalistic concept of confidentiality which is grounded not only in law but in medical ethics governing a doctor's obligations to his patients.

Confidentiality is an old medical ideal which has a basis in the Hippocratic oath and is time-honored in medical practice. Medical privilege on the other hand is a comparatively new legal concept. It is not found in the common law but has been conferred by statutes which only date back to the New York statute of 1828 (14). Unlike standards of confidentiality, which are applicable wherever the concept of the Hippocratic oath is accepted as a part of medicine, privilege applies only to courtroom testimony. It varies from jurisdiction to jurisdiction in accordance with the presence or absence of state laws, the precedents set by earlier cases, and the breadth or narrowness of the construction of applicable laws by the court.

With an increasing need for paramedical and nonmedical personnel to perform therapy and with treatment records increasingly available to insurance companies, community mental health personnel, state agencies, federal agencies, and others, the concept of confidentiality becomes more difficult to uphold than it has been in the familiar one-to-one doctor-patient relationship.

An adult enters a therapeutic relationship by his own choice. A child is almost always brought to the treatment situation by interested adults. Once he is in treatment the therapist decides how much of what the patient discloses should be passed on to parents, school, juvenile court authorities, or other interested third parties. Malmquist (22) has said that the question of privacy for the child, particularly the right of the child not to have his family informed of communications to the therapist, takes on wider implications when it becomes a question of how much of the material may be routinely released to others in the community. In many cases the child and his parents have little knowledge or control over this. Parents may have signed a general consent slip which has been modeled after the sharing of information between two physicians. In the mental health area this may allow disclosure of what the patient has discussed to all sorts of community agencies. Conferences and reports regarding the child thus may be open to school personnel, social workers, representatives of county welfare boards, or private community agencies. Malmquist describes a case where material was pooled at a conference attended by personnel from the community clinic and public agencies. Following this conference, a summary by one of the persons was sent to the school which felt entitled to the report since it had initiated the referral of the patient to the clinic. The patient later dropped out of school and gave as his reason the fact that material in the report had been "used against me."

Malmquist disagrees with the position of the Group for the Advancement of Psychiatry which stated in its report that problems of confidentiality with children in psychiatric treatment resemble confidentiality problems with psychotic adults (18). This position leads to the conclusion that information must be shared with parties who are more responsible, in the interest of the patient. Malmquist says that in reality this position is appropriate only with a small minority of children and that particularly with adolescents the question of the child's right to privacy from the remainder of the family may be very real.

A 17 year old "minor" at a child guidance clinic may not wish to have the information about him released even though his parents have signed a blanket consent slip, and he also may not wish the parents themselves to know. In many cases it becomes a Herculean task of clinical judgment to decide what and how to share with parents, who still have responsibility for a child.

Malmquist also deals with the confused situation that arises because a person undergoing an evaluation by a physician may see the relationship in terms of the patient-doctor relationship although the doctor may be an employee of an agency, may consider his primary responsibility to be to that agency, and may not consider himself bound by the traditional doctor-patient model. One of his conclusions is that the same degree of confidentiality that we accord to "affluent delinquents" should also be accorded to the less affluent children who are evaluated by order of a court or on request of a school rather than in response to their family's initiation.

Ross (34) has described a change in his own attitude on this question over an eight-year period. He says of his earlier (33) thoughts, referring to an article he wrote in 1958:

My original thesis was that the need for confidentiality was crucial in the treatment of a child. Most children, I stated, have experiences in which they confide in an adult only to have the confidences betrayed; and these experiences, I thought, cause children to generalize that adults cannot be trusted. . . . I wrote that confidentiality in the child's session is of paramount importance at the beginning of treatment. . . I proposed that he be told, "Everything you do and say in your hour with me is strictly between the two of us, and I won't tell your mother about it."

In 1966 he had come to the conclusion that only some children needed or would be helped by this degree of confidentiality and he recommended that confidentiality be discussed with the child in the first interview only in those cases in which the therapist feels the child requires such assurance. The question of confidentiality, Ross believes, should be individualized and left to the judgment of the therapist except when a child specifically asks that a piece of information be held in confidence.

When a patient invokes confidentiality under such circumstances, the therapist must, of course, honor this agreement.

This raises the question of what to do when the child has invoked confidentiality and the therapist considers communication to the parent of vital importance; for example, when the child has convinced the therapist that he plans to engage in dangerous, antisocial, or self-destructive behavior. When this is the case, the issue must be dealt with in the context of treatment, the therapist working toward helping the child alter his decision either with respect to his intentions or with respect to his not wanting his parents to know. If the therapist is unsuccessful in either of these attempts, he must recognize that he really does not have a workable therapeutic relationship with the patient, so that a violation of confidentiality by notifying the parents (after telling the child of his intentions) can hardly disrupt a treatment relationship.

Although Ross and others have written about the effect on treatment when confidentiality is breached, there has been little or no attention to the question of the legal rights of child patients. Do child patients understand the confidential nature of the therapy situation? Do they understand that the treatment of minors involves more than a one-to-one relationship and thus deviates from the normal evaluatory or therapy situation? Have they consented to the sharing of information? What is the validity of their consent? Is the parents' consent to the breach of confidentiality all that is needed for the therapist to share information or is the child's consent also needed? All of these very complicated legal questions go unanswered largely because breach of confidentiality does not usually lead to legal action. Although it *can* give rise to a legal action, this legal right has more of the quality of fiction than of fact. Particularly in the case of a minor (even though the release of confidential material may damage him in many ways in future years, including entrance to college, employment opportunities, positions with such federal agencies as the Peace Corps) it is hard to imagine a situation where he could recover damages. Part of the minor's problem is that the adult who authorized treatment for him would not be likely to bring suit for breach of confidentiality in his behalf. Another part of the problem is that the damages he may suffer from breach of confidentiality may not occur for many years and may be extremely difficult to prove. But the major part of the problem is that United States courts pay only lip service to the concept of confidentiality of the doctor-patient relationship and in practice allow physicians a great deal of latitude when they disclose confidential information even when this information was secured in the therapy of a responsible adult.

A leading case on the divulging of information by a psychiatrist in the course of treating a patient is *Berry* v. *Moench* (6). Here a treating physician gratuitously gave information to a physician who had asked him if a former patient would be a good marital risk. Dr. Moench not only furnished confidential information—much of the information he furnished was incorrect or was based on hearsay from prejudiced observers, such as the family of the patient's former wife—but Dr. Moench advised the physician to warn the girl against his former patient: "My suggestion to the infatuated girl would be to run as fast and as far as she possibly could in any direction away from him." In this leading case the court ruled that in spite of the doctor's reliance on hearsay, his failure to identify the sources of some of the derogatory information he had furnished, his seven-year-long lack of contact with the patient with a resulting lack of information about Berry's psychiatric status, and the great breach of confidentiality, such considerations were outweighed by the doctor's duty to "protect the happiness" of the young girl (although the doctor had had a contractual relationship with his former patient but had no relationship with those making the inquiry). The court said that if four criteria are met—good faith, fair reporting, conveying only such information as is necessary to accomplish the purpose of protecting a third party, and giving information only to persons necessary to accomplish the purpose of protection—the patient cannot recover for breach of confidence. In a similar case where the treating physician was held guiltless for divulging prejudicial information, the New York State Supreme Court held that the physician was justified in disclosing to the Air Force that the patient, a civilian employee of the Air Force, had been absent from work because of alcoholism although the patient had not been willing to have this information divulged (12). The physician had contended, and the court found this contention to be a good defense to the patient's suit, that whatever his obligation of confidentiality to the patient, the physician's overriding duty was to make the disclosure because it would benefit a branch of the government.

In spite of the fact that the law decrees that physicians do have civil liability for damages directly caused by the violation of a confidence, few American cases deal directly with this issue and recovery by the patient is almost unheard of—indicating that this protection against unauthorized disclosure is rarely invoked and when it is invoked rarely succeeds. If this is the fate of the adult plaintiff, the opportunity of the minor plaintiff to be compensated for a breach of confidentiality would be even more remote.

Not the possibility of legal redress but the feeling that confidentiality is the essence of the doctor-patient relationship and that therapy cannot function without confidentiality is the main impetus to maintenance of confidentiality in adult treatment. In child treatment, as Ross has indicated, great breaches of the principle of confidentiality occur and are taken for granted.

New therapy modes contribute to the problem. Confidentiality in a one-to-one relationship is of course much easier to maintain than it is in group therapy situations where other members of the group are privy to information. The special problems of family group therapy have been dealt with by Grosser and Paul in a discussion of ethical issues in family group therapy, but legal considerations are largely overlooked (16).

The community mental health center will generate confidentiality problems all its own. Part of the problem is the social-work principle of sharing of information and the concept of problem families who will over the course of their lifetimes make a number of contacts with various facilities, making a central file of social-work information a help to many professionals who will in the short and long term come in contact with these people. Lewis, in a paper on confidentiality in the community mental health center, notes that

the common practice of sending out photostat copies of complete records is deplorable from the point of view of confidentiality, however expedient it may be administratively. Nor is the issue evaded by conveying the material orally, in person or by telephone, instead of in writing. On the contrary, the most insidious breaches in confidentiality occur during the casual discussion of patients that all too frequently take place (20).

He recommends that insurance companies require only a general statement of the patient's illness—such as "emotional problems" or "psychological difficulties"—and that only relevant information—never information merely desired "for the record"—should be released and this only with the full understanding and consent of patient, parent, or guardian. Few therapy facilities have attempted to meet this standard.

Information to and from colleges frequently breaches the ideal of confidentiality. Private psychiatrists are reluctant to turn down a college request for information on their patients; college psychiatrists are in the difficult position of agents of a third party, working for the patient but also in the service of the employing student health facility. One of those urging that college admissions officers not be furnished details of prior psychiatric treatment—or even furnished information that the patient *has been* in psychiatric treatment—is Dr. Dana Farnsworth, director of University Health Services at Harvard. Speaking at a meeting of the Association of College Admission Counselors, he urged that they stop giving consideration to or asking questions about prior psychiatric treatment of college applicants (29). "The fact that an applicant has or has not had psychiatric treatment should be irrelevant to the admissions process. Whether or not the applicant has the intellectual capacity to do the work that will be required of him and the emotional maturity and motivation to use his intelligence effectively is of central importance." He recommended that admission personnel delete from their application forms the question about prior psychiatric treatment. Requiring such information is "essentially an invasion of privacy" and the knowledge he will have to divulge such information on college application and job application forms may "discourage a person from seeking help when he needs it and could most effectively profit from it."

Dr. Farnsworth in his role as head of a student mental health service has himself been the object of attack on the ground that such health services do not protect the confidentiality of student communications. One controversy was initiated by Dr. Thomas Szasz whose name is a bad word in some psychiatric circles because of his thesis that psychiatrists use their position and power to manipulate people and in the process deprive them of civil rights. Unpopular with psychiatrists, Dr. Szasz is considered by lawyers as the chief exponent of protection of the civil rights of psychiatric patients. In a sociological journal he devotes himself to the question of the ambiguous role of the college psychiatrist under the arresting title "The Psychiatrist as Double Agent" (36). He says of the college psychiatrist:

Toward the students . . . he is a compassionate counselor and therapist who promises to be a faithful conspirator with the student in his struggle for liberation. . . . Toward the institution . . . he shows the other side of his face: He . . . will select and control students and inform about them as the needs of the school and the community require.

His is the kind of false representation of the college psychiatrist's role and function that, if practiced by the police, industry, or medical establishments, would be denounced by critics and condemned by the courts. The same deception practiced in the name of mental health has, however, so far escaped both public criticism and judicial prohibition.

The question of divulgence of information by college health service doctors was raised in two celebrated instances, the first when the Peace Corps raised the threat of legal action against college physicians who would not help them in the evaluation of Peace Corps applicants who had received psychiatric service at college (25) (this threat was countered by a strong stand in favor of the confidentiality of the student's therapy session content by Dr. Robert Arnstein, of the Yale University Student Health Service, who was willing to have a test case brought against him [1]) and the second when a University of Texas psychiatrist released the contents of a psychiatric interview with Charles J. Whitman after Whitman's death in order to provide light on the seventeen murders and the wounding of twenty-six more victims committed by sniping from the university tower.

Although the release of the content of Whitman's session was condemned at the time, Robitscher has raised the question of whether a patient who thrusts himself into the light of either notoriety or fame cannot be discussed after his death in order to provide information that the public has a right to know (32). He would add this special situation as a fifth exception to the four recognized exceptions to the rule of confidentiality—when the patient has given prior assent to the breach of confidentiality, when the disclosure is required by statute or court order, when there is a necessity to disclose for the benefit or welfare of the patient, and when the information is essential for the protection of society in general.

William Curran, visiting professor of health law at Harvard University, has reported on the replies to questionnaires on maintenance of confidentiality in the student health service sent out to 488 members of the American College Health Association (12). Although most schools had no printed set of general policies, they seemed aware of the values to be gained in respecting the therapeutic relationship. Parents are not routinely informed of contacts for consultation, counseling, or short-term, out-patient, crisis-oriented treatment. In all schools information about psychiatric referrals and treatment was not generally available to members of the college administration. Some of the schools kept psychiatric records separate from general medical records and the majority of schools would not reveal information without consent of students or parents. Curran's conclusion, which is at variance with that of many psychiatric observers, is that most breaches of confidence occur only when necessary to protect the welfare of the individual or community. He does not deal with two crucial questions—whether parents have a right to know if their children are receiving psychiatric evaluation or treatment, and whether the consent of patients or parents to have information released should be binding on health service physicians or whether the physician can make an independent judgment concerning the usefulness of the disclosure.

Turning from the subject of confidentiality to the statutory right of privilege which enables a patient to silence his physician in a courtroom situation where without such statute the physician would be forced to testify, privilege statutes are not uniform from jurisdiction to jurisdiction. Privilege statutes do not exist in nine states. They have only very limited application, such as only preventing the disclosure of information about venereal disease, in other jurisdictions. In many jurisdictions they apply only to physicians and not to nurses, social workers, psychologists, and others who may be in a therapeutic relationship to the patient. In recent years a paradoxical situation has arisen. In one state a psychologist doing the identical kind of treatment sometimes performed by psychiatrists is not accorded the right to have privileged communications made to him because the statute only gives this right to physicians, while in the neighboring state legislative action has given the psychologist this right but in the absence of a physician's privilege statute the doctor can be compelled to disclose what went on in the treatment session (31). Some commentators believe that even in jurisdictions which do not have good privilege statutes, a therapist who refuses to divulge confidential information in court will usually be treated respectfully by the court. In one such instance, the court said that even in the absence of a doctor-patient privilege statute it would not compel the psychiatrist to testify because the psychiatrist-patient relationship is "unique and not at all similar to the relationship between physician and patient" and thus is more deserving of privilege than the ordinary doctor-patient relationship (7).

## Consent and Informed Consent

Until the last decade, physicians, although dependent on the consent of the patient before they can legally initiate or carry out treatment, have not had to worry greatly over the formal requirements of consent. The mere fact that the patient is in treatment and stays in treatment carries with it the implication that he consents to the treatment. Hospitals often felt that they were well protected by loosely worded forms by which a patient agreed in advance that he consented to anything that was done to him while in the hospital. When patients were dissatisfied with the results of their treatment, when they suffered untoward side effects which had not been anticipated, their recourse was to commence a malpractice proceeding against the doctor. These actions were often very difficult to win, partly because the criteria of what constitutes acceptable medical practice are often vague and partly because even when doctors have been guilty of negligence in their care of patients, proof that will satisfy a court of law, usually dependent on the testimony of other physicians, is difficult for the plaintiff to secure.

Lawyers have always known that for consent to be valid it must be an "informed consent." If a patient consents to an operation but has no idea concerning what he is assenting to, the consent is not valid. Like the old doctrine in the law of contracts that there is no contract without a "meeting of the minds," a mutual understanding on the terms of the contract by the parties to the contract is necessary for the agreement to be valid. Since the law tells us that a person has a right to do what he wishes or have done according to his wishes as far as his own person is concerned, any interference with this right constitutes a battery, an unlawful attack. If a patient in a general hospital does not agree to some procedure that is proposed, he can refuse the procedure. If the procedure is performed against his wishes, a battery has been committed on his person. In the case of minors who are brought to treatment not because of their own wishes but because of the wishes of their parents or parent substitutes, the patients concerned are usually considered incompetent to accede to or refuse procedures, and someone else—the closest relative in some cases or some person delegated by law such as the superintendent of a mental hospital when a patient has been committed—provides the consent for the patient.

The concept that consent must be based on a real understanding of the procedures involved and that the patient must be familiar with possible effects and major side effects has come into prominence in the last decade. This has been due to the development of an expanded legal doctrine of informed consent and also because of increased concern for the subjects of medical research experiments.

Tracing the growth of a legal doctrine can illustrate how chance occurrences can influence that growth. In 1958 in an unremarkable decision in the Bang case, the Supreme Court of Minnesota held that it was a proper question for jury determination whether the plaintiff had consented to the performance of an operation which resulted in the severance of his spermatic cords (3). The plaintiff, who had consented to a transurethral prostatic resection, testified that nothing had been said concerning the fact that he would be rendered sterile by the operation. The defendant hospital presented evidence, which was not contradicted, that bilateral section of the spermatic cords and ligation of the vas deferens was routine in elderly patients because their reproductive years are considered over and the possibility of infection is reduced. Although the plaintiff's case was dismissed in the lower court, on appeal the Supreme Court of Minnesota held that, in the absence of an emergency, the patient should have been informed before the operation that the plan was to sever his spermatic cords, that if this plan was carried out he would be rendered sterile, but if it was not carried out there would be an increased possibility of infection; the case was therefore remanded for a new trial. Two years later under a very different factual situation the language of the Bang case was used to support a ruling regarding informed consent which has now been followed in many jurisdictions and which greatly increases the liability of physicians. In this case the plaintiff alleged not that a procedure was performed which she had not understood would be performed, which would be analogous to the Bang case, but that the procedure when performed had produced deleterious side effects and if she had understood that these side effects might have occurred, she would never have consented to the treatment. Ever since this landmark case of *Natanson v. Kline* (26), the plaintiff has had two turns at bat when he wants to proceed against his physician. He can sue on the grounds that the physician was negligent and he can at the same time sue because of his lack of understanding of possible deleterious effects even in the absence of any negligence by the physician. The patient was receiving cobalt irradiation treatment to prevent the recurrence of a malignancy. She contended that if she had understood all the possible side effects of this treatment she would not have given consent to the treatment. Like the Bang case, the Natanson case does not appear too remarkable if it is remembered that at the time the plaintiff had her treatment, cobalt irradiation was a new and somewhat experimental type of therapy. But courts in most jurisdictions have relied on the reasoning of this case in order to make physicians liable for many bad results and many side effects if these could have been anticipated by the physician but were not explained to the patient.

Psychiatrists are given more leniency than other physicians in explaining the possible consequences of treatment to patients if they feel that explaining all the effects of treatment would have a bad effect on the patient's psychiatric condition. In a case where a patient gave consent to an electric shock treatment but was not warned that there was a risk of fracture, the court held that a jury might well think that when a doctor deals with a mentally sick patient and has a strong belief that the patient's only hope of cure is from electric shock treatment, the doctor would not be liable if in the belief that dangers involved were minimal he did not stress these dangers to the patient (8).

The expansion of the doctrine of informed consent leaves many unanswered questions. One of the most difficult questions to answer is how remote must a possibility of a bad effect be before a doctor is not obliged to mention it to the patient. A Florida court has held that if the possibility of a bad effect is only one in 500 cases, the disclosure does not have to be made (14). Various courts are now going through the process of determining for their own jurisdictions what degrees of possibility or probability need be discussed. Another question that will have to be settled in courts of law is that concerning the side effects of medication which are often so varied and so numerous that physicians would have a very difficult time explaining them all to their patients.

Patients who are under legal disability, such as those committed to mental hospitals or who are wards of a court under guardianship estates, are not considered to have any capacity to give or refuse consent for treatment. Consent must be given by the entity controlling the incompetent person. This entity may be a court, it may be a legal guardian, it may be the closest relative, or it may in some cases be a hospital superintendent. Minors are similarly special persons in the eyes of the law and cannot on their own volition consent to treatment, except when an emergency dictates—as when an appendectomy must be done and the parent is not available—or when a child is considered emancipated. The concept of emancipation cannot be clearly and concisely defined. An emancipated person is a minor who is separated from his home or parents and who wholly and completely supports himself and directs his own destiny. Under this definition of emancipation, college students who are sometimes considered emancipated by student health authorities should not be considered emancipated unless they have made such a break from home as to be fully independent.

Right in the middle, between the two situations of a minor who clearly does not have the capacity to understand the nature of treatment and must have someone supply consent for him and the emancipated minor who is close to majority, is independent of home, and is obviously capable of making his own decisions, there is the mature minor who appears old enough and capable enough to appreciate and understand the consequences of the treatment. The age and the circumstances that make a minor mature enough to give consent are a question for the court to decide in each individual case. Courts have held that seventeen- and eighteen-year-olds were sufficiently mature to give a valid consent in the absence of parental consent (2). Paul Lieberman, in a Medicolegal Monograph of the Law Department of the American Medical Association, discusses the situation where parents give consent to a treatment (an example might be a therapeutic abortion) but the mature minor refuses to give consent (21). In this case, says Lieberman, the physician might be found guilty of a battery and he suggests that "it is good practice, if not essential, to get the consent of both the minor and the parents whenever treating a child over fifteen."

In psychiatric practice, the continued attendance of the minor patient implies his consent to the treatment. His parents must also give assent to the treatment unless the child is emancipated, although in some instances mature children may be held to be capable of giving their own consent. If drugs or somatic therapies are used, the consent is not valid unless full information is given on which consent must be based. This information is to be given to the minor if his consent is considered necessary and to the parent or parent-substitute if the minor's consent is held insufficient. The information must include common side effects of drugs and common ill consequences of treatment. Even in cases where the mental state of the minor—such as severe depression or psychosis—persuades the therapist that disclosure of possible ill effects would not be in the best interest of the minor, the disclosures must be made to the parent for a consent that is informed.

One of the difficult situations concerning minors is the question of surgical sterilization which is sometimes recommended for promiscuity, particularly in retarded girls, and has been recommended in the case of severely retarded girls because they are not able to manage the hygienic material, sanitary napkins and the like, that absorb blood flow. In the latter case physicians would be reluctant to perform surgery in the absence of law on the subject; in the case of the promiscuous retardate who is

often maintained in an institution solely because of the possibility of pregnancy outside the institution (although figures show there has been an
increase of pregnancies in institutionalized patients in recent years—so
institutionalization alone is not always a complete contraceptive), the
recommendation has been made that sterilization offers an alternative to
commitment (4).

The reason that the topics of confidentiality and consent become irretrievably intertwined is that in a number of situations the minor seeks
medical treatment but does not want his parents to know that he feels
the need of such treatment, whether it is treatment for venereal disease,
an illegitimate pregnancy, the prescribing of contraceptives, or merely, as
in the case of some minors with psychiatric problems, psychotherapy on
the basis of a self-referral.

Legislative action to allow minors to secure treatment without parents'
consent is of recent origin and is confined almost entirely to the field of
treatment of venereal disease. A Massachusetts law passed in 1954 states,
referring to State Venereal Disease Clinics, that "physical examination
and treatment by a registered physician or surgeon acting under the
authority of the department of public health upon the person of a minor
who voluntarily appears therefor, shall not constitute an assault or an
assault and battery upon such a person" (24). In 1967 a similar law was
passed in Connecticut (11). A broader exception to the requirement of
parental consent for the treatment of a minor has been set forth in a new
Maryland law, passed in 1967, which has been called the first of its kind
in the United States (23) and which has served as a model for a more
recent New Jersey law; these laws specifically allow physicians to examine
and treat minors for venereal disease without consent of the parents or
guardians. The Nebraska legislature has also recently passed a bill allowing for treatment of venereal disease on the written consent of the minor
alone (27), and similar legislation is being considered in a number of
other states. Writing in the *New England Journal of Medicine*, Dr. Donald Hayes Russell points out that (35) the Maryland law seems a model
statute because it is designed to see that venereal infections, which are
rapidly increasing in teenagers, will receive the earliest possible treatment,
but that this legislation places the physician in the place of the parent and
leaves him with difficult decisions to make. For instance, if the doctor
feels that it is in the best interest of the patient to confide in his parent,
but the patient refuses to allow such divulgence, should the doctor refuse
to treat the patient? And if in such a case the doctor does refuse to treat
the patient, would the doctor be liable for damages in a suit brought
against him by the parents of the minor? If the parent has not given consent for the treatment and the minor is without funds, who is to pay the
doctor? (Some insurance companies have refused medical compensation
for procedures performed on a minor without parental consent.) Is the
Maryland law a violation of parental rights? The argument can be made

that parents cannot discharge their responsibilities to their children if essential knowledge is withheld from them. Parental rights frequently involve moral and religious issues that may be a part of the traditional framework within which parents seek to perform their responsibilities.

The Maryland law also allows examination and treatment of the illegitimately pregnant minor without parental consent or disclosure.

The question of whether the nonpregnant teenager who seeks to prevent pregnancy should be considered mature and therefore be considered capable of consenting to the prescription of contraceptive medication or the insertion of an intrauterine contraceptive device or the fitting of a diaphragm has never been decided legally. Unmarried sexually active girls have been given contraceptive information or devices with the consent of their parents in some jurisdictions. Dr. J. F. Hulka, Associate Professor of Obstetrics and Gynecology and Maternal and Child Health at the University of North Carolina School of Public Health, has asked in a letter, also in the *New England Journal of Medicine*:

Should not the non-pregnant teen-ager who seeks to prevent pregnancy be considered mature? Whatever her psychologic reasons for sexual activity, certainly her concern for preventing pregnancy is that of a reasonable woman. Perhaps if pregnancy were morally or medically as easy to cure as venereal disease, there would be no need for discussing the rights of minors to have access to means of preventing pregnancies. But in our present state of the art, the question of pills without parental consent for sexually active teen-agers must be raised vis-a-vis our apparent acceptance of pregnancy and venereal disease as conditions conferring legal maturity upon our teen-agers (19).

In addition to impetus given to the doctrine of informed consent by court decisions of the last decade, attention has been focused on the question of consent because of medical and public interest in organ transplants, particularly kidney and heart, in recent years. A mentally incompetent donor or a minor donor may not realize the risk of an operation or the consequences of living out the remainder of a life with only one kidney. On the other hand either may be under great pressure to serve as a donor because he may be a close relative of the prospective donee and his kidney may be considered to have a maximum chance of continuing to function in the new host. The retarded have also been described by some Orwellian physicians as sources of all kinds of organs and grafts and it has been said that these people can be "farmed" and their tissues and organs can be "harvested." There has also been the life-and-death decisions in recent years of the appropriateness of organ transplant to an unproductive member of society, a child and more particularly a mentally deficient child, when other more productive members of society might make better use of their greater longevity that would result from the transplant. Similar types of questions have arisen when efficacious drugs have been in very short supply and the physician must determine which patient is to receive the treatment or when a complicated technical procedure such as dialysis can only be furnished to selected patients. The physician finds himself making ethical and sociological judgments such as predicting the chance that the patient will be able to assume a useful place in society. A Denver team of three surgeons who worked together on kidney transplants states that children, whose social worth is not yet known, are reasonable subjects for kidney transplants but mental defectives, mental incompetents, and unwilling patients will not be given transplants (37).

Turning from the recipient to the donor, Paul Freund, professor at the Harvard Law School, has commented on the "special problem of subjects not possessed of full capacity to consent, in particular the problem of children" (15).

The law here is that parents may consent for the child if the invasion of the child's body is for the child's welfare or benefit. This has become familiar through the kidney-transplant cases, in which the Massachusetts Supreme Judicial Court was asked to render an advisory opinion. Benefit was found to exist in the psychic welfare of the normal donor brother because, after considerable interrogation of the normal child, it was concluded that he would be suffering under some feeling of inadequacy if he did not make the donation, and so the transplants were judicially approved. But what of unrelated donors who will become more important as transplants between strangers become more feasible? Shall children be ineligible, since it would be hard to find any benefit to the donor child in the transplant with a stranger and the parent seems legally incapable of giving consent in the absence of benefit to the child? It may be that the result is that children will be ineligible as donors for transplants, unless, perhaps—and here we have some variables—the risk is relatively slight. Might benefit be found on the monetary side?

Coming to that, what of the giving of payment as it may affect the reality of consent? I would suggest that the amounts paid should not be so large as to constitute undue influence—that is, so large as to obscure an appreciation of the risk and weaken the will to self-preservation. We ought not to be put into the business of buying lives.

Other aspects of the renewed interest in informed consent have to do with research and experimental medicine. One of these aspects is the use of patients and nonpatients as experimental subjects in situations where the subjects do not understand the implications of the experiments or even know that an experiment is being conducted. Dr. Henry Beecher, Harvard professor of research in anesthesia, originally passed doubts on such experiments by pointing out instances where in order to achieve a balanced research design patients have not been given treatment that they expected to receive—for example, patients have received placebos instead of antibiotics—and an extension of his ideas has focused attention on captive populations such as prison inmates or the mentally retarded who are used as experimental subjects in situations where either their consent is given under pressure or is not even asked (5). The other aspect of experimental medicine dealing with consent is invasion by behavioral scientists into areas which are traditionally considered private but where the needs or desires of the researcher or the needs of the research design have persuaded the researcher not to fully inform the experimental subject or to secure experimental participation from incompetents. In *Privacy and Behavioral Research*, a report prepared for the Office of Science and Technology, Executive Office of the President of the United States (28), examples are given of research procedures that may harm the participant through a violation of his rights, particularly by an invasion of his privacy without his consent. These include such research procedures as asking a child to report his parents' disciplinary methods, experimental projects done in classrooms in which children were asked to report about various aspects of the personality of their peers, and experiments in which subjects are provoked into anger or depressed moods in order to study their reactions. The study asks many questions. In a research project designed to discover the relationship between level of anxiety and the need to be with someone, the investigator induced an anxiety state by deceiving his subjects. Is such deception warranted? How is consent to participate in the experiment nullified by such a deception? In a study to discover how well a family can survive in an extended stay in a fall-out shelter, the investigator recorded all conversation during the interval without the family's prior knowledge or consent. What, if any, sanctions are there to such intrusion on privacy?

The report notes that an individual has an inalienable right to dignity, self-respect, and freedom to determine his own thoughts and actions within the broad limits set forth by the requirements of society. The essential element in privacy and self-determination is the privilege of making one's own decision concerning the extent to which one will reveal thoughts, feelings, and actions. "When a person consents freely and fully to share himself with others—with a scientist, an employer, or credit investigator—there is no invasion of privacy, regardless of the quality or nature of the information revealed."

But in drug testing, where the placebo effect may be important, in experiments where the influence of the observer if known will affect the behavior of the observed, and in many other situations the informed consent of the subject may be considered the nullification of the experiment. The report states, referring to consent to invasion of privacy but in terms that apply to all manipulations:

Informed consent has little meaning when children are involved. Consent is normally obtained after providing adequate information to adults who serve as surrogates for the children. These may be parents, school principal, or the school board. Exceptions even to this form of consent are occasionally justified by the over-riding social value of the experiment, the unavailability of other means of accomplishing its purpose, and reduction to a minimum of the impact on the subject's privacy.

Although the question of securing informed consent becomes more complicated rather than less complicated the more it is discussed, a few conclusions that can be made safely are that the use of captive subjects—in particular, convicts, institutionalized mental patients, the institutionalized retarded, and even populations subject to less extreme types of coercion such as "volunteer" soldier or college student participants—as research subjects is hard to justify because the validity of the consent is difficult to prove. Another conclusion that can be drawn is that the cautious researcher will proceed to have his experimental design and his method for procuring consent checked out by an appropriate panel or board connected with his institution or with the agency sponsoring the research, rather than deciding on his own if the rights of his experimental subjects are adequately safeguarded.

Recent studies are typical of the experiments going on today in which consent of older and younger child subjects raises questions. One hundred and sixty Swedish teenagers ranging from eleven to eighteen years old were shown seven movies filled with scenes of rape, mob killings, sadistic beatings, sexual excesses, and orgies of brutality as part of an experiment to judge the emotional impact of the movies. The films had all been banned by the Swedish government's board of censors (30). Brown University researchers have frustrated newborn infants by depriving them of liquids unless they learn to suck through a straw. The experiment showed that after a certain period of time the newborn infants were adaptable enough so that they could learn to suck through a straw (9). The questions of whether such experiments are of any benefit to the experimental subject, whether experiment is in the best interest of the subject, and whether the consent of the parent is valid remain to be answerd. Bernard Hirsh, director of the Law Division of the American Medical Association, states that use of children or mentally incompetent persons as subjects in experiments involving risk or injury without medical benefit to themselves is of questionable legality even if the prior consent of parent or guardian is obtained. "The courts have made it clear that the child is not the property of its parents and may not be dealt with without regard for his best interest" (18).

# 20

## Theoretical Considerations in Child Psychotherapy

HERMAN S. BELMONT, M.D.

A consideration of psychotherapy of children must be related to an adequate concept of mental health. Deviations from mental health call for various sociomedical measures; one of the most important is psychotherapy. Treatment approaches should also be related to a workable system of diagnostic classification based on etiology and psychodynamics, since any rational approach to therapy must select the type of therapy most appropriate and effective for a particular psychodynamic picture. In addition, psychotherapy must be rooted in a theoretical rationale which is reasonably consistent with and related to a theory of psychic development and psychopathology.

Without these, we find ourselves only too easily in the muddle of indiscriminately using various therapeutic approaches for those conditions presented to us, not on the basis of what is to our best knowledge the most appropriate therapeutic approach, nor with any clear concept of therapeutic goal. Rather, the therapeutic method is more likely determined by what personnel may be more readily available at the moment or more easily trained, for example, or on the basis of attending to large numbers at one time, or using a type of treatment in which we have a prejudiced investment. Similarly, we may be tempted to apply to all conditions a form of treatment found highly effective through our past experience in the treatment of a very specialized category. Without carefully working within a reasonably scientific frame of reference embodying concepts of etiology, pathology, diagnosis, and therapy, we may easily succumb to substituting wish for reality in selection of treatment approach. Thus a form of treatment that attends to large numbers of children at one time, or one that focuses on purely environmental handling for all cases rather than a more painstaking approach, may be adopted as an almost universal therapeutic technique, not on the basis of what is to the best of our knowledge indicated realistically but what we would like to be indicated. In an area such as psychotherapy, where immediate results are not likely to be dramatic, where treatment is sometimes costly and demanding of very limited personnel, the temptation to confuse these issues is very great. And often, in evaluating effectiveness of treatment methods, the therapist's bias is more than matched by the patient's or family's, especially in the more immediate reporting of progress and results.

## Toward a Concept of Mental Health

A definition of mental health which comprehends all possible theoretical objections and is at the same time practical and useful in evaluating adjustment and maladjustment is not easy to reach. Such a definition must be sufficiently flexible and all-encompassing to allow for infinite individual variations while still retaining a qualitatively specific statement of principles. Such a flexibility should take into account developmental progression in the child's changing personality and therefore cannot be based on absolute values. Another reason for flexibility is the common objection that mental health is very susceptible to definition in terms of value judgments. Personal values, particular investment or experience in one or another sociocultural group, or professional experience with certain theoretical orientations, may color our objective delineation of mental health criteria. We would like a definition bound as little as possible by limitations of specialized value judgments. A further caution is the need to make sufficient allowance for longitudinal vicissitudes and deviations in development which if evaluated cross-sectionally at any moment in time would appear pathological. Sometimes too close a scrutiny of behavior at any one point in time, instead of enabling a more accurate appraisal of behavior, leads to a distorted one.

It is frequently suggested that what is a good definition of mental health in one situation would not be considered adequate in another. Such an orientation feels that a definition of mental health will vary depending on sociocultural milieu, physical handicaps, psychological stresses to which an individual is being exposed, and so on. Accordingly, therefore, we are not to use the same definition for mental health in the ghetto as in an upper-middle-class suburb. Those who support such a double standard of mental health confuse freedom from social deviation and maladjustment with good mental health. Such an orientation also confuses understandable poor mental health with good mental health. A child raised in a broken home in a disadvantaged environment may be openly hostile to all authority for understandable reasons. However, this does not reduce the significance of serious characterologic problems. The same would hold true even if a sizable proportion of his peers shared his attitude toward authority.

All individuals who deviate from a particular range of behavior in a given social situation are not necessarily sick at all. Sociologically, they may constitute a problem but from a psychiatric point of view they may not be sick. The strength of their psychic structures, their dynamic interrelationships, their maturity and potential for further development, etc., may be quite adequate; and yet on the basis of certain aspects of developmental experience these individuals may deviate from certain standards of behavior in a particular social situation and not be psychiatrically sick. A child reared in the Warsaw ghetto will perhaps be deviant for a time in an upper-middle-class American suburb, but not necessarily in poor mental health. On the other hand, a child suffering the effects of painful neurotic obsessional neurosis, quite miserably uncomfortable and deviant from one definition of mental health, may appear entirely adequate in adjustment to the demands of school and home and socially no problem at all, for the present.

An important differentiation which has to be understood, therefore, in deliberating the choice of therapeutic approach, is the distinction between a dynamic definition of mental health and a sociological concern with behavior in a social situation. A second area of potential confusion has to do with poor mental health which is easily explainable on the basis of the negative influence of a very poor social environment on a child's personality development. The fact that the poor mental health is understandable leads then to the position that this is not poor mental health at all but good mental health considering the developmental background. That some children, having grown up in a particularly depriving milieu, understandably are able to invest little feeling in object relationships or understandably have poor reality testing does not change the fact that they fall short of good mental health, that certain basic functions of the personality are seriously at fault. The fact that these characteristics, as far as the children are concerned, may not cause them a problem which they want to solve is also beside the point. This does not bring these children any closer to mental health. Nor does the fact that certain sociological measures may be instituted which protect them from the further consequences of these characteristics.

A dynamic concept of mental health, to be useful in understanding therapeutic efforts, has to be based on the nature of the individual's personality structure and potential for function, in terms which will be more fully defined below. Thus an individual with given personality resources will have the same resources wherever he is. It is true, however, that sociological factors will play a crucial role developmentally in determining the degree of mental health a child can achieve at any particular age. That is, sociological factors certainly play an etiologic contributory role. Furthermore, at any particular point in development and given a particular degree of mental health, sociological factors are highly significant in terms of the degree of burden they place on the child's personality resources and the degree of opportunity allowed for the most effective utilization of inner personality adjustment in relation to the child's environment.

There is a growing tendency to think of mental health in situational terms; if an individual functions in a particular situation with the help of whatever adjuncts are available to him, then considerations of his state of mental health are deemed superfluous and irrelevant for all practical purposes. The primary goal here is to help the individual function in his immediate situation by minimum necessary adjustments in his situation, sometimes with shotgun approaches to adverse environment. A restless hyperactivity may derive from not enough to eat and a situational adjustment providing sufficient food allays the symptomatology. But this does not mean that all restless hyperactivity can be so easily corrected by a situational modification, let alone this particular form of environmental change. The hyperactivity may instead, for example, be a consequence of insufficiently controlled aggressive drives, now discharged in aimless motor activity. Let us assume that stricter external controls of motor activity in the form of punishments are imposed. Then the motor activity may temporarily be less in evidence in this situation, but the underlying anxiety and weak and threatened internal controls persist. This orientation is sometimes extended further, where an individual is not functioning well in his particular situation because of basic defects in his personality structure. His malfunction is understandable and explainable, and even commonplace, on the basis of certain adverse circumstances of life. Then this is not termed a problem of mental health, but simply a sociological phenomenon. Such an orientation to mental health may be the most practicable immediate basis for coping with the overall sociological adjustment of large numbers of our people. This, however, should not be allowed to confuse the issue of what is and what is not mental health. The above approach to a definition of mental health, though there are those who may justify it by social necessity or limited funds or large numbers, has the limitation inherent in an immediate adjustment criterion and does not include overriding general principles of total longitudinal life adjustment. Restriction of diagnosis and treatment to this level has the same limitations.

A definition of mental health cannot be so constricting that it is based on the use of specific methods of adaptation to the inner and outer demands of life. Every subculture accepts certain forms of behavior as satisfactory solutions to the problems peculiar to it. In many cases, such "solutions" are unacceptable by the standards of another culture. Consider petty stealing, lying, or delinquent gang activities. It is true that the very special demands of a particular society or culture may require specialized methods of adjustment peculiarly adaptive to that culture, a ghetto culture for example. Such special methods of adjustment, just because they may manifestly appear foreign and different from those more characteristically observed in upper-middle-class society, are not necessarily evidence of poor mental health. They may be or they may not be, but this depends on basic concepts of intrapsychic dynamics and the strengths and resources of the personality. In certain instances, they may constitute the most adaptive adjustment to a difficult situation. The particular methods used to solve the problem of an immediate adjustment to a particular situation are no more necessarily an evidence of good mental health than is the use of specific and apparently deviant measures of adjustment in a realistically stressful environment necessarily an evidence of poor mental health. The specific measures of adjustment used are a product of intrapsychic resources measured against a particular situation. We cannot form an assessment of mental health by measuring behavior against a preconceived standard of blacklisted specifics, especially when the standard is devised by one group, and colored by its particular prejudices, to evaluate behavior within another group.

This leads us to question what kind of definition of mental health can encompass these various theoretical considerations. Such a definition while covering the import of concepts, such as the psychoanalytic term "ego strength," must be couched in words which do not rely too heavily on specific theoretical terms in order to convey concepts which are universally acceptable.

The GAP Child Psychiatry Committee (3) defined

the mature and healthy person as one who actively, flexibly, and rationally masters his environment most of the time; shows a unity and integrity of personality; is able to perceive the world and himself, including his own feelings, in essentially correct proportions; can postpone immediate gratifications in favor of more long-term goals; exhibits the capacities for love, work and play; enjoys a certain sense of mental well-being; and possesses a set of values which permit him to organize his life and work while also tolerating the values of others. The truly mature individual may at times forsake adjustment and conformity for the less certain and more painful, but ultimately more rewarding and constructive, experience of attempting to alter or influence his world in a creative fashion. He also possesses the capacity for further personality development throughout adult life.

The various elements comprising this definition are essentially those functions which the psychoanalyst has assigned to the theoretical structure of the personality designated as ego. Norms for these functions at progressive levels of development of the ever-changing child have been laid down in a now extensive and ever-growing body of child development studies from many different vantage points (A. Freud, B. Bornstein, Piaget, Gesell, Escalona, Sontag, Erikson, and many others). Such functions are the capacity for self-preservation, sense of identity, object relations, reality testing, concept formation, memory and acquisition of knowledge, action and trial action (thinking), perceptual-motor function, avoidance of excessive stimuli, control and regulation of drive discharge, postponement of immediate satisfaction for future gain, experiencing of anxiety and adaptive use of mechanisms of defense, integration and synthesis of stimuli from all sources, including those from the various personality structures and the external environment, and finally the effective utilization of all these resources for adaptation to and making changes in the external world. One should emphasize particularly the concept of age appropriateness in these areas and stress more the multiple criteria of mental health. Adjustment to a particular environment, especially one in which the child has not been reared, is but one of many contributing factors that enter into an assessment of mental health. Thus the expression in the GAP definition, " . . . one who actively, flexibly and rationally masters his environment most of the time," unnecessarily restricts the definition.

The range of psychopathological disorders in the latency age child can be understood as failures in the achievement of one or another criterion of this definition of mental health. Classification of the disorder, to be defined comprehensively, must include an assessment of what normally expected functions are interfered with (the degree, scope, duration, acute or chronic, remitting or continuous, etc.), the relative strength of the other personality structures and functions, the various symptomatic manifestations of the malfunction, and, most importantly, what is the nature and interplay of all the etiologic factors in the disorder. Obviously, to effectively make these assessments requires a comprehensive understanding of such concepts as the relationship of somatic and psychological factors, developmental change, not only in the form of progressive behavioral manifestations but also in terms of intrapsychic phenomena, and psychosocial concepts. The child's environment has to be considered in relation to his psychological state, both developmentally and in terms of current interplay with the personality structure.

Thus, for a satisfactory understanding of child mental health and in order to classify child psychopathology, it is necessary to keep in mind at the same time, both cross-sectionally and longitudinally, several different concepts. These include the child's hereditary endowments, his constitutional inclinations (for example, the alternative of mastery or retreat in the face of an obstacle), his built-in maturational timetable, the variety, intensity, and timing of his experiences in the form of social interactions, physical and psychological stimuli, and the resultant nature of his overall developmental progression. All of these factors, in turn, mutually and continuously influence one another. A composite assessment of all of these factors, in multiple dimensions, makes possible an educated evaluation of the nature and degree of the child's difficulties at any point. This may be a maturational variation or an understandable and adaptive though disturbed reaction to a severely stressful environment. It may be an intrapsychic conflict now only precipitated by a minimal environmental stimulus, though resulting from earlier untoward influences of cumulative environmental interactions with the developing personality, or it may be a phasic developmental adjustment problem, or it may appear as some form of psychosomatic disorder. Whatever the nature of the difficulty, only through a familiarity with the many psychodynamic factors contributing to it can we really claim to have an understanding of the psychopathology. This is as different from classifying childhood psychological disturbances by symptom lists (on the assumption, frequently, that all problems with the same symptoms have the same etiology) as sophisticated dream analysis is different from interpreting dreams by substitution lists of symbol meanings. Only with such an understanding can one begin intelligent treatment planning.

## Problems of Community Mental Health

When we consider this orientation to mental health, and classification and diagnosis of psychopathology, we can see that the appropriate management of the infinite variety of disorders calls for a broad spectrum of therapeutic approaches, each aimed at best coping, for an individual, with a particular combination of contributory factors and intrapsychic processes which have interfered with the achievement of our goals of mental health. With the increasing interest and activity of government agencies in mental health, with the prospect of more government funding for the purpose of building, maintaining, and restoring mental health, certain basic questions of methodology have arisen which bear a close relation to all that has been said above. Some maintain that the approach, in the face of all of the variables involved, must be a massive extension in number, scope, and sophistication of diagnostic and treatment centers aimed at careful individualized study and treatment of large numbers of children initially referred mainly from home and school because of question about their mental health adjustments.

Others are repelled by the enormity of this task in the face of such objections as tremendous financial burden, limitation of skilled personnel, the exclusion of low socio-economic group children because they do not fit a static middle-class model of a "good patient," and, finally, questions about the longitudinal effectiveness of such measures. They feel that the greatest good can be served by a predominantly mass approach through environmental measures. To achieve prevention, through more favorable development, to maintain and restore mental health, they indicate that the largest number of individuals in this age period can best be taken care of by applying all resources to the creation of a more favorable home, school, and social environment. They are thinking of various milieu approaches, including neighborhood reform, family counseling, increased parent and family education, group play and work programs, day care programs, group therapy programs, increased psychoeducational or school ego building programs, and flexible programs of substitute child care. They reason that a large number of children, particularly those in low socio-economic circumstances, falling short of our goals of mental health, and an equally large number threatening to do so, of all the many etiologic factors listed as contributing to disorders of mental health, are responding first and foremost to adverse environmental circumstances.

Therefore a shotgun attack on the contributions of environment to psychopathology has been recommended in the hope that large numbers of problems will thus be corrected or prevented.

A more extreme position is taken by those who advocate a purely ecological approach to the child in a child guidance setting. They feel that the focus of treatment cannot be directed to the child as an individual. The child's symptoms are usually described in some such catchphrase as "part of the process of interchange between people." Symptoms are not accounted for in psychodynamic terms and Freud's insights regarding psychological development are regarded as more of a hindrance than a help in understanding behavior. In fact, the one-to-one relationship of the child therapy situation is seen as potentially disruptive to the totality of family life.

This type of orientation has all of the disadvantages and limitations of the two major positions already reviewed. While the approach is geared to the individual, and has all the limitations inherent in an individual approach, it does not take into account nor does it utilize the full spectrum of psychopathology and therapeutic measures available. While it focuses on the role of environment, in this respect it is also subject to its own criticisms of the intrapsychic therapies in that it is a rather limited and circumscribed approach to the total child, ignoring many of the more far-reaching aspects of intrapsychic factors.

What needs to be clearly understood is that no one type of therapeutic approach to all child psychopathology can be reasonably opposed to all others. For each clinical entity there is a form of treatment which according to our present state of knowledge and experience is the most effective. For certain problems where a child's capacity to function adaptively is crucially disrupted at least in considerable degree by serious environmental handicaps, acute reactive disorders for example, environmental modification is not only helpful but required, whereas intensive individual psychotherapy would here be limited in its usefulness. Such a problem is not one of intrapsychic pathology or poor mental health, but of environment. Where the lifelong experience of adverse environment has contributed to a disorder in development of basic personality structures, while environmental manipulation could have had preventive value earlier, it now can no longer lead to a complete reversal of deficits accumulated through the years.

If my wife mixes a cake batter but does not mix it quite as well as the recipe requires, and if she has failed to add the eggs to the batter, then after the cake is baked it will do little good to start mixing the cake or even to add a raw egg to it. Depending on the severity and duration of the environmental deficiencies or interferences, the resulting personality disturbances will be so integrally incorporated in the total personality that correction of the etiologic environmental factors is not going to reverse the damage already done. At best, one can hope that environmental modification will arrest further progression of the pathological development. Here, if the problem is one of a history of marked poverty of stimulation, the child may show a flattened and barren outlook on life. With a deficiency of warm, loving, and dependable objects during the early years, there may be an insufficient fusion of aggressive and libidinal drives, with a resulting hostile outlook on society and uninhibited rage reactions in response to small frustrations. Such personality disturbances are solidly rooted in the matrix of the personality of the child and such a child when placed now in a more favorable environment does not easily, if ever, reverse his pathological behavior. It is more likely that he will soon draw his environment into still another repetition of its previous unfortunate treatment of him. Under such circumstances, long and patient and carefully prescribed living experience may in some measure ameliorate the difficulties, and specific educational experience may be helpful in developing compensations for the deficiency.

If the personality development has led to intrapsychic conflictual problems, as for example conflicts about sexual role or a need for punishment, individual psychotherapy is indicated, perhaps supplemented by other measures in the child's current life situation. There are disturbances of mental health in which the pathology resides predominantly intrapsychically, as, for example, in certain neurotic conditions like anxiety hysteria or obsessional neurosis, and where the current environment has little to do with the nature of the psychopathology, although past experiences have played an etiologic role. These require more specialized dynamic psychotherapy or psychoanalysis, whereas environmental approaches do little to alter the basic pathology.

A problem arises when we wish to offer any one psychotherapeutic approach as the solution to all problems regardless of their peculiar distinguishing characteristics. The difficulty is augmented when advocates of particular approaches are motivated by various reasons, ranging from limited experience with a sufficient variety of psychopathology, to prejudiced theoretical conviction, to an idealistic urge to solve all of man's problems. What results is a denial of the many complex factors that play a role in mental health and illness and the assumption of an oversimplified and overgeneralized approach to all of the emotional disorders of childhood.

There is no objection to a carefully considered massive program aimed at an improvement of clearly known and established contributions to the child's development and life situation. Moreover, it is even desirable, since better neighborhoods, work and play opportunities, better schooling, and social progress, etc., can contribute to the opportunity for healthier psychological development of many children and ameliorate some of the emotional problems of many others. However, while this is undoubtedly true, it would be a mistake to believe that this is what is needed to prevent or treat all types of childhood psychological disorders. Assume that such a massive shotgun approach has been undertaken and has alleviated a major portion of these general environmental contributions to emotional problems. Then, more than ever, it is necessary that adequate diagnostic resources as well as an entire spectrum of therapeutic measures be available for the range of psychological problems other than those which will respond purely to environmental intervention.

## Diagnostic Considerations

For some reason, in the field of child psychiatry, there is a temptation to overgeneralize in assigning to a symptom complex only one limited psychodynamic explanation and then to proceed therapeutically on that basis. Only after a considerable period does it become evident that the etiology and therapy for the symptom complex do not always lie in one direction, nor always in the other. Rather, as might be expected, multiple etiologic factors and dynamics may exist for the same symptomatic picture in many different combinations. I once (1) attempted to show how several isolated positions concerning the etiology (and therefore the therapeutic approach) of severe ego disturbance of childhood actually participated jointly in a complemental relationship in every case. Elsewhere (2) I presented a summary review of a number of different causes for the basic problem of learning disorder. Here, there were many varieties of interference with the ego's function, each resulting in a disorder of learning. In turn, each variety of psychopathology calls for an appropriate therapeutic approach, regardless of the fact that we are dealing with one principal symptom complex. The choice of therapy cannot be a matter of devout loyalty to one and only one type of therapy, or another. Unfortunately, however, this is what has often evolved, so that at times we find an almost patriotic zeal determining therapeutic recommendation, while the more realistic indications for choice of therapy are overlooked.

Aside from establishing a rational relationship between psychopathology and therapy of choice, some may empirically use other methods of treatment that seem to have been effective elsewhere. There can be no objection to this if such projects are undertaken on a limited scale, and thoroughly studied and researched before being utilized on a wholesale basis. While it is true that many of our more widely used therapies have themselves not been sufficiently subjected to the same rigid research, at the same time their continued use as the treatments of choice pending adequate research is at least supported by cumulative clinical impression and an extensive body of theoretical rationale.

Much of the confusion about choice of therapy derives from differences in understanding of the concept of internalization of conflict. There are some who minimize intrapsychic factors because they do not believe there is any diagnostic entity in the school-age child which cannot be treated if only appropriate and adequate changes can be made in the child's environment. We believe such a position is inconsistent with numerous and intensive clinical observations which demonstrate that the personality structure of the school-age child is in certain fundamental ways quite different from that of the preschool child. Anna Freud made this distinction clear in her discussion of types of anxiety (5). The young child, before age six, experiences largely objective anxiety. Such controls as he imposes on his instinctual wishes are determined predominantly by expectations, prohibitions, and threats of the world around him. For the young child, of course, the parents constitute the principal representatives of the external world. During this period of the child's development, for example, it is readily evident that to a considerable degree changes in the parental attitudes and expectations are rather quickly and easily reflected in changes in the child's behavior. This situation, diagrammatically and with much simplification, could be represented by an open U-tube, in which adding or removing fluid from one side readily affects the level on the other side; usually the immediate behavioral response is quite predictable from the particular change in the external environment. To some extent, even in these early years, and especially in cases of precocious development, there are evidences that the personality of the child has begun to take over some of the function of regulating and controlling his instinctual wishes, but even here such controls still bear a close relationship with the external world. They are less firmly established, more readily influenced from without, and require continuing support from the outside in order to be maintained.

By the time a child has reached first grade, if he has been developing normally, we find a different situation. It is as though there is no longer free and direct interchange between the two sides of the U-tube, as though a cork has been placed at its base. At best, there is a very slow leak around the cork. Now the child has taken over within his own psychic structure many of the prohibitions and controls previously derived from sources in the external world. This is the consequence of developmental changes during the latter part of the preschool period, culminating in the establishment of firm identifications with important child-rearing figures. These changes are best explained by the psychoanalytic theory of the resolution of the oedipal conflict. As a part of the termination of the oedipal conflict, there is laid down a new psychic structure in the child's personality, the superego. The child's ego now mediates the emergence of instinctual wishes with one eye on the superego, so to speak, responding now to the threat of superego anxiety where it previously responded almost exclusively to external danger, objective anxiety. While, in addition, external threats will continue to influence behavior throughout life, from this time on there continues to operate a potent intrapsychic factor which will significantly figure in the child's conflicts with his wishes. This superego structure retains those characteristics of the external prohibitions as the child saw them, not only on the basis of what he had experienced but also in terms of the intensity of his own drives at that crucial time when he took those prohibitions over and made them his own. Once this development has taken place, the child's behavior will be determined by both real external dangers and also by a powerful intrapsychic agent. The superego continues to retain the qualities and characteristics which it held at the time it was laid down. Therefore it becomes understandable that such a personality is capable of developing a conflict which cannot be easily resolved and which manifests itself in pathological symptomatology at a time when one cannot rationally understand the conflict in terms of current environmental circumstances. Such a conflict is intrapsychic between several personality structures and the pathology cannot be resolved by altering the current environment, as evidenced by its continued existence in the face of even optimal environmental circumstances.

Furthermore, it should be stated that these intrapsychic processes are entirely unconscious and for this reason are not amenable to outside influence or the reasoning process under ordinary circumstances. Psychoanalysis is a form of psychotherapy with which it is possible to make these unconscious processes conscious and subject them to understanding and reason. This is probably the main way in which psychoanalysis differs from conditioning, family therapy, group therapy, etc.

It is true that children will also develop symptomatology when confronted with an overly stressful current environment and will improve in such a case if the environment is changed for the better. However, these are two different situations and must not be confused inasmuch as the therapeutic approach is different in each case. Undoubtedly, because the child continues to develop and is very much dependent on his environment, there may be considerable overlap and interplay between intrapsychic and environmental factors, and attention to both factors may be necessary but for entirely different reasons. Just as excessive intrapsychic determinants of pathology will preclude a successful environmental approach, so will continuing adverse environment in other cases interfere with efforts to resolve intrapsychic pathology.

An area of confusion is the failure to distinguish properly between past and present environmental influence on the child. The fact that there has in the past been a developmental interference, deriving from qualitative or quantitative environmental disturbance, does not mean that now, in the present, all the consequences can be erased by simple compensatory modification of the child's environment today. If we accept the epigenetic concept of the child's development, with each new experience in the child's life contributing to qualitative dynamic growth changes, it is self-evident that timing of experience is of basic importance. To attempt to correct the consequences of intense and overly severe disciplinary training at age two by more reality oriented and understanding expectations at age ten is a gross oversimplification of both theory of development and therapy.

All the multiple factors discussed above are a part of a rationale for diagnostic classification and psychotherapy of the school age child. This is not the place to attempt to systematize in one or another classification the many diagnostic categories based on these factors. The previously referred-to GAP report No. 62 (June 1966) contains an appendix with a comprehensive outline for dynamic-genetic diagnostic formulation and also a number of the systems of classification which have been offered by child psychiatrists. The strengths of most of these classifications have been extracted and utilized in the GAP's comprehensive proposal. With a thorough dynamic-genetic formulation as a basis, we can then better ascertain the therapy or combinations of types of therapy most appropriate. The choice will be related also to treatment goal, whether we are aiming for extensive personality reorganization or symptomatic change, whether for circumscribed and limited changes in the present or projected long-range goals. The methods in working toward such goals, depending on the formulation, will include the various forms of psychotherapy, other medical approaches involving pharmacologic, biochemical, and physical rehabilitative efforts, and the many forms of environmental modification.

## The Therapies of Childhood

Psychotherapy may be administered by one person almost exclusively or by a team of therapists, sometimes of different disciplines working together. The background of the therapist is usually primarily medicine, social work, psychology, or education. The child may be seen alone, or as one of a group of varying scope, or together with his family. The child may be seen alone and the parents alone by the same therapist or by different therapists, in varying degrees of cooperation and communication with one another. The length and frequency of visits vary as well, from very short in duration to several hours at a time, from five or six visits a week to infrequent contact. The child may see the therapist in an office setting, an institutional setting such as a day school, residential center, or hospital, or in the child's own home.

Various medical approaches may be utilized as a primary method of treatment and exclusive of other treatment approaches, or as a supplement to psychotherapeutic or environmental methods.

Treatment efforts through modification of environment are equally varied in scope. One form of environmental approach to a child's problems, for example, is the effort to alter the parents' behavior and attitudes in some way. Such an attempt, again, may take the form of any of the several approaches used with the child, a form of psychotherapy,

or medical or environmental measures. The overall social or physical nature of the child's or his family's environment may be modified by
broad sociological measures or by efforts more specifically focused on a
particular child, his family, or interactions within the family. The child's
milieu may be changed by full- or part-time placement in another home,
school, hospital, or residential center, or by special educational and activities programs in or outside the home.

Psychotherapy of children, even if provided on an individual one-to-
one basis, takes many forms. In some cases the total diagnostic evaluation will indicate clear-cut and extensive intrapsychic pathology calling for
intensive analytic investigation of the personality dynamics, as in a firmly
established case of anxiety hysteria. This does not mean that the treatment for such a case will always be directed toward this goal. Other
less desirable goals (in the estimation of some) for the same case are
for various reasons sometimes sought, such as symptomatic relief without
insight or varying degrees of readjustment of the underlying personality
structure and its conflicts. Then a different treatment approach will be
used. Here, the goals should be clearly differentiated and stated and a
basis offered for not selecting the goal and treatment of choice. Furthermore, the effectiveness of such methods of treatment should not be
compared with intensive insight therapies without taking into account at
the same time the difference in underlying goals. In other cases, such as
temporary situational crises or developmental interferences, for example,
more intensive insight therapies would in fact be contraindicated whereas
brief supportive, abreactive, educational, or limited insight therapy, together with some environmental modification, might be the indicated
treatment.

This point is well illustrated by therapeutic approaches to several types
of nocturnal enuresis in school age children. A four-year-old who has had
continuous uninterrupted nocturnal enuresis, largely on the basis of maternal compliance and failure to train, does not require intensive insight
therapy any more than a child with encopresis on the basis of fecal
impaction. A more effective approach is to work with the parents and
child toward enabling the child to take over the responsibility for sphincter control. This might involve helping the parents to understand better
their role in relation to the child and ultimately to establish and communicate more consistent expectations. With the child, it might involve
allowing him, through various measures, first to experience some success,
and finally to establish more adequate controls for maintaining the success, via his interaction with his parents as well as re-educational efforts
in therapy. On the other hand, a case of recent regressive onset of nocturnal enuresis following hospitalization for surgery, if evaluated as predominantly reactive to the threats of surgery and hospitalization, might
well respond to an opportunity for abreactive ventilation, a mastery of
the stress situation by working it through repetitively in play and verbal-

ization, and some opportunity for insight. In still another case, where a regressive enuresis of several years' duration is but one symptom of a neurosis, an anxiety hysteria with elaborate paralyzing anxiety about forbidden sexual fantasies, the treatment of choice would likely be psychoanalysis. This form of treatment differs from others in focusing on the child's unconscious fantasies in relation to his overall personality structure and environment.

Here, as summed up years ago by Erik Erikson (4), the then chairman of the Committee on the Psychoanalysis of Children and Adolescents of the American Psychoanalytic Association, there is a "systematic investigation of unconscious, or as yet unverbalized pathogenic associations between certain facts, fantasies and affects," and an investigation of the "defense mechanisms developed or rigidified in the attempt to deal with these associations." There is a "systematic selective communication to the child of the results of such investigation" in a way that he can understand and assimilate. Then there is a systematic follow-up that investigates secondary fantasies, affects, and defenses resulting from the treatment effort. "The systematic check of the therapeutic situation continues until there is evidence that the child's ego mastery has become more adequate for his age."

The principal types of individual treatment of the child have been described previously by many other authors (4a) and the following summary is not in any way original. There are a few major categories. Psychoanalytic treatment is the most intensive and effective one for those disorders which are predominantly intrapsychic and in which there is a severe unrealistic superego and a relatively strong ego (4a). Generally, the indications for child psychoanalysis are the classical neuroses, anxiety hysteria, conversion hysteria, and obsessive-compulsive neurosis. Many cases which do not initially appear so, with careful diagnostic evaluation are often found to be cases of classical neurosis. Briefly these include:

1. Children who show inhibition in ego functions or reactions, or who show marked ego restrictions.
2. Cases in which a regression in psychosexual development has occurred at a specific time.
3. Cases in which the child wishes consciously to be, or acts in his behavior as if he were, of the opposite sex.
4. When antisocial behavior is caused by an unconscious need for punishment, as the result of a strong sense of guilt (either conscious or unconscious).
5. Pregenital conversion syndromes—prolonged tics or stuttering.
6. Cases whose main presenting symptom is a sexual perversion.

Many other diverse symptom pictures often will be found to reflect the underlying dynamic picture of the neurosis, with intrapsychic conflict at the core, and as such are best treated psychoanalytically.

Another category of individual psychotherapy is primarily educational. Here the effort is directed at achieving improvement through development of controls or intensification of already existing defenses. Where the educational approach helps evolve or reinforce necessary ego controls, the treatment is used to supplement development deficits. Where the treatment aims at intensification of an already present neurotic defense, through increased reaction-formation or counterphobic attitudes, for example, while there may be symptomatic improvement, increasing quantities of energy are being bound up in the maintenance of the defense and the treatment cannot be considered a valid approach to the underlying problem. Such is the nature of moralistic admonition or efforts to counter inappropriate behavior for unconscious causes by emphasizing reality, such as, "There is no reason to be afraid of the dog. He has never in five years hurt anyone." Similarly, avoidance of problem areas by encouragement of diversionary activity or compensatory development again misses the point. A child has a character trait of chronic provocative behavior, resulting in his being regularly beat up by his peers, on the basis of a problem with effective discharge of his aggressive drives. While it may be symptomatically helpful to train the child in the use of karate, his basic problem remains. On the other hand, a child may be benefited by helping him to accept his drives and to discharge them in suitable outlets, utilizing available channels for instinctual gratification.

Education through provision of intellectual insights may offer a child some relief by giving him a prop, but again unless the insight is worked through and felt as consistent with emotions, in effect the spontaneous adaptive discharge of drives is impaired.

Many types of conditioning therapies fall into the category of educational approaches. To the extent the symptoms thus alleviated are bound up in basic intrapsychic conflicts which remain unresolved and continue to damage the child's mental health, to this extent they fall short of matching therapy to psychopathology. Such an approach would attribute to the symptom the significance of the underlying pathology.

Conditioning therapies can remove symptoms. However, it is important that one understand the role of symptom removal in any one case, as a part of the total psychodynamic picture. This type of therapy is not a substitute for other therapies. Silberstein (6), in a knowledgeable approach to treatment of enuresis in children never before bladder trained, utilized conditioning techniques to interrupt the symptom. However, he was prepared to work concurrently with parents and child and, in certain instances, to undertake intensive psychotherapy of the child when the underlying dynamics indicated the need.

Various types of suggestion also constitute a form of education in psychotherapy. Under the strong influence of the relationship with the therapist, symptoms are given up. Just as in hypnosis the subject relinquishes his own wishes and behavioral manifestations in accordance with the expectations of the hypnotist, so does the patient relinquish his symptom manifestations in compliance with the suggestions and wishes of the therapist. This takes many forms and is reinforced by assorted supplementary aids, ranging from the reputation and authority of the therapist, magical gestures, rituals of therapy, concrete props, placebos, to the reputation of a type of therapy.

Educational aspects of therapy generally aim more or less in the direction of establishing controls. The development of these controls may be very necessary to maintain effective function, or may simply be temporary and superficial devices for removal or concealment of symptoms. Abreaction in psychotherapy, on the other hand, operates in the opposite direction. This aspect of psychotherapy aims at achieving release and discharge. The patient is encouraged, through provision of a permissive atmosphere, to communicate thoughts and feelings ordinarily kept in control. The opening up may be general and nonspecific or may be related to more specific conflict areas. In either case there is at least some temporary relief through the discharge of feelings which had previously been contained only at the cost of great energy. Where the ventilation provides an opportunity for working through and mastering an isolated conflict area or an acute trauma which had been passively experienced, it is evident that abreaction and mastery may have permanent therapeutic effect. Where the abreactive treatment encourages discharge of anxiety deriving from a basic underlying unresolved conflict, this offers only temporary relief. Where the abreaction consists of discharge of impulses which are otherwise engaged in a basic intrapsychic conflict with severe prohibitions, perhaps even drives at a developmentally regressed level, such discharge does not in any way alter the psychopathology. In fact, it may only serve to intensify the punitive, guilt-producing, and controlling functions of the personality.

It is only when such measures are utilized with appropriate regard for the specific needs of the patient that they will be most helpful. When they are used to deal with established intrapsychic conflict, in order to be used properly and effectively they must fit into the context of a systematic treatment approach which respects the genetic, structural, and dynamic aspects of the personality.

These basic psychotherapeutic principles and methods operate, in varying combination with the medical and environmental approaches, in every form of therapy for every child treated for a psychiatric problem. Whereas it is at times difficult to achieve an understanding of how these many factors interrelate in treating those children who can be seen individually, this is tremendously compounded when children are treated in groups, or simultaneously with other members of the family, or with multiple therapeutic personnel. It becomes that much more difficult to tailor therapeutic efforts to particular needs while at the same time more variables are introduced. A further potential difficulty results from the tendency to be less exacting in individual diagnostic evaluation when treating patients en masse, whereas it would appear the exact reverse should hold. Group and milieu approaches generally would seem to have their greatest potential usefulness for cases which tend to be developmental or current environmental and situational in nature. Also, where the treatment goal is more limited, and primarily symptom amelioration or better adjustment in a specific situation is desired, such approaches would appear more in order. Here opportunities for ventilation and abreaction, for education and control, for suggestion and persuasion, seemingly serve the purpose of the goals. On the other hand, where children of school age with firmly established intrapsychic conflicts are so treated, we must recognize that it is highly unlikely that such therapeutic methods can at this stage in their development achieve a systematic fundamental resolution of the basic pathology.

Thus, considering the infinite variety of contributory variables in a child's mental health and social adjustment, alongside of the already currently utilized numerous forms of treatment, and all of the backgrounds, skills, and personalities of psychotherapists, the probability of inappropriate or ineffectual treatment efforts is great. The potential solution for this unsatisfactory state of affairs lies in several directions. There is a distinct need for training of those personnel of all disciplines concerned with treatment of children, not only in the dynamics and genetics of the entire range of diagnostic categories, but also the entire range of treatment methods. Where realistic limitations prevent such extensive training for all involved personnel, then certainly it should be required for those who have the authority of executing mental health programs, for the individuals who have final responsibility for planning diagnosis and treatment recommendations.

Further, there must be some kind of rationale of diagnosis and treatment so that we can get away from a tubular vision approach to psychopathology. Random and aimless expenditure of effort with poorly defined goals cannot be considered an adequate basis for treatment innovations.

Each form of treatment, and especially innovations, should have funding tied inseparably to well-planned clinical or action research designs which will clearly provide directions for further research and some basis for evaluation of previous efforts. Especially there should be extensive financial support for further study and use of that body of theory of psychopathology and technique which has made available to us the most systematic and comprehensive knowledge in this area to date. Psychoanalytic theory as developed from psychoanalytic treatment of children and adults and study of normal development has provided us with many basic and universally acknowledged concepts. Isolated segments of psychoanalytic theory have been borrowed and utilized, sometimes out of context or with limited understanding, to serve as the foundation for certain specialized treatment forms. Other parts of psychoanalytic theory, either regarded in isolation or extracted from long since modified earlier writings in the field, have been subjected to bitter criticism. At times the entire body of psychoanalytic theory is erroneously equated with the more specifically indicated and highly specialized psychoanalytic treatment method. Then the value of analytic theory is derogated as limited and worthless for all practical purposes on the basis that psychoanalysis as a form of treatment is not appropriate for a wide range of disorders which do not fulfill the necessary indications. For certain types of disorders, psychoanalytic treatment is still the treatment of choice. Its further study is certainly one of the most promising areas for investment of research effort available today in the field of psychopathology and is a sine qua non alongside of research of other methods for treating problems where psychoanalytic treatment would be quite inappropriate. Hopefully, the selection of other treatment methods for thorough study will, as well, be more on the basis of careful rationale than expediency.

## CHAPTER 1
### An Overview of Child Psychiatry

1. Freud, A. *Normality and Pathology in Childhood* (New York: International Universities Press, 1963).
2. ———. *Psychoanalytic Study of the Child*, Vol. 8 (New York: International Universities Press, 1953).
3. ———. *Psychoanalytic Study of the Child*, Vol. 17 (New York: International Universities Press, 1962).
4. ———. *The Psychoanalytic Treatment of Children* (London: Imago Publishing, 1946).
5. Freud, S. "Analysis of a Phobia in a Five-Year-Old Boy," in J. Strachey (ed.), *The Standard Edition of the Complete Psychological Works of Sigmund Freud*, Vol. 10 (London: Hogarth Press, 1955).
6. ———. "The Interpretation of Dreams," in J. Strachey (ed.), *The Standard Edition of the Complete Psychological Works of Sigmund Freud*, Vols. 5 and 6 (London: Hogarth Press, 1953).
7. ———. "Three Essays on the Theory of Sexuality," in J. Strachey (ed.), *The Standard Edition of the Complete Psychological Works of Sigmund Freud*, Vol. 10 (London: Hogarth Press, 1955).
8. Kanner, L. *American Journal of Orthopsychiatry* 19 (1949).
9. ———. *Child Psychiatry* (Springfield, Ill.: Charles Thomas, 1966).
10. Kolansky, H. *Psychoanalytic Study of the Child*, Vol. 22 (New York: International Universities Press, 1967).
11. ——— and Stennis, W. *Journal of the Albert Einstein Medical Center* 16, no. 1 (Spring 1968).
12. Mahler, M.; Settlage, C.; and others. "Severe Emotional Disturbances in Childhood: Psychoses," in S. Arieti (ed.), *American Handbook of Psychiatry* (New York: Basic Books, 1959).
13. Pearson, G. H. J. *Bulletin of the Philadelphia Association for Psychoanalysis* 5, no. 1 (May 1955).
14. Weil, A. M. *Psychoanalytic Study of the Child*, Vol. 8 (New York: International Universities Press, 1953).

## CHAPTER 2
### Disturbances in Development and Childhood Neurosis

1. Bornstein, B. *Psychoanalytic Quarterly* 4 (1935): 93–119.
2. ———. *Psychoanalytic Study of the Child*, Vols. 3 and 4 (New York: International Universities Press, 1949), p. 194.

3. ———. *Psychoanalytic Study of the Child*, Vol. 6 (New York: International Universities Press, 1951), pp. 279–285.
4. ———. *Psychoanalytic Study of the Child*, Vol. 8 (New York: International Universities Press, 1953), p. 68.
5. Brody, S. *Psychoanalytic Study of the Child*, Vol. 16 (New York: International Universities Press, 1961), pp. 251–274.
6. Freud, A. *The Ego and the Mechanisms of Defense* (New York: International Universities Press, 1946), pp. 117–131.
7. ———. "Indications and Contraindications for Child Analysis." Summarized by S. Shapiro. *Bulletin of the Philadelphia Association for Psychoanalysis* 18 (1968): 217–220.
8. ———. *Normality and Pathology in Childhood* (New York: International Universities Press, 1965), pp. 154–155. 8a. p. 155; 8b. p. 18; 8c. p. 161; 8d. p. 68; 8e. p. 163.
9. ———. *Psychoanalytic Study of the Child*, Vol. 1 (New York: International Universities Press, 1945), pp. 127–149.
10. ———. *Psychoanalytic Study of the Child*, Vol. 21 (New York: International Universities Press, 1963), pp. 245–265.
11. Freud, S. "Analysis of a Phobia in a Five-Year-Old Boy," J. Strachey (ed.), *The Standard Edition of the Complete Psychological Works of Sigmund Freud*, Vol. 10 (London: Hogarth Press, 1955).
12. ———. "An Outline of Psychoanalysis," in J. Strachey (ed.), *The Standard Edition of the Complete Psychological Works of Sigmund Freud*, Vol. 23 (London: Hogarth Press, 1964), p. 184.
13. Fries, M., and Woolf, P. *Psychoanalytic Study of the Child*, Vol. 8 (New York: International Universities Press, 1953), pp. 48–62.
14. Greenacre, P. *Psychoanalytic Study of the Child*, Vol. 9 (New York: International Universities Press, 1954), p. 20.
15. Hartmann, H. *Psychoanalytic Study of the Child*, Vol. 5 (New York: International Universities Press, 1950), pp. 74–96.
16. Mahler, M. *Psychoanalytic Study of the Child*, Vol. 7 (New York: International Universities Press, 1952), pp. 286–305.
17. Nagera, H. *Early Childhood Disturbances, the Infantile Neurosis, and the Adulthood Disturbances* (New York: International Universities Press, 1966). 17a. p. 57.
18. Pearson, G. H. J. *Bulletin of the Philadelphia Association for Psychoanalysis* 5 (1955): 9–14.
19. Peller, L. Personal communication.
20. Provence, S., and Lipton, R. C. *Infants in Institutions* (New York: International Universities Press, 1962).
21. Spitz, R. *No and Yes* (New York: International Universities Press, 1957).
22. ———. *Psychoanalytic Study of the Child*, Vol. 1 (New York: International Universities Press, 1945), pp. 53–74.
23. Waelder, R. *Psychoanalytic Study of the Child*, Vol. 9 (New York: International Universities Press, 1954), p. 56.
24. Winnicott, D. W. "Transitional Objects and Transitional Phenomena," *Collected Papers* (New York: Basic Books, 1958).

## CHAPTER 3
*Ego Disturbances in Children*

1. American Psychiatric Association. *Diagnostic and Statistical Manual of Mental Disorders*, 2d ed. (Washington, D.C., 1968).
2. Bonaparte, M.; Freud, A.; and Kris, E. (eds.). *The Origins of Psychoanalysis* (New York: Doubleday Anchor Books, 1957), p. 26.
3. Freud, A. *The Ego and the Mechanisms of Defense* (New York: International Universities Press, 1946).
4. Freud, S. "Analysis Terminable and Interminable," in J. Strachey (ed.), *The Standard Edition of the Complete Psychological Works of Sigmund Freud*, Vol. 23 (London: Hogarth Press, 1964), p. 216.
5. ———. "An Outline of Psychoanalysis," in J. Strachey (ed.), *The Standard Edition of the Complete Psychological Works of Sigmund Freud*, Vol. 13 (London: Hogarth Press, 1964), pp. 145–146.
6. Geleerd, E. *Psychoanalytic Study of the Child*, Vols. 3 and 4 (New York: International Universities Press, 1949), pp. 311–332.
7. Goldfarb, W. *Archives of General Psychiatry* 11 (1964): 620–634.
8. Harlow, H. *Science* 130 (1959): 421.
9. Itard, J. *The Wild Boy of Aveyron* (New York: Appleton-Century-Crofts, 1962), p. 10.
10. Kanner, L. *American Journal of Orthopsychiatry* 19 (1949): 416–426.
11. Mahler, M. *Psychoanalytic Study of the Child*, Vol. 7 (New York: International Universities Press, 1952), pp. 286–305.
12. *The New Testament in Modern English*. Trans. J. B. Phillips (New York: The Macmillan Co., 1968), p. 391.
13. Nunberg, H. *Principles of Psychoanalysis* (New York: International Universities Press, 1955), pp. 150–151.
14. Piaget, J. *The Construction of Reality in the Child* (New York: Basic Books, 1954), pp. 219–319.
15. Spitz, R. *A Genetic Field Theory of Ego Development* (New York: International Universities Press, 1959).
16. ———. *No and Yes* (New York: International Universities Press, 1957).
17. Weil, A. *Psychoanalytic Study of the Child*, Vol. 8 (New York: International Universities Press, 1953), p. 271.

## CHAPTER 4
*Vicissitudes of Adolescence*

1. Bernfeld, S. "Über eine typische Form der mannlichen Pubertät." Quoted in A. Freud, reference 4, p. 257.
2. Blos, P. *American Journal of Orthopsychiatry* 24 (1954): 733.
3. ———. *On Adolescence: A Psychoanalytic Interpretation* (New York: Free Press, 1962), p. 5. 3a. p. 54; 3b. p. 220.
4. Freud, A. *Psychoanalytic Study of the Child*, Vol. 13 (New York: International Universities Press, 1958), p. 264.
5. ———. *Psychoanalytic Study of the Child*, Vol. 18 (New York: International Universities Press, 1963), pp. 245–265.
6. Grinspoon, L. *Marijuana Reconsidered* (Cambridge, Mass.: Harvard University Press, 1971), p. 323.

7. Katan, A. *International Journal of Psychoanalysis* 32 (1951): 69. Quoted in P. Blos, reference 3, p. 5.
8. Kolansky, H., and Moore, W. *Journal of the American Medical Association* 216, no. 3 (1971): 486–492.
9. Nagera, H. *Early Childhood Disturbances, the Infantile Neurosis and the Adult Disturbances* (New York: International Universities Press, 1966).
10. Spiegel, L. *Psychoanalytic Study of the Child*, Vol. 13 (New York: International Universities Press, 1958), p. 302.

## CHAPTER 5

*Juvenile Delinquency*

1. Adelson, E. T.; Sugar, C.; and Wortis, B. *American Journal of Psychiatry* 105 (1949): 620.
2. Bakwin, H. *American Journal of Diseases of the Child* 89 (1955): 368.
3. Banar, R. *American Journal of Psychiatry* 111 (1954): 242.
4. Becher, P. W. *Psychological Reports* 16 (1965): 276.
5. Berman, S. *American Journal of Orthopsychiatry* 29 (1959): 613.
6. Bernabeu, E. P. *Psychoanalytic Quarterly* 27 (1958): 386–387.
7. Berninghausen, D., and Faunce, R. *Journal of Experimental Education* 33 (1964): 164–165.
8. Bettelheim, B., and Sylvester, E. *Psychoanalytic Study of the Child*, Vol. 5 (New York: International Universities Press, 1950), pp. 340–341. 8a. p. 106.
9. Blos, P. *Psychoanalytic Study of the Child*, Vol 12 (New York: International Universities Press, 1957), p. 231. 9a. p. 239.
10. Brigham, J. C.; Ricketts, J. L.; and others. *Journal of Consulting Psychology* 31 (1967): 420.
11. Butler, F. O. *American Journal of Mental Deficiency* 53 (1948): 79.
12. Cowden, J. E., and Pacht, A. R. *Journal of Consulting Psychology* 31 (1967): 381.
13. Dana, R. A., and others. *Journal of Clinical Psychology* 19 (1963): 355.
14. Eissler, K. R. *Psychoanalytic Study of the Child*, Vol. 5 (New York: International Universities Press, 1950), pp. 107–108. 14a. p. 99.
15. Falstein, E. I. *American Journal of Orthopsychiatry* 28 (1958): 616.
16. Fenichel, O. *The Psychoanalytic Theory of Neurosis* (New York: W. W. Norton, 1945), p. 505.
17. Galdston, I. *Mental Hygiene* 32 (1948): 529–530.
18. Gatling, F. P. *Journal of Abnormal and Social Psychology* 45 (1950): 751.
19. Glueck, S., and Glueck, E. *Delinquents in the Making: Paths to Prevention* (New York: Harper & Bros., 1952), p. 17.
20. Gregory, J. *Archives of General Psychiatry* 13 (1965): 103. 20a. p. 107.
21. Harrington, R., and Davis, R. *Child Development* 24 (1953): 286.
22. Henning, J. J., and Levy, R. H. *Journal of Clinical Psychology* 23 (1967): 164.
23. Hirschberg, J. C., and Noshpitz, J. *American Journal of Diseases of the Child* 89 (1955): 361.
24. Hobbes, Thomas. *Leviathan* (Chicago: Encyclopedia Britannica, 1952), p. 139.
25. Johnson, A. M. *American Journal of Diseases of the Child* 89 (1955): 472.
26. ———, and Szurek, S. A. *Psychoanalytic Quarterly* 21 (1952): 330.

27. Kaplan, M.; Ryan, J.; and others. *American Journal of Psychiatry* 113 (1957): 1109.
28. Karpman, B., and others. *American Journal of Orthopsychiatry* 20 (1950): 245. 28a. p. 233; 28b. p. 227; 28c. pp. 262–263.
29. Kaufman, I., and Heims, L. *American Journal of Orthopsychiatry* 28 (1958): 146.
30. King, C. H., and Rabinowitz, C. *American Journal of Orthopsychiatry* 35 (1965): 610.
31. Kirkwood, J. W. *Nervous Child* 11 (1955): 28.
32. Knight, J. A. *American Journal of Orthopsychiatry* 30 (1960): 422.
33. Lively, E., and others. *American Journal of Orthopsychiatry* 32 (1962): 160.
34. Loomis, S. D., and others. *Archives of General Psychiatry* 17 (1967): 494.
35. Madoff, J. M. *Journal of Consulting Psychology* 23 (1959): 519.
36. Mann, A. *American Journal of Mental Deficiency* 56 (1951): 414.
37. Massimo, J. L., and Shore, M. F. *Psychiatry* 30 (1967): 230.
38. Pearson, G. H. J. (ed.). *A Handbook of Child Psychoanalysis* (New York: Basic Books, 1968), pp. 59–60.
39. Ricks, D., and others. *Journal of Abnormal and Social Psychology* 69 (1964): 688.
40. Schulman, I. *International Journal of Group Psychotherapy* 2 (1952): 337. 40a. p. 343.
41. ———. *Nervous Child* 11 (1955): 35.
42. Shore, M. F., and Massimo, J. L. *Journal of Consulting Psychology* 29 (1965): 214.
43. Shore, M. F., and others. *Journal of Clinical Psychology* 21 (1965): 212.
44. Stabenau, J. R.; Tupin, J.; and others. *Psychiatry* 28 (1965): 55.
45. Stallak, G. E., and Guerney, B. *Journal of Clinical Psychology* 20 (1964): 281.
46. Tappan, P. W. *American Journal of Psychiatry* 108 (1952): 682.
47. Telson, S. *Journal of Rehabilitation* 30 (1964): 10.
48. Wagner, E. E., and Hawkins, R. *Journal of Projective Techniques and Personal Assessment* 28 (1964): 364.
49. Wolk, R. L., and Reid, R. *Group Psychotherapy* 17 (1964): 59.
50. Young, D. J., and Alverson, P. J. *Philadelphia Sunday Bulletin,* March 9, 1969, p. 7.
51. Zivan, M., and Jones, N. A. *Personnel and Guidance Journal* 43 (1965): 462. 51a. p. 465.

## CHAPTER 6

### *Drug Addiction*

1. Balter, M. B., and Levine, J. *Psychopharmacology Bulletin* 5 (1969): 3–13.
2. Connell, P. H. *Maudsley Monograph,* no. 5 (London: Oxford University Press, 1958).
3. Conrad, J. *Youth,* in *Three Short Novels* (New York: Bantam Books, 1960).
4. *Drugs and the Young* (New York: Times-Life Books, 1970).
5. Farnsworth, N. R. *Science* 162 (1968): 1086–1091.
6. Freud, A. *The Psychoanalytic Treatment of Children* (New York: International Universities Press, 1946).

7. Goodman, I., and Gilman, A. *The Pharmacological Basis of Therapeutics* (New York: The Macmillan Co., 1967).

8. Horn, D. Presentation at World Conference on Smoking and Health, New York, September 11, 1967.

9. Lewis, E. Personal communication (Bureau of Narcotics, U.S. Department of Justice).

10. Louria, D. *The Drug Scene* (New York: McGraw-Hill, 1968).

11. Lourie, R. S., and Werkman, S. L. "Technical Problems in the Diagnosis and Treatment of Adolescents," in G. Caplan and S. Lebovici (eds.), *Psychiatric Approaches to Adolescence* (New York: Excerpta Medica Foundation, 1966).

12. *Marijuana and Health: A Report to the Congress from the Secretary, Department of Health, Education and Welfare* (Washington, D.C.: U.S. Government Printing Office, 1971).

13. Mizner, G.; Barter, J.; and Werme, H. *American Journal of Psychiatry* 127 (1970): 15–24.

14. National Clearinghouse for Drug Abuse Information. *Answers to Most Frequently Asked Questions About Drug Abuse* (Bethesda, Md., 1970).

15. Sadusk, J. F. *Journal of the American Medical Association* 196 (1966): 707–709.

16. Scher, J. *Archives of General Psychiatry* 15 (1966): 539–551.

17. Smith, Kline and French Laboratories. *Drug Abuse: Escape to Nowhere* (Philadelphia, 1967).

18. Tinklenberg, J. Personal communication.

19. Weil, A. T.; Zinberg, N. E.; and Nelson, J. M. *Science* 162 (1968): 1234–1242.

20. Werkman, S. L. *Clinical Proceedings of Children's Hospital* 26 (1970): 235–242.

21. ———. *Rocky Mountain Medical Journal* 66 (1969): 32–36.

## CHAPTER 7

*Suicide and Attempted Suicide in Children and Adolescents*

1. Adler, A.; Freud, S.; Friedjung, J. D.; Molitor, K.; Reitler, R.; Sadger, J.; and Stekel, W. "About Suicide, Especially of High School Students," *Diskussionen des Wiener Psychoanalytischen Vereins* (Wiesbaden: J. F. Bergman, 1910).

2. Balser, B. H., and Masterson, J. F. *American Journal of Psychiatry* 116 (1959): 400–404.

3. Bender, L., and Schilder, P. *American Journal of Orthopsychiatry* 7 (1937): 225–234.

4. Bollea, G., and Mayer, R. *The International Journal of Child Psychiatry* 35 (1968): 336–344.

5. Borges, Jorge Luis. *Labyrinths: Selected Stories and Other Writings* (New York: New Directions, 1964), p. 114.

6. Breed, W. A. *The Practitioner* 120 (1919): 401.

7. Camus, Albert. *The Myth of Sisyphus and Other Essays* (New York: Vintage, 1955).

8. Caplan, G. *Manual for Psychiatrists Participating in the Peace Corps Program* (Washington, D.C.: Medical Program Division, Peace Corps, 1962), p. 82.

9. ———. *Prevention of Mental Disorders in Children* (New York: Basic Books, 1961), p. 13.
10. Cerny, L., and Cerna, M. *Cesko. Psychiat.* 58, no. 3 (1962): 162–169.
11. Cohen, A. Y. "L.S.D. and the Student: Approaches to Educational Strategies" (unpublished ms., University of California Counseling Center, Berkeley, 1967).
12. Dublin, L. I. *Suicide: Sociological and Statistical Study* (New York: Ronald Press, 1963).
13. Durkheim, Emile. *Suicide* (Glencoe, Ill.: Free Press, 1951).
14. Erikson, Erik. *Journal of the American Psychoanalytic Association* 4 (1956): 1.
15. Erkkila, S. *Duodecim* 53 (1937): 536–547.
16. ———. *Ugesk f. laeger* (Finland) 97 (1935): 305–309.
17. Ford, R. *Journal of Forensic Sciences* 2, no. 2 (1950): 171–176.
18. Freud, A. *Psychoanalytic Study of the Child*, Vol. 13 (New York: International Universities Press, 1958), pp. 255–279.
19. Freud, Sigmund. *Collected Papers*, trans. J. Rivera (London: Hogarth Press, 1925), p. 13.
20. ———. "On Narcissism (1914)," in J. Strachey (ed.), *The Standard Edition of the Complete Psychological Works of Sigmund Freud*, Vol. 14 (London: Hogarth Press, 1957), pp. 73–91.
21. Hall, G. S. *Adolescence*, Vol. 2 (Boston: D. Appleton, 1964).
22. Hartmann, H. *Essays on Ego Psychology* (New York: International Universities Press, 1964).
23. Hendin, H. *Suicide and Scandinavia* (New York: Grune & Stratton, 1964).
24. Jaconziner, H. *Journal of the American Medical Association* 191 (1965): 1.
25. Kielberg, Sarah. *Bibliot. f. laeger* 129 (May–June 1937): 137–176, 177–240.
26. ———. *Nord. med. tidskr.* 12 (1936): 1193–1199.
27. Krenberger, S. *Eos* 20 (1928): 122.
28. Lewin, B. *The Psychoanalysis of Elation* (New York: W. W. Norton, 1950).
29. Lourie, R. *Texas Medicine* 63, no. 11 (1967): 58–63.
30. MacDonald, A. *Publications of the American Statistical Association* 10 (1906–1907).
31. Mapes, C. C. *Medical Age* 21 (1903): 289–295.
32. Maria, G. *Rass. int. Clin. Ter.* 42 (1962): 985–993.
33. *Medical World News*, March 28, 1969.
34. Mooney, W. E. *Psychoanalytic Quarterly* 37, no. 1 (1968): 80.
35. Mulcock, D. *Medical Officer* 94 (1955): 155–160.
36. O'Dea, J. J. *Suicide (Including Children's Suicide)* (London, 1882).
37. Parish, I. *American Journal of Medical Science* 21 (1837): 258.
38. Pressler, C. *J. de Medecine de Strasbourg* 477 (1929): 511.
39. Rochlin, G. *Psychoanalytic Study of the Child*, Vol. 16 (New York: International Universities Press, 1961).
40. Saroyan, William. *The William Saroyan Reader* (New York: George Braziller, 1958), p. 13.
41. Schmidt, G. *Allgemeine Zeitschrift fur Psychiat.* 112 (1939): 32–43.
42. Schneer, H. I., and Kay, P. In S. Lorand and H. Schneer (eds.), *Adolescents* (New York: Paul Hoeber, 1962), pp. 180–201.
43. Schneidman, E. "Orientation toward Death: A Vital Aspect of the Study of Lives," in R. W. White (ed.), *Essays on Personality in Honor of Henry A. Murray* (New York: Atherton Press, 1963).

44. Schwalbe, J. *Deutsche Med. Wochenschr.* 55 (1929): 1007–1009.
45. Seeger, M. *Intern. Ztschr. f. Individualpsychol.* 11 (1933): 152–153.
46. Seiden, R. H. "Youthful Suicide: A Review of the Literature," unpublished report prepared for the Joint Commission on Mental Health of Children, New York, 1967.
47. Serin, S. *Mental Hygiene* 22 (1927): 33–37.
48. Sexton, Ann. *Live or Die* (Boston: Houghton Mifflin, 1966), p. vii.
49. Shankel, L. W., and Carr, A. C. *Psychiatric Quarterly* 30, no. 1 (1956): 478–493.
50. Shapiro, L. B. *Journal of Nerv. and Mental Dis.* 81 (1935): 547–553.
51. Tobben, H. *Deutsche Zeitschrift f. d. ges. gerichtl. Med.* 14 (1930): 499–516.
52. Von Obermuller, W. *Ztschr. f. Kinderforsch.* 45 (1936): 149–156.
53. Winslow, J. *Anatomy of Suicide* (London, 1840).
54. Wolfgang, M. E. *Clinical Exp. Psychopathol. Quart. Rev. Psychiat. Neurol.* 20 (1959): 335–349.
55. Zilboorg, G. *American Journal of Orthopsychiatry* 7 (1937): 15–31.
56. ———. *Archives of Neurology and Psychiatry* 35 (1936): 270–291.

## CHAPTER 8

### *The Psychosocial Dynamics of Today's Youth*

1. Berke, J. *Counter Culture* (London: Peter Owen, 1970).
2. Blos, P. *Psychoanalytic Study of the Child,* Vol. 23 (New York: International Universities Press, 1968), pp. 245–264.
3. Bronfenbrenner, U. Quoted in D. McDonald, *The Center Magazine* 3, no. 4 (July 1970): 31.
4. Cobb, R. Cartoon in *The Open Conspiracy* (New York: Avon, 1971), p. 133.
5. Darlington, J. *Evolution of Man and Society* (New York: Simon & Schuster, 1970).
6. De Chardin, P. *The Phenomenon of Man* (New York: Harper & Bros., 1955).
7. Erikson, E. Quoted in D. McDonald, *The Center Magazine* 3, no. 4 (July 1970): 30–31.
8. Esalen Institute, Big Sur, California.
9. *Evergreen Review* (New York: Grove Press, 1970).
10. Farber, J. *The Student as Nigger* (New York: Simon & Schuster, 1969).
11. Frankenstein, C. *Psychodynamics of Externalization* (Baltimore: Williams & Wilkins, 1968).
12. Friedenberg, Edgar. *Social Issues,* 25, no. 2 (Spring 1969).
13. ———. *The Open Conspiracy* (New York: Avon, 1971), frontispiece.
14. Fromm, E. *The Sane Society* (New York: Rinehart, 1955).
15. Gioscia, V. "Groovin' on Time: Fragments of a Sociology of the Psychedelic Experience," *Psychedelic Drugs* (New York: Grune & Stratton, 1969), pp. 167–177.
16. Gordon, J. *Atlantic Monthly* (January 1971): 51–66.
17. Halleck, S. Quoted in D. McDonald, *The Center Magazine* 3, no. 4 (July 1970): 25.
18. Hedgepath, W. *The Alternative* (New York: The Macmillan Co., 1970).
19. Joyce, J. *Finnegan's Wake* (New York: Viking Press, 1939).
20. Keniston, K. *The Uncommitted* (New York: Dell, 1965).

21. Kerouac, J. *On the Road* (New York: Viking Press, 1955).
22. Kierkegaard, S. *The Present Age* (New York: Harper & Row, 1962).
23. Laing, R. D. *The Politics of Experience* (New York: Random House, 1967).
24. Lederer, W. *Psychological Issues* 15 (1964).
25. Lifton, R. "Protean Man," *History and Human Survival* (New York: Random House, 1970).
26. Marx, K. Discussed in F. Pappenheim, *The Alienation of Modern Man* (New York: Monthly Review Press, 1959), pp. 116–118.
27. Marcuse, H. *One-Dimensional Man* (Boston: Beacon Press, 1964).
28. McDonald, D. *The Center Magazine* 3, no. 4 (July 1970): 22–33.
29. McLuhan, M. *Understanding Media: The Extensions of Man* (New York: McGraw-Hill, 1966).
30. Mead, M. *Culture and Commitment* (New York: Doubleday, 1970).
31. Morris, D. *The Naked Ape* (New York: McGraw-Hill, 1967).
32. Mumford, L. *The Pentagon of Power* (New York: Harcourt Brace Jovanovich, 1970).
33. Novak, M. *The Experience of Nothingness* (New York: Harper & Row, 1970).
34. Reich, C. *The Greening of America* (New York: Random House, 1970).
35. Rieff, P. *The Triumph of the Therapeutic* (New York: Harper & Row, 1966).
36. Riesman, D. *The Lonely Crowd* (New Haven, Conn.: Yale University Press, 1950).
37. Roszak, T. *The Making of a Counter Culture* (New York: Doubleday, 1968).
38. Slater, P. *The Pursuit of Loneliness* (Boston: Beacon Press, 1970).
39. Sorokin, P. *Social and Cultural Dynamics*, Vol. 1 (New York: The Bedminster Press, 1962), p. 73.
40. Steiner, C. *The Radical Therapist* 1, no. 2 (June–July 1970).
41. Thoreau, H. Quoted in *Generation Gap* (New York: Dell, 1971), p. 70.
42. Toffler, A. *Future Shock* (New York: Random House, 1970).
43. Tönnies, F. Discussed in F. Pappenheim, *The Alienation of Modern Man* (New York: Monthly Review Press, 1959), pp. 64–103.
44. Yablonsky, L. *Synanon: The Tunnel Back* (New York: The Macmillan Co., 1967).

## CHAPTER 9

*Cultural Disadvantage: A Psychosocial Phenomenon*

1. Edwards, T. J. *Disadvantaged Child,* Vol. 1 (Seattle, Wash.: Special Child Publications, 1967).
2. ———. *Forging Ahead in Reading,* Proceedings of the Twelfth Annual Convention, International Reading Association (Newark, Del.: International Reading Association, 1968).
3. ———. *Journal of Reading* 11 (October 1967): 10–13.
4. ———. *Reading and Inquiry,* Proceedings of the Ninth Annual Convention of the International Reading Association (Newark, Del.: International Reading Association, 1965), pp. 256–261.
5. Goodman, M. E. *Race Awareness in Young Children* (Cambridge, Mass.: Addison-Wesley Press, 1952).

6. Grier, W. H., and Cobbs, P. M. *Black-Rage* (New York: Basic Books, 1968).
7. Kardiner, A., and Ovesey, L. *Mark of Oppression* (Cleveland, Ohio: Meridian, 1963).
8. Lomax, L. E. *Negro Revolt* (New York: Harper & Row, 1962).
9. May, E. *Wasted Americans* (New York: Harper & Row, 1964).
10. Passow, H. A. (ed.). *Education in Depressed Areas* (New York: Teachers College Press, 1963).
11. Powledge, F. *Black Power—White Resistance* (New York: World Publishing, 1967).
12. Raph, J.; Goldberg, M. L.; and Passow, H. A. *Bright Underachievers* (New York: Teachers College Press, 1966).
13. Silberman, C. H. *Crisis in Black and White* (New York: Random House, 1964).
14. White, M. A., and Chanry, J. (eds.). *School Disorder, Intelligence and Social Class* (New York: Teachers College Press, 1966).

## CHAPTER 10

*Psychosomatic Disorders of Childhood*

1. Abramson, H. A. In H. I. Schneer (ed.), *The Asthmatic Child* (New York: Hoeber, 1963), p. 27.
2. Agle, D. P., and Ratnoff, O. D. *Archives of Internal Medicine* 109 (1962): 685.
3. ———. *Psychosomatic Medicine* 29 (1967): 491.
4. Alexander, F. *Psychosomatic Medicine* 5 (1943): 205.
5. ———. *Psychosomatic Medicine* (New York: W. W. Norton, 1950), p. 139.
6. American Psychiatric Association. *Diagnostic and Statistical Manual of Mental Disorders* (Washington, D.C.: American Psychiatric Association, 1968), p. 46.
7. Apley, J. *The Child with Abdominal Pains* (Oxford: Blackwell Scientific Publications, 1959).
8. ———. *Proceedings of the Royal Society of Medicine* 51 (1958): 1023.
9. ———, and MacKeith, R. *The Child and His Symptoms* (Philadelphia: F. A. Davis Co., 1968). 9a. p. 61; 9b. p. 49; 9c. pp. 61–65; 9d. p. 63; 9e. p. 65; 9f. pp. 42–43.
10. ———, and Naish, J. M. In D. F. O'Neill (ed.), *Modern Trends in Psychosomatic Medicine* (London: Butterworths, 1955), p. 81.
11. Bettelheim, Bruno. *American Journal of Orthopsychiatry* 18 (1948): 649.
12. ———, and Sylvester, E. *Psychoanalytic Study of the Child*, Vols. 3–4 (New York: International Universities Press, 1949), p. 353.
13. Blank, H., and Brody, M. W. *Psychosomatic Medicine* 12 (1950): 254.
14. Block, J.; Jennings, P. H.; Harvey, E.; and Simpson, E. *Psychosomatic Medicine* 26 (1964): 307.
15. Bowlby, J. *Maternal Care and Mental Health*, Monograph Series, No. 2 (Geneva: World Health Organization, 1951).
16. Breuer, J., and Freud, S. "Studies on Hysteria," in J. Strachey (ed.), *The Standard Edition of the Complete Psychological Works of Sigmund Freud*, Vol. 2 (London: Hogarth Press, 1953), p. 1.
17. Bykov, K. M. *The Cerebral Cortex and the Internal Organs*, trans. by W. H. Gantt (New York: Chemical Publishing Co., 1957).

18. Chapman, L. F.; Goodell, H.; and Wolff, H. G. *Federation Proceedings* 16, 1 (1957): 22.
19. Dekker, E.; Barendregt, J. T.; and deVries, K. In A. Jores and H. Freyburger (eds.), *Advances in Psychosomatic Medicine* (New York: R. Brunner, 1961), p. 235.
20. Duncan, C. H.; Stevenson, I. P.; and Ripley, H. S. *Psychosomatic Medicine* 12 (1950): 23.
21. Engel, G. L. *American Journal of Digestive Diseases* 3 (1958): 315.
22. ————. *American Journal of Medicine* 19 (1955): 231.
23. ————. *American Journal of Psychiatry* 114 (1958): 1076.
24. ————. *Gastroenterology* 40 (1961): 313.
25. ————. *Journal of the American Medical Association* 215 (1971): 1135.
26. ————. In J. Marmor (ed.), *Modern Psychoanalysis* (New York: Basic Books, 1968). 26a. p. 251.
27. ————. *Proceedings of the Royal Society of Medicine* 6ſ (1967): 553.
28. ————. *Psychological Development in Health and Disease* (Philadelphia: W. B. Saunders, 1962).
29. ————. *Psychosomatic Medicine* 16 (1954): 496.
30. ————, and Reichsman, F. *Journal of the American Psychoanalytic Association* 4 (1956): 428.
31. ————, and Schmale, A. H. *Journal of the American Psychoanalytic Association* 15 (1967): 344.
32. ————, and Segal, H. L. *Psychosomatic Medicine* 18 (1956): 374.
33. ————. *Journal of Psychosomatic Research* 11 ( 1967): 3.
34. Falstein, E. I., and Rosenblum, A. H. *Journal of the American Academy of Child Psychiatry* 1 (1962): 246. 34a. p. 261; 34b. p. 263.
35. Fenichel, O. *The Psychoanalytic Theory of Neurosis* (New York: W. W. Norton, 1945), p. 236. 35a. p. 237.
36. Finch, S. M., and Hess, J. H. *American Journal of Psychiatry* 118 (1962): 819.
37. Freud, A. *Psychoanalytic Study of the Child*, Vol. 7 (New York: International Universities Press, 1952), p. 69.
38. ————. *Psychoanalytic Study of the Child*, Vol. 17 (New York: International Universities Press, 1962), p. 149, and Vol. 18 (New York: International Universities Press, 1963), p. 245.
39. ————. Preface in R. Spitz, *The First Year of Life*. (New York: International Universities Press, 1965), p. vii.
40. Freud, S. "Psychical (or Mental) Treatment," in J. Strachey (ed.), *The Standard Edition of the Complete Psychological Works of Sigmund Freud*, Vol. 7 (London: Hogarth Press, 1953), p. 287.
41. ————. "The Psycho-Analytic View of Psychogenic Disturbance of Vision," in J. Strachey (ed.), *The Standard Edition of the Complete Psychological Works of Sigmund Freud*, Vol. 11 (London: Hogarth Press, 1955), p. 211.
42. Fried, R., and Mayer, M. F. *Journal of Pediatrics* 33 (1948): 444.
43. Furman, R. A., and Katan, A. (eds.). *The Therapeutic Nursery School* (New York: International Universities Press, 1969). 43a. p. 262; 43b. pp. 257ff; 43c. pp. 234 ff.
44. Gallagher, J. R. *Medical Care of the Adolescent* (New York: Appleton-Century-Crofts, 1966), pp. 6–15.
45. Garner, A., and Werner, C. *The Mother-Child Interaction in Psychosomatic Disorders* (Urbana, Ill.: University of Illinois Press, 1959).
46. Gerard, M. In F. Deutsch (ed.), *The Psychomatic Concept in Psychoanalysis* (New York: International Universities Press, 1953), p. 82.

47. Gitelson, M. *Bulletin of the Menninger Clinic* 23 (1959): 165.
48. Glaser, J. *Allergy in Childhood* (Springfield, Ill.: Charles C Thomas, 1956), p. 6.
49. Greene, W. A., Jr., and Miller, G. *Psychosomatic Medicine* 20 (1958): 124.
50. Jacobson, E. *The Self and the Object World* (New York: International Universities Press, 1964), p. 17. 50a. p. 16.
51. Jessner, L.; Lamont, J.; Long, R.; Rollins, N.; Whipple, B.; and Prentice, N. *Psychoanalytic Study of the Child*, Vol. 10 (New York: International Universities Press, 1951), p. 353.
52. Kaplan, S. M.; Gottschalk, L. A.; and Fleming, D. F. *Archives of Neurology and Psychiatry* 78 (1957): 656.
53. Katan, A. *Psychoanalytic Study of the Child*, Vol. 16 (New York: International Universities Press, 1961), p. 184.
54. Kaufman, M. R. In F. Deutsch (ed.), *The Psychosomatic Concept in Psychoanalysis* (New York: International Universities Press, 1953), pp. 124ff.
55. Kierland, R. R. *Journal of Pediatrics* 66 (1965): 203.
56. Knapp, P. H. In H. I. Schneer (ed.), *The Asthmatic Child* (New York: Hoeber, 1963), p. 250.
57. Leider, M. *Practical Pediatric Dermatology* (St. Louis: C. V. Mosby and Co., 1956).
58. Lipton, E. L.; Steinschneider, A.; and Richmond, J. B. In L. W. Hoffman and M. L. Hoffman (eds.), *Review of Child Development Research*, Vol. 2 (New York: Russell Sage Foundation, 1966), p. 190. 58a. p. 176.
59. Long, R. T.; Lamont, J. H.; Whipple, B.; Bandler, L.; Blom, G.; Burgin, L.; and Jessner, L. *American Journal of Psychiatry* 114 (1958): 890.
60. Margolin, S. G. "Anaclitic Therapy of Organic Diseases," paper read at the Midwinter Meeting of the American Psychoanalytic Association, New York, December 1951.
61. ———, and Kaufman, M. R. *Medical Clinics of North America* (Philadelphia: W. B. Saunders, 1948), p. 609.
62. Marmor, M., and Kert, M. *California Medicine* 88 (1958): 325.
63. McDermott, J. F., and Finch, S. M. *Journal of the American Academy of Child Psychiatry* 6 (1967): 512. 63a. p. 522; 63b. p. 518.
64. Meara, R. H. *British Journal of Dermatology* 67 (1955): 60.
65. Meyer, J., and Haggerty, R. J. *Pediatrics* 29 (1962): 539.
66. Miller, N. E. *Annals of the New York Academy of Science* 159 (1969): 1025.
67. ———. *Circulation Research* 27, suppl. 1 (1970): 3.
68. ———. *Science* 163 (1969): 434.
69. Mohr, G. J.; Josselyn, I. M.; Spurlock, J.; and Barron, S. H. *American Journal of Psychiatry* 114 (1958): 1067. 69a. p. 1072.
70. Mohr, G. J.; Tausend, H.; Selesnick, S.; and Augenbraun, B. *Journal of the American Academy of Child Psychiatry* 2 (1963): 271.
71. Pasternack, B. *Journal of Pediatrics* 66 (1965): 164.
72. Peshkin, M. In H. I. Schneer (ed.), *The Asthmatic Child* (New York: Hoeber, 1963), pp. 1–15. 72a. p. 1.
73. Provence, S. A., and Lipton, R. *Infants in Institutions* (New York: International Universities Press, 1962).
74. Prugh, D. G. *Gastroenterology* 18 (1951): 339. 74a. p. 341; 74b. p. 354.
75. ———. In A. J. Solnit and S. A. Provence (eds.), *Modern Perspectives in Child Development* (New York: International Universities Press, 1963), p. 246.

76. Purcell, K.; Bernstein, L.; and Bukantz, S. *Psychosomatic Medicine* 23 (1961): 305.
77. Purcell, K., and Metz, J. R. *Journal of Psychosomatic Research* 6 (1962): 251.
78. Purcell, K.; Turnbull, J. W.; and Bernstein, L. *Journal of Psychosomatic Research* 6 (1962): 283.
79. ————. *Pediatrics* 31 (1963): 486.
80. Ratner, B., and Silberman, A. E. *Journal of Allergy* 24 (1953): 371.
81. Recs, L. *Journal of Psychosomatic Research* 7 (1964): 253.
82. Renbourne, E. T. *Journal of Psychosomatic Research* 4 (1960): 149.
83. Rosenbaum, M. *American Journal of Orthopsychiatry* 29 (1960): 762.
84. Rosenthal, M. J. *Pediatrics* 10 (1952): 581.
85. Rothman, S. *Physiology and Biochemistry of the Skin* (Chicago: University of Chicago Press, 1954).
86. Sandler, J. *British Journal of Medical Psychology* 31 (1958): 19.
87. Saul, L. J. *International Journal of Psychoanalysis* 19 (1938): 451.
88. Schmale, A. H. *Psychosomatic Medicine* 20 (1958): 259.
89. Schur, M. In R. M. Loewenstein (ed.), *Drives, Affects, Behavior* (New York: International Universities Press, 1953), p. 67.
90. ————. *Psychoanalytic Study of the Child*, Vol. 10 (New York: International Universities Press, 1955), p. 119. 90a. p. 160.
91. ————. *Psychoanalytic Study of the Child*, Vol. 13 (New York: International Universities Press, 1958), p. 190.
92. Sedlis, E. *Journal of Pediatrics* 66 (1965): 158.
93. Seitz, P. F. D. *Psychosomatic Medicine* 15 (1953): 405.
94. Shapiro, D.; Tursky, B.; Gershon, W.; and Stern, M. *Science* 163 (1969): 588.
95. Sperling, M. *International Journal of Psychoanalysis* 38 (1957): 341.
96. ————. *Journal of the American Academy of Child Psychiatry* 7 (1968): 44. 96a. p. 47.
97. ————. *Journal of the American Academy of Child Psychiatry* 8 (1969): 336.
98. ————. *Psychoanalytic Quarterly* 15 (1946): 302.
99. ————. *Psychoanalytic Study of the Child*, Vol. 7 (New York: International Universities Press, 1952), p. 115.
100. Spitz, R. *Psychoanalytic Study of the Child*, Vol. 1 (New York: International Universities Press, 1945), p. 53.
101. ————. *Psychoanalytic Study of the Child*, Vol. 6 (New York: International Universities Press, 1951), p. 271.
102. Spock, B. *Baby and Child Care* (New York: Pocket Books, 1957), p. 174.
103. Ullman, M. *Psychosomatic Medicine* 21 (1959): 473.
104. ————, and Dudek, S. *Psychosomatic Medicine* 22 (1960): 68.
105. Van der Bogert, F., and Moravec, C. L. *Journal of Pediatrics* 10 (1937): 466.
106. Wessel, M. A.; Cobb, J. C.; Jackson, E. B.; Harris, G. S.; and Detewiler, A. C. *Pediatrics* 14 (1954): 421. 106a. p. 432; 106b, p. 431.
107. White, K. L., and Long, W. N. *Journal of Chronic Diseases* 8 (1958): 567.
108. Wise, F., and Wolfe, J. *Journal-Lancet* 56 (1936): 441.

## CHAPTER 11

*Mental Retardation*

1. Atkinson, R. C. *American Psychologist* 23 (1968): 225–239.
2. Baller, W. R. *Genetic Psychology Monographs* 18 (1936): 165–244.
3. Bass, M. S. *Mental Retardation* 2 (1964): 198–202.
4. Baumeister, A. A. (ed.). *Mental Retardation: Appraisal, Education, Rehabilitation* (Chicago: Aldine Publishing, 1967).
5. Bijou, S. W. "Functional Analysis of Retarded Development," in N. R. Ellis (ed.), *International Review of Research in Mental Retardation*, Vol. 1 (New York: Academic Press, 1966), pp. 1–19. 5a. p. 2.
6. Charles, D. C. *Genetic Psychology Monographs* 47 (1953): 3–71.
7. Clark, G. R., Kivitz, M. S., and Rosen, M. *A Transitional Program for Institutionalized Adult Retarded*, Project No. RD 1275P, Vocational Rehabilitation Administration, Division of Research and Demonstrations (Washington, D.C.: Department of Health, Education and Welfare, 1968).
8. Cromwell, R. L. "A Social Learning Approach to Mental Retardation," in N. R. Ellis (ed.), *Handbook of Mental Deficiency* (New York: McGraw-Hill, 1963), pp. 41–91.
9. Denny, M. R. "Research in Learning and Performance," in H. A. Stevens and R. Heber (eds.), *Mental Retardation: A Review of Research* (Chicago: University of Chicago Press, 1964). 9a. p. 136.
10. Dentler, R. A., and Macker, B. *Psychological Bulletin* 59 (1962): 273–283.
11. Descoeudres, A. *The Education of Mentally Defective Children* (Boston: Heath, 1928).
12. Dugdale, R. C. *The Jukes* (New York: Putnams, 1910).
13. Ellis, N. R. "The Stimulus Trace and Behavioral Inadequacy," in N. R. Ellis (ed.), *Handbook of Mental Deficiency* (New York: McGraw-Hill, 1963), pp. 134–158.
14. Frostig, M.; Lefever, D.; and Whittlesey, J. *Perceptual and Motor Skills* 12 (1961): 383–394.
15. Goddard, H. H. *The Kallikak Family* (New York: Macmillan, 1914).
16. Goffman, E. "Characteristics of Total Institutions," in *Symposium of Preventive and Social Psychiatry* (Washington, D.C.: Walter Reed Army Institute of Research, 1957), pp. 43–84.
17. Hays, W. *American Journal of Mental Deficiency* 56 (1951): 198–203.
18. Heber, R. (ed.). *A Manual on Terminology and Classification in Mental Retardation*, monograph suppl., *American Journal of Mental Deficiency* (1961): 3. 18a. p. 4.
19. Holland, J. G., and Skinner, B. F. *The Analysis of Behavior* (New York: McGraw-Hill, 1961).
20. Itard, J. *De l'education d'un homme sauvage* (Paris, 1801).
21. Johnson, G. O. *American Journal of Mental Deficiency* 55 (1950): 60–89.
22. Kantor, J. R. *Interbehavioral Psychology*, rev. ed. (Bloomington, Ind.: Principis Press, 1959).
23. Kennedy, R. J. *A Connecticut Community Revisited*, Project No. 655, Office of Vocational Rehabilitation (Washington, D.C.: Department of Health, Education and Welfare, 1966).
24. Kirk, S. A. *Early Education of the Mentally Retarded* (Urbana, Ill.: University of Illinois Press, 1958).

25. ———. "Research in Education," in H. A. Stevens and R. Heber (eds.), *Mental Retardation: A Review of Research* (Chicago: University of Chicago Press, 1964), pp. 57–99.
26. Kugel, R. B., and Wolfensberger, W. (eds.). *Changing Patterns in Residential Services for the Mentally Retarded* (Washington, D.C.: President's Committee on Mental Retardation, 1969).
27. Lovaas, O. I., and others. *Science* 151 (1966): 705–707.
28. Mardin, P. W., and Farber, B. *Social Problems* 8, no. 4 (1961): 300–302.
29. McCarthy, J. J., and Kirk, S. A. *Illinois Test of Psycholinguistic Abilities: Experimental Edition,* Institute for Research on Exceptional Children (Urbana, Ill.: University of Illinois Press, 1961).
30. Montessori, M. *The Montessori Method* (New York: Stokes, 1912).
31. Patterson, G. R., and Gullion, M. *Living with Children* (Champaign, Ill.: Research Press, 1968).
32. Pestalozzi, J. *How Gertrude Teaches Her Children* (London: Allen & Unwin, 1915).
33. President's Committee on Mental Retardation. *MR: 69 toward Progress: The Story of a Decade* (Washington, D.C.: U.S. Government Printing Office, 1969), p. 6.
34. Seguin, E. *Traitement moral, hygiene, et education des idiots* (Paris, 1846).
35. Seligman, M.; Maier, S.; and Solomon, R. "Unpredictable and Uncontrollable Aversive Events," in F. R. Brush (ed.), *Aversive Conditioning and Learning* (New York: Academic Press, 1969).
36. Skeels, H. M., and Dye, H. B. *Proceedings of the American Association for Mental Deficiency* 44 (1939): 114–136.
37. Smith, Kline & French Laboratories. *Reinforcement Therapy* (Philadelphia, 1966).
38. Sparks, H. L., and Blackman, L. J. *Exceptional Children* 31 (1965): 242–246.
39. Spitz, H. H. "Field Theory in Mental Deficiency," in N. R. Ellis (ed.), *Handbook of Mental Deficiency* (New York: McGraw-Hill, 1963), pp. 11–40.
40. Sutherland, J., and others. *American Journal of Mental Deficiency* 59 (1954): 266–271.
41. Tredgold, R. F., and Soddy, K. *A Text-Book of Mental Deficiency* (Baltimore: Williams & Wilkins, 1956).
42. Windle, C.; Stewart, E.; and Brown, S. *American Journal of Mental Deficiency* 66 (1961): 213–217.
43. Zigler, E. *Science* 155 (1967): 292–298. 43a. p. 298.

## CHAPTER 12

### The Displaced Child: Problems of the Adopted Child,

### Single-Parent Child, and Stepchild

1. Blos, P. *Psychoanalytic Study of the Child,* Vol. 23 (New York: International Universities Press, 1968), pp. 245–263.
2. Bowlby, J. *Child Care and the Growth of Love* (London: Penguin Books, 1953), p. 53.
3. Eisendorfer, A. *Psychoanalytic Quarterly* 12 (1943).
4. Freud, Anna, and Burlingham, D. *Infants Without Families* (New York: International Universities Press, 1944).

5. Freud, Sigmund. "Three Essays on the Theory of Sexuality," in J. Strachey (ed.), *The Standard Edition of the Complete Psychological Works of Sigmund Freud*, Vol. 7 (London: Hogarth Press, 1953).
6. Isaacs, S. *Fatherless Children—Childhood and After* (New York: International Universities Press, 1945).
7. Lederer, W. *Psychological Issues* 4, no. 3 (1964).
8. Menlove, F. R. *Child Development* 36 (1965): 519–532.
9. Neubauer, P. *Psychoanalytic Study of the Child*, Vol. 15 (New York: International Universities Press, 1960), pp. 286–309.
10. Ostrovsky, E. S. *Children Without Men* (New York: Collier Books, 1962).
11. Peller, L. *Bulletin of the Philadelphia Association for Psychoanalysis* 11 (1961): 145–154.
12. ———. *Bulletin of the Philadelphia Association for Psychoanalysis* 13 (1963): 1–14.
13. Reich, A. *Journal of the American Psychoanalytic Association* 2 (1954).
14. Schechter, M. *Journal of the American Psychoanalytic Association* 15, no. 3 (1967): 695–708.
15. Simon, M., and Centuria, A. C. *Journal of the American Psychiatric Association* 122, no. 8 (1966): 858–868.
16. Spock, B. *Baby and Child Care* (New York: Pocket Books, 1957).
17. Wieder, H., and Kaplan, E. H. *Psychoanalytic Study of the Child*, Vol. 24 (New York: International Universities Press, 1969), pp. 399–431.

## CHAPTER 13

### *Learning Disabilities*

1. *Bender Visual-Motor-Gestalt Test* (New York: Psychological Corporation, 1938).
2. Betts, E. A. *The Foundations of Reading Instruction* (New York: American Book Company, 1946).
3. Blanchard, P. *Psychoanalytic Study of the Child*, Vol. 2 (New York: International Universities Press, 1946), pp. 163–187.
4. Bricklin, B., and Bricklin, P. M. *Strong Family, Strong Child* (New York: Delacorte Press, 1970).
5. *Detroit Tests of Learning Aptitude* (Indianapolis, Ind.: Test Division of the Bobbs-Merrill Co., 1941).
6. Fernald, G. M. *Remedial Techniques in Basic School Subjects* (New York: McGraw-Hill, 1943), p. 7.
7. Freud, Sigmund. *The Problem of Anxiety* (New York: W. W. Norton, 1936).
8. Frostig, M. *Frostig Developmental Test of Visual Perception* (Palo Alto, Calif.: Consulting Psychologists Press, 1963).
9. ———, and Horne, D. *The Frostig Program for the Development of Visual Perception* (Chicago: Follett, 1964).
10. Gates, A. I. *Journal of Genetic Psychology* 59 (1941): 77–83.
11. *Gates Associative Learning Test* (Philadelphia: The Reading Clinic, Temple University, 1928).
12. Harris, I. D. *Emotional Blocks to Learning* (New York: Free Press, 1961), pp. 13–25.
13. *Harris Tests of Lateral Dominance* (New York: Psychological Corporation, 1956).

14. Hartmann, H.; Kris, E.; and Loewenstein, R. M. *Psychoanalytic Study of the Child*, Vol. 2 (New York: International Universities Press, 1946), pp. 11–30.
15. *Illinois Test of Psycholinguistic Abilities* (Urbana, Ill.: University of Illinois, 1968).
16. Kass, C. "Some Psychological Correlates of Severe Reading Disability" (unpublished doctoral dissertation University of Illinois, 1962).
17. Kephart, N. C. *The Slow Learner in the Classroom* (Columbus, Ohio: Charles E. Merrill, 1960).
18. Klein, E. *Psychoanalytic Study of the Child*, Vols. 3 and 4 (New York: International Universities Press, 1949), 369–390.
19. Orton, S. *Reading, Writing and Speech Problems of Children* (New York: W. W. Norton, 1937).
20. Pearson, G. H. J. *Psychoanalysis and the Education of the Child* (New York: W. W. Norton, 1954), pp. 23–82.
21. ———. *Psychoanalytic Study of the Child*, Vol. 7 (New York: International Universities Press, 1952), pp. 322–386.
22. Rappaport, D. *Diagnostic Psychological Testing*, Vol. 1 (Chicago: The Yearbook Publisher, 1946).
23. Rappaport, S. R. *Psychoanalytic Study of the Child*, Vol. 16 (New York: International Universities Press, 1961), pp. 423–450.
24. Robinson, H. M. *Why Pupils Fail in Reading* (Chicago: University of Chicago Press, 1946), pp. 88–89.
25. Smith, L. *Journal of Experimental Education* 18 (1950): 321–329.
26. Stauffer, R. G. *Journal of Education Research* 41 (1948): 436–452.
27. *Van Wagenen Reading Readiness Test* (Minneapolis: Van Wagenen Psycho-Educational Research Laboratories, University of Minnesota, 1938).
28. Waldman, M. *The Reading Teacher* 23, no. 4 (January 1970): 325–330.
29. *Wechsler Memory Scale* (New York: Psychological Corporation, 1942).

## CHAPTER 14

### Audiological Disorders

1. Davis, H., and Silverman, S. *Hearing and Deafness*, 3d ed. (New York: Holt, Rinehart & Winston, 1970).
2. Downs, M., and Sterritt, G. A. M. A. *Archives of Otolaryngology* 85 (1967): 15–22.
3. Jerger, J. *Modern Developments in Audiology* (New York: Academic Press, 1963).
4. Lenneberg, E. *Biological Foundations of Language* (New York: John Wiley and Sons, 1967).
5. McConnell, F., and Ward, P. *Deafness in Childhood* (Nashville, Tenn.: Vanderbilt University Press, 1967).
6. McGann, M. *American Journal of Roentgenology* 88 (1962): 1183–1186.
7. Myklebust, H. *Auditory Disorders in Children* (New York: Grune & Stratton, 1954).
8. ———. *The Psychology of Deafness* (New York: Grune & Stratton, 1960).
9. Newby, H. *Audiology*, 2d ed. (New York: Appleton-Century-Crofts, 1964).

10. Rosenberg, P. *Journal of Speech and Hearing Disorders* 31, no. 3 (1966): 279–283.
11. ———, and Toglia, J. *Journal of Speech and Hearing Disorders* 32, no. 2 (1967): 170–176.
12. Stevens, S. S., and Warshofsky, F. *Sound and Hearing* (New York: Time, Inc., 1965).
13. Travis, L. E. *Handbook of Speech Pathology* (New York: Appleton Century-Crofts, 1957).

## CHAPTER 15

### Speech Pathology

1. Affeld, J. E., and Hansen, J. E. *Nursing World* 128 (1954): 10.
2. American Speech and Hearing Association Committee of the Midcentury White House Conference. *Journal of Speech and Hearing Disorders* 17 (1952): 129.
3. Bangs, J. Personal communication, Speech and Hearing Center, Houston, Texas.
4. Eisenson, J. *Examining for Aphasia*, rev. ed. (New York: Psychological Corporation, 1954).
5. Gens, G. W. *Training School Bulletin* 46 (1949): 49.
6. ———. *Training School Bulletin* 47 (1950): 32.
7. ———. *Training School Bulletin* 48 (1951): 19.
8. ———, and Bibey, M. L. *Journal of Speech and Hearing Disorders* 17 (1952): 32.
9. Johnson, W., and others. *Speech Handicapped School Children* (New York: Harper & Row, 1967).
10. Karlin, I. W., and Strazulla, M. *Journal of Speech and Hearing Disorders* 17 (1952): 268.
11. Kastein, S., and Fowler, E. P. *Archives of Otolaryngology* 60 (1954): 468.
12. Meader, C. L., and Muyskens, J. H. In H. Weller (ed.), *A Handbook of Biolinguistics* (Toledo, Ohio, 1950).
13. Morley, D. E. *Journal of Speech and Hearing Disorders* 17 (1952): 25.
14. Morris, J. V. *American Journal of Mental Deficiency* 57 (1953): 661.
15. Strauss, A. A. *American Journal of Physical Medicine* 33 (1954): 93.
16. Sugar, O. *Journal of Speech and Hearing Disorders* 17 (1952): 301.
17. Van Gelder, D. W., and Kennedy, L. *Pediatrics* 9 (1952): 48.
18. Van Riper, C. *Speech Correction: Principles and Methods* (Englewood Cliffs, N.J.: Prentice-Hall, 1963).
19. ———. *Speech Therapy: A Book of Readings* (Englewood Cliffs, N.J.: Prentice-Hall, 1953).
20. ———. In J. Eisenson (ed.), *Stuttering: A Symposium* (New York: Harper & Row, 1958), pp. 275–390.
21. Weinstock, J. J. *Journal of Speech and Hearing Disorders* 33 (1968): 15.
22. Weiss, D. A. *Cluttering* (Englewood Cliffs, N.J.: Prentice-Hall, 1964).
23. Wepman, J. *Journal of Speech and Hearing Disorders* 18 (1953): 4.

## CHAPTER 16

*The Physically Handicapped Child*

1. Anderson, E. E., and others. *Journal of the American Medical Association* 216 (1971): 1023.
2. Apgar, V. *Anesthesia and Analgesia* 47 (1968): 325.
3. Baker, C. J., and Rudolph, A. J. *American Journal of Diseases of Children* 121 (1971): 393.
4. Bloomfield, D. K. *American Journal of Obstetrics and Gynecology* 107 (1970): 883.
4a. Blyth, H., and Carter, C. "A Guide to Genetic Prognosis in Pediatrics," in *Developmental Medicine and Child Neurology*, suppl. no. 18 (1969): 35.
5. Brady, R. O., Jr. Reported in *Medical World News*, November 13, 1970, p. 64.
6. Buchheit, W. A., and others. *New England Journal of Medicine* 280 (1969): 938.
7. Burlingham, D. *Psychoanalytic Study of the Child*, Vol. 16 (New York: International Universities Press, 1961), p. 121.
8. ———. *Psychoanalytic Study of the Child*, Vol. 20 (New York: International Universities Press, 1965), p. 194.
9. Commoner, B. *Science and Survival* (New York: Viking Press, 1967), p. 150.
10. Cooke, R. E. Presentation at the Second International Conference on Congenital Malformations, reported in *Medical World News*, August 16, 1963, pp. 44–45.
11. Deeths, T. M., and Breeden, J. T. *Journal of Pediatrics* 78 (1971): 299.
12. Elizan, T. S., and Fabiyi, A. *American Journal of Obstetrics and Gynecology* 106 (1970): 147.
13. Emich, J. P. Reported in *Medical World News*, May 14, 1971, pp. 20–22.
14. Erikson, E. H. *Identity and the Life Cycle* (New York: International Universities Press, 1959), p. 171.
15. Ermert, A. Z. *Kinderheilk* 105 (1969): 1; abstract #1592 in *Exerpta Medica* 22 (1969): 285.
16. Finkel, A. J. *Journal of the American Medical Association* 216 (1971): 1018.
17. Fishbein, L., and others. *Chemical Mutagens* (New York: Academic Press, 1970), p. 364.
18. Fraiberg, S. *Psychoanalytic Study of the Child*, Vol. 23 (New York: International Universities Press, 1968), p. 264. 18a. p. 266; 18b. p. 278; 18c. p. 298.
19. Fraser, F. C. In A. Rubin (ed.), "Etiological Agents: II. Physical and Chemical Agents," *Handbook of Congenital Malformations* (Philadelphia: Saunders, 1967), p. 398.
20. Freeman, R. D. In S. Chess and A. Thomas (eds.), "Emotional Reactions of Handicapped Children," *Annual Progress in Child Psychiatry and Development* (New York: Brunner/Mazel, 1968), p. 565.
21. Freud, A. *Psychoanalytic Study of the Child*, Vol. 7 (New York: International Universities Press, 1952), p. 69.
22. Galston, A. W. *Science* 167 (1970): 237.
23. Garb, S., and others. *Pharmacology and Patient Care*, 3d ed. (New York: Springer, 1970), p. 598. 23a. p. 69.

24. Garfunkel, J. M. Personal communication, May 1971.
25. Goodman, L. S., and Gillman, A. *The Pharmacological Basis of Therapeutics*, 4th ed. (New York: The Macmillan Co., 1970), p. 1794.
26. Graham, F., Jr. *Since Silent Spring* (Boston: Houghton Mifflin, 1970), p. 333.
27. Gray, M. J. *Clinical Obstetrics and Gynecology* 11 (1968): 568.
28. See reference 61a.
29. See reference 4a.
30. Gustafson, S. R., and Coursin, D. B. (eds.). *The Pediatric Patient* (Philadelphia: Lippincott, 1964), p. 160.
31. Hartmann, H. *Ego Psychology and the Problem of Adaptation* (New York: International Universities Press, 1958), p. 121.
32. Heys, R. E., and others. *Obstetrics and Gynecology* 33 (1969): 390.
33. *Hospital Formulary Management* 4, no. 6 (1969): 26.
34. Inhorn, S. L., and Meisner, L. F. *Science* 166 (1969): 685.
35. Jacobson, E. *The Self and the Object World* (New York: International Universities Press, 1964), p. 250.
36. Jansen, K. *Royal College of Surgeons of England* 40 (1967): 237.
37. Kaback, M. M. "Mass Screening for Tay-Sachs Carriers," *Medical World News*, May 14, 1971.
38. Karnofsky, D. A. *Annual Review of Pharmacology* 5 (1965): 447.
39. Laurence, K. M., and Carter, C. O. "Some Environmental Factors in the Incidence of C. N. S. Malformations in South Wales," abstracted in *Developmental Medicine and Child Neurology Suppl.* 15 (1968): 83.
40. Lipton, E. L. *Psychoanalytic Study of the Child*, Vol. 25 (New York: International Universities Press, 1970), p. 146. 40a. p. 156; 40b. p. 157; 40c. p. 160.
41. Lubs, H. A., and Ruddle, F. H. *Science* 169 (1970): 495.
42. Mahler, M. S. In M. Schur (ed.), "On the Significance of the Normal Separation-Individuation Phase," *Drives, Affects, Behavior*, Vol. 2 (New York: International Universities Press, 1965), p. 502.
43. ———. *On Human Symbiosis and the Vicissitudes of Individuation*, Vol. 1 (New York: International Universities Press, 1968), p. 271.
44. Masland, R. L. In G. Caplan (ed.), "Researches into the Prenatal Factors that Lead to Neuropsychiatric Sequelae in Childhood," *Prevention of Mental Disorders in Children* (New York: Basic Books, 1961), p. 425.
45. ———. Statement to the House Appropriations Subcommittee on NIH Funding, reported in *Medical World News*, May 26, 1961, p. 24.
46. McIntosh, R., and others. *Pediatrics* 14 (1954): 505.
47. Milunsky, A., and others. *Journal of Pediatrics* 72 (1965): 790.
48. Mirkin, B. L. *Journal of Pediatrics* 78 (1971): 329.
49. ———. *Postgraduate Medicine* 47 (1970): 91.
50. Mulcahy, R. *American Journal of Obstetrics and Gynecology* 101 (1968): 844.
51. Nagera, H., and Colonna, A. B. *Psychoanalytic Study of the Child*, Vol 20 (New York: International Universities Press, 1965), p. 267.
52. Neel, J. V., and Schull, W. J. "The Effect of Exposure to the Atomic Bomb on Pregnancy Termination in Hiroshima and Nagasaki." National Academy of Sciences, National Research Council Publication no. 461 (Washington, D.C., 1956).
53. Nelson, B. *Science* 166 (1969): 977.
54. Nelson, M. M., and Forfar, J. O. *Developmental Medicine and Child Neurology* 11 (1969): 3.
55. Newton, M., and Norris, L. A. *Science* 168 (1970): 1606.

56. Nicholson, H. O. *Journal of Obstetrics and Gynecology of the British Commonwealth* 75 (1968): 307.
57. Niederland, W. G. *Psychoanalytic Study of the Child*, Vol. 20 (New York: International Universities Press, 1965), p. 518. 57a. page 521; 57b. page 522.
58. O'Brien, J. S., and others. *Science* 172 (1971): 61.
59. Perlstein, M. A., and Hood, P. N. *Journal of the American Medical Association* 188 (1964): 850.
60. Pitkin, R. M. *Illinois Medical Journal* 134 (1968): 265.
61. Polani, P. E. In M. Fishbein (ed.), "Incidence of Congenital Defects," *Birth Defects* (Philadelphia: Lippincott, 1963), p. 335.
61a. Queenan, J. T., and Gadow, E. C. *Obstetrics and Gynecology* 35 (1970): 648.
62. Reed, S. C. *Counseling in Medical Genetics* (Philadelphia: Saunders, 1963), p. 278.
63. Reynolds, J. W. *Journal of Pediatrics* 76 (1970): 464.
64. Rubin, A. (ed.). *Handbook of Congenital Malformations* (Philadelphia: Saunders, 1967), p. 398.
65. Schiff, D., and others. *Journal of Pediatrics* 77 (1970): 457.
66. Schwartz, A. D., and Pearson, H. A. *Journal of Pediatrics* 78 (1971): 558.
67. Shere, E., and Kastenbaum, R. *Genetic Psychology Monographs* 73 (1966): 255.
68. Smith, D. W. *Recognizable Patterns of Human Malformation* (Philadelphia: Saunders, 1970), p. 368. 68a. p. 1.
69. Smithells, R. W. *Advances in Teratology* 1 (1966): 251.
70. South, M. A., and others. *Journal of Pediatrics* 75 (1969): 13.
71. Spitz, R. A. *Psychoanalytic Study of the Child*, Vol. 1 (New York: International Universities Press, 1945), 53.
72. Stern, H., and Williams, B. M. *Lancet* 1 (1966): 293.
73. Stuart, D. M. *Pharmacological Index* 8 (1966): 4.
74. Sutherland, J. M., and Light, I. J. *Pediatric Clinics of North America* 12 (1965): 781.
75. Swift, P. N. *Developmental Medicine and Child Neurology* 10 (1968): 237.
76. Totterman, L. E., and Saxen, L. *Acta Obstetrica Gynecologica et Scandanavia* 48 (1969): 542.
77. Vollman, R. F., and others. Paper read at the American Association of Anatomists, Kansas City, Mo., April 4–7, 1967. Abstracted in *Anatomical Record* 157 (1967): 337.
78. Warkany, J., and Takacs, E. *American Journal of Pathology* 35 (1959): 315.
79. White, L. R., and Sever, J. L. In A. Rubin (ed.), "Etiological Agents. I. Infectious Agents," *Handbook of Congenital Malformations* (Philadelphia: Saunders, 1967), p. 398. 79a. p. 356.
80. Winnicott, D. W. *International Journal of Psycho-Analysis* 34 (1953): 89.

CHAPTER 17
*Milieu Therapy*

1. Cumming, J., and Cumming, E. *Ego and Milieu* (New York: Atherton Press, 1962), pp. 1 and 5.
2. French, E. L., and Scott, J. C. *How You Can Help Your Retarded Child* (Philadelphia: Lippincott, 1967), pp. 93–107.

3. Goertzel, V., and Goertzel, M. C. *Cradles of Eminence* (Boston: Little, Brown, 1962).
4. Menninger, W. C. *Southern Medical Journal* 32 (1939): 348.
5. Redl, F. *When We Deal with Children* (New York: Free Press, 1966), pp. 68–94.
6. Stanton, A., and Schwartz, M. *The Mental Hospital* (New York: Basic Books, 1954).
7. Sullivan, H. *American Journal of Psychiatry* 10 (1931): 977.

## CHAPTER 18

### Child Psychiatry in the School

1. Aichorn, A. *Wayward Youth* (New York: Viking Press, 1935).
2. Allensmith, W., and Goethals, G. W. *The Role of the Schools in Mental Health* (New York: Basic Books, 1962), pp. 5, 141–146.
3. American Psychiatric Association. *Planning Psychiatric Services for Children* (Washington, D.C., 1964), p. 3.
4. Cruikshank, W. *A Teaching Method for Brain Injured and Hyperactive Children* (Syracuse, N.Y.: Syracuse University Press, 1961).
5. Erikson, E. H. *Childhood and Society* (New York: W. W. Norton, 1950), p. 227.
6. Frostig, M. *Developmental Test of Visual Perception*, 3d ed. (Palo Alto, Calif.: Consulting Psychologists Press, 1961).
7. Golding, William. *Lord of the Flies* (New York: Capricorn Books, 1959).
8. Gross, R. *The Teacher and the Taught* (New York: Dell, 1963), p. ix.
9. Institute for Research on Exceptional Children, *Illinois Test of Psycholinguistic Abilities* (Urbana, Ill.: University of Illinois Press, 1961).
10. Itard, J. *The Wild Boy of Aveyron* (New York: Appleton-Century-Crofts, 1962), pp. xxiii, 5, 6, 10–11.
11. Kephart, N. C. *The Slow Learner in the Classroom* (Columbus, Ohio: Charles F. Merrill Books, 1960).
12. Margolin, Sidney. Personal communications.
13. Peller, L. Personal communications.
14. Stennis, W. *Aspects of the Neurological Examination*, film produced by Bucks County Schools, Doylestown, Pennsylvania, 1968.
15. ———. "Emotional Development of Children—The Evolution and Application of a Systematic Method of Classification within a School Setting." Paper presented at the Annual Meeting of the American Academy of Child Psychiatry, Denver, Colorado, October 1970.
16. ———; Houlihan, R.; and Green, P. *Diagnostic Educational Grouping* (Doylestown, Pa.: Bucks County Schools, July 1970).
17. Waelder, Robert. Personal communications.

## CHAPTER 19

### Child Psychiatry and the Law

1. Arnstein, R. *American Journal of Psychiatry* 122 (1965): 644.
2. *Bakker v. Welsh*, 108 N.W. 94 (1906); *Lacey v. Laird*, 139 N.E.2d 25 (1956); see L. Lasagna, *Daedalus* (Spring 1969): 457.

3. *Bang v. Charles T. Miller Hospital,* 88 N.W.2d 186 (1958).
4. Bass, M. S. *Mental Retardation* 2 (1964): 198.
5. Beecher, H. K. *New England Journal of Medicine* 274 (1966): 1354; *Daedalus* (Spring 1968): 275.
6. *Berry v. Moench,* 331 P.2d 814 (1959).
7. *Binder v. Ruvell,* Civil Docket 52C2535, Circuit Court of Cook County, Ill., June 24, 1952; this case has been commented on, *inter alia,* in M. S. Guttmacher and H. Weihofen, *Psychiatry and the Law* (New York: Norton, 1952), Comment 47 *Northwestern University Law Review* 384 (1952), and J. Robitscher, *Pursuit of Agreement: Psychiatry and the Law* (Philadelphia: Lippincott, 1966).
8. *Bolam v. Friern Hospital,* 2 A 1 1 E.R. 118 (1957), an English decision; see comment by B. D. Hirsh, *Journal of the American Medical Association* 176 (1961): 436. There is considerable American precedent for the same point of view.
9. *Brown Alumni Monthly* (March 1969): 17.
10. *Clark v. Geraci,* 208 N.Y.S.2d 564 (1960).
11. Connecticut—Public Act No. 206 (1967), Connecticut General Statutes Annotated sections 19–89a (1973).
12. Curran, William. *AMA News* (August 12, 1968): 9; *Psychiatric News* (June 1968): 18.
13. DeWitt, C. *Privileged Communications between Physician and Patient* (Springfield, Ill.: Charles C Thomas, 1958).
14. *Ditlow v. Kaplan,* 181 So.2d 226 (1966).
15. Freund, P. A. *New England Journal of Medicine* 273 (1965): 687.
16. Grosser, G. H., and Paul, N. L. *American Journal of Orthopsychiatry* 34 (1964): 875.
17. Group for the Advancement of Psychiatry, *Report,* No. 45 (1960).
18. Hirsh, B. *AMA News* (August 21, 1967): 13.
19. Hulka, J. F. *New England Journal of Medicine* 278 (1968): 1296.
20. Lewis, M. *American Journal of Orthopsychiatry* 37 (1967): 946.
21. Lieberman, P. "Caveat—Medical Treatment of Minors," mimeographed paper prepared by the Law Department of the American Medical Association, Washington, D.C.
22. Malmquist, C. P. *American Journal of Orthopsychiatry* 35 (1965): 787.
23. *Maryland Annotated Code,* art. 438, 149D (1968); *New Jersey Statutes Annotated,* title 9, chap. 17A–4, 17A–5 (1968).
24. *Massachusetts General Laws,* chap. III, sec. 117 (1967).
25. Menninger, W. W., and English, J. T. *American Journal of Psychiatry* 122 (1965): 638.
26. *Natanson v. Kline,* 350 P.2d 1093 (1960).
27. *Nebraska Revised Statutes Supplement,* art. 11, 71–1119, 71–1120 (1967).
28. *Privacy and Behavioral Research* (Washington, D.C.: U.S. Government Printing Office, February 1967).
29. *Psychiatric News* (November 1967): 2.
30. *Psychiatric News* (July 1968): 20.
31. *Ritt v. Ritt,* 238 A.2d 196 (1967), held that the psychologist's privilege granted by New Jersey statute did not apply to psychiatrists who at that time were not covered by a privilege statute.
32. Robitscher, J. *Journal of the American Medical Association* 202 (1967): 398; 17 *Cleveland-Marshall Law Review* 200 (1968).
33. Ross, A. O. *Mental Hygiene* 42 (1958): 60.
34. ———. *Mental Hygiene* 50 (1966): 360.

35. Russell, D. H. *New England Journal of Medicine* 278 (1968): 35.
36. Szasz, T. *Trans-Action* 4 (1967): 16.
37. Starzl, T. E.; Waddell, W. R.; and Marchioro, T. L. Quoted in *Medical Tribune*, April 25–26, 1964, p. 9.

## CHAPTER 20

### Theoretical Considerations in Child Psychotherapy

1. Belmont, H. *Bulletin of the Philadelphia Association for Psychoanalysis* 5 (1955): 80–91.
2. ———. *Proceedings of the Twenty-First Annual Reading Institute at Temple University*, Vol. 3 (Philadelphia: The Reading Clinic, Temple University, 1964).
3. Committee on Child Psychiatry of the Group for the Advancement of Psychiatry. "Psychopathological Disorders in Childhood; Theoretical Considerations and a Proposed Classification," *Report* 6, no. 62 (June 1966).
4. Erikson, E. In G. H. J. Pearson (ed.), *Handbook of Child Psychoanalysis* (New York: Basic Books, 1968), pp. 371–372. 4a. pp. 41–62.
5. Freud, A. *The Ego and the Mechanisms of Defense* (New York: International Universities Press, 1955).
6. Silberstein, R. M. *Bulletin of the Philadelphia Association for Psychoanalysis* 12, no. 4 (1962), 137–148.

# Index